CONTEMPORARY TOPICS IN MOLECULAR IMMUNOLOGY

VOLUME 2

CONTEMPORARY TOPICS IN MOLECULAR IMMUNOLOGY

(Formerly: Contemporary Topics in Immunochemistry)

CONTEMPORARY TOPICS IN MOLECULAR IMMUNOLOGY

VOLUME 2

EDITED BY

R. A. REISFELD

Department of Experimental Pathology
Scripps Clinic and Research Foundation
La Jolla, California

and

W. J. MANDY

Department of Microbiology
University of Texas
Austin, Texas

SPRINGER SCIENCE+BUSINESS MEDIA, LLC 1973

Library of Congress Catalog Card Number 73-186260
ISBN 978-1-4684-7775-7   ISBN 978-1-4684-7773-3 (eBook)
DOI 10.1007/978-1-4684-7773-3

© Springer Science+Business Media New York 1973
Originally published by Plenum Press, New York 1973
Softcover reprint of the hardcover 1st edition 1973

CONTRIBUTORS TO THIS VOLUME

Ettore Apella *Laboratory of Cell Biology*
National Cancer Institute
and
Laboratory of Immunology
National Institute of Allergy
  and Infectious Diseases
National Institutes of Health
Bethesda, Maryland

Neil R. Cooper *Department of Experimental Pathology*
Scripps Clinic and Research Foundation
La Jolla, California

Thomas S. Edgington *Division of Clinical Pathology*
Scripps Clinic and Research Foundation
La Jolla, California

S. Ferrone *Department of Experimental Pathology*
Scripps Clinic and Research Foundation
La Jolla, California

David Givol *Department of Chemical Immunology*
The Weizmann Institute of Science
Rehovot, Israel

John K. Inman *Laboratory of Cell Biology*
National Cancer Institute
and
Laboratory of Immunology
National Institute of Allergy
  and Infectious Diseases
National Institutes of Health
Bethesda, Maryland

Simonetta Landucci-Tosi *Osservatorio di Genetica Animale*
Via Pastrengo 28
Turin, Italy

Alfred Nisonoff *Department of Biological Chemistry*
University of Illinois College of Medicine
Chicago, Illinois

M. A. Pellegrino *Department of Experimental Pathology*
Scripps Clinic and Research Foundation
La Jolla, California

Edward F. Plow *Division of Clinical Pathology*
Scripps Clinic and Research Foundation
La Jolla, California

Roberto J. Poljak *Department of Biophysics*
Johns Hopkins University School of Medicine
Baltimore, Maryland

Ludmila Prokěsová *Department of Immunology*
Institute of Microbiology
Czechoslovak Academy of Science
Prague, Czechoslovakia

Jaroslav Rejnek *Department of Immunology*
Institute of Microbiology
Czechoslovak Academy of Science
Prague, Czechoslovakia

Susan Spring-Stewart *Department of Biological Chemistry*
University of Illinois College of Medicine
Chicago, Illinois

Roberto Tosi *Laboratorio di Biologia Cellulare del C.N.R.*
Via Romagnosi 18A
Rome, Italy

Foreword

This series was originally entitled *Contemporary Topics in Immunochemistry,* and Volume 1 bearing that name was published. Upon its editorial review and while charting the development of future volumes, the editors began to sense that the word "Immunochemistry" was somewhat restrictive according to its present interpretation. Accompanying the expansion of knowledge in immuno-biology is a demand for explanations in molecular terms. Since the intent of the series is to focus attention on research at the molecular level in any aspect of immunology, the editors and publisher felt the term "Immunochemistry" should be replaced with "Molecular Immunology." Thus, the series now bears a revised appellation, *Contemporary Topics in Molecular Immunology.* The editors feel this more accurately reflects the intended breath of the series.

An apology is offered to writers, librarians, and other catalogers for the inconvenience this change will cause.

F. P. Inman
General Editor

Athens, Georgia
March, 1973

Preface

The earliest explorers into immunology were at once confronted by myriad molecular riddles which became increasingly complex as immunochemical techniques resolved one question only to raise scores of others. Even as our knowledge of cellular immunology was growing remarkably fast, during the past two decades exciting experiments delineated the molecular structure of immunoglobulins. These joint advances not only shaped the *Gestalt* of present-day immunology, but paved the way for an incisive molecular approach to the challenges of research.

The articles in this volume mirror some of these molecular approaches to the structure of immunoglobulins and their genetically segregating allotypic specificities. Thus, R. Poljak brings into focus some highlights of X-ray crystallographic studies of immunoglobulins. Undoubtedly, further refinements in this approach will soon provide an even more concise picture of the topography of the antigen-binding site. In this context, D. Givol describes the elegant approach of affinity labeling to elucidate the chemical and molecular nature of the antigen-binding site. He provides a model of the structure of the antigen-binding site involving the unique complementation of the light and heavy polypeptide chains of the immunoglobulin molecule. S. Spring-Stewart and A. Nisonoff deal with a special problem in immunochemistry, i.e., that of individual antigenic specificities of idiotypes associated with antibody molecules. These authors focus primarily on the potential of idiotypes as markers for clones of antibody-producing cells to follow certain events occurring in immunologically-competent lymphoid cell populations.

Two articles deal with immunoglobulin allotypes. The one by E. Appella and J. K. Inman details the structure of immunoglobulin light chains as deduced from the amino acid sequence analyses of these polypeptide chains of mice and rabbits. Such analyses provide the basis for discussions on certain allotype-related sequence variations. The related work of R. Tosi and S. Landucci-Tosi focuses mainly on refinements in techniques utilizing cross-linked antisera for the detection and quantitation of subtle allotypic determinants in rabbits.

Unlike other review series, this volume does not provide comprehensive coverage of only one subject. Thus, consideration was given to some research

ix

which, in the editors' opinions, warrants special focus and attention. A case in point is the article by J. Rejnek and L. Prokesová who have organized an impressive collection of data illustrating why germfree piglets represent an ideal model with which to study nonantibody immunoglobulins as well as dynamics of antibody formation. A molecular approach to a fascinating system of great biologic significance is delineated by N. R. Cooper who describes the activation of the human complement system. Various mechanisms and the extensive series of steps in the activation process are considered and critically discussed, including activators and enzymes required to trigger the complement system in the absence of antigen and specific antibody. An intricate and biologically relevant system of genetically determined cell surface markers is discussed by S. Ferrone and M. A. Pellegrino who focus on the complex reactivities of histocompatibility (HL-A) antigens, their alloantibodies, and complement in the lymphocytotoxic reaction. This article also offers critical and detailed discussions of the cellular distribution, cell surface expression, and cross-reactivity of HL-A antigens and the serologic evaluation of soluble HL-A cell surface markers. Finally, T. S. Edgington and E. F. Plow look at antibodies as biological probes of the structure and functional molecular anatomy of fibrinogen. These authors elaborate immunochemical approaches to the structure and conformation of fibrinogen and its multiple physiological derivatives and describe molecular events which modulate the expression of native antigens and control the emergence and expression of neoantigens by complex molecules.

One might wonder from the title of this series how many aspects of the broad discipline of immunology could and should be considered contemporary. If we select topics that indicate present-day progress and that evoke thought leading to tomorrow's research designs, we hope to have kept the promise of that title. The choices of subject by our coeditors in subsequent volumes will continue to expand the meaning of "contemporary immunology" and will rectify any of our obvious omissions in this volume.

R. A. Reisfeld
W. J. Mandy

Contents

Immunoglobulins and Antibodies in Pigs
Jaroslav Rejnek and Ludmila Prokesová

Activation of the Complement System
Neil R. Cooper

HL-A Antigens, Antibody, and Complement in the Lymphocytotoxic Reaction

Functional Molecular Anatomy of Fibrinogen: Antibodies as Biological Probes of Structure

Chapter 1

X-Ray Crystallographic Studies
of Immunoglobulins

Roberto J. Poljak

Department of Biophysics
Johns Hopkins University School of Medicine
Baltimore, Maryland

I. INTRODUCTION

The techniques of X-ray crystallography have been successfully applied to the study of complex biological polymers such as nucleic acids and proteins. These studies have provided structural models from which we have tried to explain the mechanisms of DNA replication, of enzyme action, and of other biological phenomena. The determination of the structure of several crystalline enzymes, achieved within the last ten years, is an outstanding example of this approach. As a result of such efforts, models have been obtained for the highly specific interactions between enzymes and their substrates. Development of methods and techniques has reached the point at which it is now possible to attempt the determination of more complex structures such as those of immunoglobulins. It is hoped that a knowledge of the three-dimensional structure of immunoglobulins will provide a useful model for the correlation of their function and primary structure and the genetic control of variability and specificity of antibodies. This article is a review of the first models of immunoglobulin structure obtained by X-ray crystallographic methods. A brief outline of some aspects of the structure and properties of immunoglobulins and the theoretical and practical aspects of protein crystallography will be presented first. The most detailed account to be given in this review will be that of the Fab structure which is currently under study in the author's laboratory.

II. STRUCTURE AND PROPERTIES OF IMMUNOGLOBULINS

In the course of an adaptive immune response, vertebrates can selectively neutralize foreign antigens. Large numbers of natural and synthetic antigens have been shown to elicit the synthesis of specific glycoprotein molecules called antibodies, which are present in the γ electrophoretic component of serum. Antibodies against specific antigens and the other glycoproteins present in the γ electrophoretic component of serum share a number of structural features and are generically called immunoglobulins (Ig). Immunoglobulins can be divided into three major classes called IgM (macroglobulins, mol. wt. approximately 900,000), IgA (mol. wt. approximately 170,000–500,000), and IgG (mol. wt. approximately 150,000). In the serum of normal individuals, IgM, IgA, and IgG are found to constitute approximately 5–10%, 10–20%, and 70–80%, respectively, of the total circulating immunoglobulin. These three classes contain carbohydrates which range from 2–3% of the total weight for IgG to about 10–12% for IgA and IgM. The covalently attached carbohydrates are largely hexose and hexosamine with smaller amounts of sialic acid and fucose. Two other minor classes of immunoglobulins called IgD and IgE have been described and characterized. The reader is referred to more extensive reviews of this subject (Immunoglobulins, Annals of the New York Academy of Sciences, Vol. 190, 1971; Edelman and Gall, 1969; Kabat, 1968; Milstein and Pink, 1970) for a detailed discussion of these two minor classes and other topics in immunology and immunochemistry.

The study of the three major classes of immunoglobulins (IgG, IgA, and IgM) is greatly facilitated by the occurrence of homogeneous pathological immunoglobulins produced by monoclonal neoplastic lymphocytic cells in mice and in humans. These myeloma proteins, associated with the spontaneous occurrence of multiple myelomatosis and other pathological lymphoproliferative disorders in man and with experimentally induced tumors in mice, have shown to be closely related to normal immunoglobulins and antibodies by a number of structural and functional properties. Myeloma proteins can be obtained in large quantities and can be readily purified to homogeneous molecular species, thus providing suitable material for detailed structural studies. In general, these myeloma proteins can be isolated as complete molecules but sometimes only a portion of the molecule is present, most frequently the "light chain" of the polypeptide structure (see below). Bence-Jones proteins are light chains (isolated from urine) which display a peculiar thermal behavior: they precipitate at 40°–60°C, redissolve at 95°–100°C, and reprecipitate on cooling. [See Humphrey and Owens (1972) for a detailed review of plasma cell dyscrasias and pathological immunoglobulins.]

The IgG class of immunoglobulins has been the most intensively studied. A diagramatic structure of a human IgG molecule is shown in Fig. 1. The molecule consists of two identical "light" (L) polypeptide chains (mol. wt.

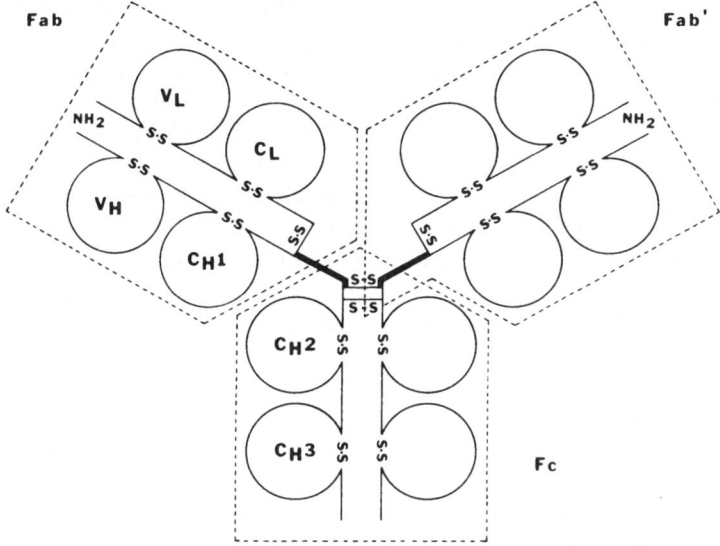

Figure 1. Diagrammatic structure of a human IgG1 molecule. The light chains are divided into two homology regions, V_L and C_L. The thicker lines in the heavy chains correspond to the "hinge" region. The four homology regions (V_H, C_H1, C_H2, and C_H3) of the heavy chains, the interchain and intrachain disulfide bonds, the N-terminal region of both chains, and the major fragments (Fab, Fab', Fc) are indicated.

20,000–25,000) and two identical "heavy" (H) polypeptide chains (mol. wt. 50,000–55,000) which are linked by interchain disulfide bonds to form a covalent arrangement of four chains. Noncovalent interactions between the H and the L chains require the use of drastic conditions (acid pH, urea, etc.) for the separation of this structure into individual polypeptide chain components after reduction of the interchain disulfide bonds. The L chains of human IgG can be antigenically classified into two classes called κ and λ, each characterized by unique sequences in their C-terminal regions. Human IgM, IgA, IgD, and IgE also include the same type of L chain (κ or λ) in their multichain structure, but their heavy chains are different and are specific to each class.

A major step in the determination of the multichain structure of IgG was taken when Porter (1959) found that controlled enzymatic digestion of rabbit IgG produces two kinds of major fragments, Fab and Fc. The Fab fragment (Fig. 1, mol. wt. 50,000) retains the antibody activity of the parent molecule except that it can only behave as a monovalent antibody. No complement fixation activity can be observed in the immune Fab-antigen complex, indicating that the Fc region is required for complement fixation. Controlled digestion of a human or rabbit IgG protein by pepsin produces a major fragment called $F(ab')_2$

(Nisonoff *et al.*, 1960). By reduction and alkylation of the inter-heavy-chain disulfide bond(s) the Fab′ fragment (Fig. 1) is readily obtained. Fab and Fab′ consist of a complete L chain and a piece (called Fd or Fd′, respectively) which is the N-terminal half of the H chain. Human Fd′ is about ten amino acid residues longer than Fd. Similar Fab fragments have been obtained by the use of other proteolytic enzymes such as trypsin. All these proteolytic enzymes split peptide bonds in a region which appears openly accessible and which has been called the "hinge" region ("flexibly") connecting Fab and Fc.

Amino acid sequence studies of the L- and H-chain components of immunoglobulins have shown that these chains possess unique structural features. When the first human myeloma L chains were sequenced it became clear that L chains of the same class (κ or λ) consist of a C-terminal half of constant amino acid sequence and an N-terminal half of variable sequence. Because of the possible genetic implications, the patterns of variability of L-chain sequences have been extensively analyzed. Thus, it has been observed that within a given class of L chains there are sequences which are very similar and can be included in one subgroup. Three subgroups have been recognized in κ chains and at least four in λ chains. All chains within a subgroup are very similar in sequence except at certain positions where a pattern of extreme variability is observed (Wu and Kabat, 1970). It is believed that these hypervariable sequences constitute the regions of the L-chain structure which come in contact with antigen, so that the presence of different sequences is correlated with the occurrence of different antibody specificities. Studies on H chains have shown that the region of constant sequence extends to about three quarters of the length of the chain beginning at the C terminal. As in the case of the L chains, the region of variable sequence occurs toward the N terminal of the molecule and spans a length of about 110 amino acid residues. The first heavy chain sequences that were determined, in the Fc region of rabbit IgG (Hill *et al.*, 1966), showed another important feature of structure: the existence of sequence homology regions. Two sequences are homologous when they contain chemically related amino acids in the same positions in the polypeptide chain (for example, serine in the first sequence and threonine at the same position in the second sequence). Another criterion for homology between two sequences is to examine amino acid differences in terms of the minimum mutational events that are necessary to change the nucleotide sequence specifying the first chain to that specifying the second polypeptide chain. If the number of mutations is smaller than can be expected from random chance then the sequences are said to be homologous. By either of the two criteria mentioned above, one can define four "homology regions": C_H1, C_H2, and C_H3 in the H chains and C_L in the L chains (Fig. 1). The N-terminal regions V_L and V_H (Fig. 1) are homologous to each other but have little or no homology with C_L, C_H1, C_H2, and C_H3. It is interesting to observe that the pattern of a single intrachain disulfide loop of similar length is present in each one of these homology regions. In addition to their genetic implications, these findings suggest that the overall three-dimensional folding of IgG molecules is determined by the existence of the homology regions. Inspired by these and other observations, several proposals were made about the folding of the H and L polypeptide chains (Singer *et al.*, 1967; Putnam *et al.*, 1967; Edelman *et al.*, 1969; Welscher, 1969; and others) which can be summarized by describing the tertiary structure of immunoglobulins as consisting of globular "domains" each corresponding to a homology region. It could be added that these domains must be packed in tetrahedral arrangements so that each homology region in the Fab of Fc parts of the molecule is in close contact with adjacent homology regions.

Electron microscopy studies have provided the first direct pictures of the general shape and structure of immunoglobulins. The elegant experiments of Valentine and Green (1967) in which a divalent hapten (bis-*N*-DNP-octamethylenediamine) was used as a link between several anti-DNP molecules provided a picture of the general shape of an IgG molecule and of the arrangement of the Fab and Fc regions (Fig. 2). When combined with antigen, the shape is that of a letter Y, with variable separations for the two arms (Fab) of the Y depending on the number of IgG molecules connected by the bis-DNP hapten. The flexibility required to obtain a variable separation is thought to reside in the "hinge" region connected Fab to Fc. Electron micrographs of an IgA protein produced by the (laboratory induced) mouse plasma cell tumor MOPC 315 (Green *et al.*, 1971) indicated that the IgA structure consists of structural units or domains. In this study on IgA, a divalent bis-DNP hapten was also used,

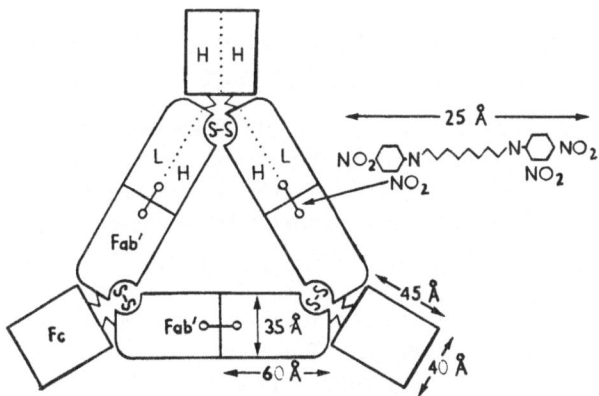

Figure 2. Diagram illustrating a hapten-linked trimer of anti-DNP rabbit IgG antibody molecules. (Reproduced from Valentine and Green (1967), with permission of Academic Press, New York.)

taking advantage of the fact that the MOPC 315 myeloma protein has the specificity of an anti-DNP antibody. No such subunits or domains have been observed in the electron micrographs of IgG.

Affinity labeling experiments have also contributed to the knowledge of the location and topography of antigen binding sites. In these experiments a haptenic group is specifically (reversibly) bound by the appropriate antibody and is then covalently attached to an amino acid side chain on the antibody molecule by means of a chemically reactive group on the hapten. In principle, amino acid side chains that are part of the reactive site of the antibody molecule or are close to it can be specifically labeled and identified. Using a number of different reactive haptens and antibodies (and also some myeloma proteins that behave like antibodies), a picture has emerged in which the antigen binding site is defined by the V_L and the V_H regions. Amino acid side chains in or close to the regions of hypervariable sequence in L and H chains have been labeled (Singer *et al.*, 1967; Haimovich *et al.*, 1970; Cebra *et al.*, 1971), thus supporting the hypothesis that these regions contribute to (or determine) the antigen binding site of antibodies. Synthetic antigens have been used as an experimental tool in analyzing the specificity of antibodies, the role of immunodeterminant groups in the antigen-antibody reaction, and the dimensions of the combining sites. With different antigens, the most exposed end of an immunodeterminant group has consistently been found to make the larger contribution to the energy of the binding reaction (Kabat, 1966; Sela, 1969; Schechter, 1971). The dimensions of the binding site have been estimated to be of the order of 35×10–15×6–10 Å by using antigenic polysaccharides (Kabat, 1966) and polypeptides (Maurer, 1964; Sage *et al.*, 1964; Haber *et al.*, 1967).

III. STUDY OF CRYSTALLINE PROTEINS BY X-RAY DIFFRACTION METHODS

Extensive, up-to-date reviews on this subject are available and the reader is referred to them (for example, Holmes and Blow, 1966; Dickerson, 1964; Cold Spring Harbor Symposium, Vol. 36: Structure and Function of Proteins at the Three-Dimensional Level, 1971) for a more extensive account of principles and methods. The present outline will be a brief, qualitative description of principles and techniques intended for immunologists and immunochemists.

X-ray diffraction has the potential for providing a high resolution picture of matter in the solid or crystalline state. This is based on the fact that X-rays with wavelengths of the order of magnitude of interatomic distances can be used to obtain diffraction patterns of crystals. There is, however, one major difficulty in producing the desired image of the atomic arrangement: The relative phase of the X-ray waves cannot be measured directly from an X-ray diffraction experiment. Since no X-ray lenses are available, reconstitution of the image from the diffraction spectra is accomplished by use of a "mathematical lens" function (a Fourier series transformation) in which both the amplitudes and phases of the diffracted rays must be known. The missing phase information can be obtained by a variety of techniques including "direct methods" in which relations between the amplitudes of the diffracted waves are analyzed mathematically to obtain the required phases. For complex molecules of the large size proteins, the only successful and widely used method of determining the phases is that of the isomorphous heavy atom substitution. When the phase of each diffracted wave has been determined, amplitudes and phases can be used to calculate a map of the electron-dense X-ray scatterers (atoms or groups of atoms) which displays their relative densities and positions. In Sections A–E a few points of the theory and practice of X-ray diffraction will be considered in more detail.

A. Crystallization

In most cases, crystals have been obtained at an advanced stage in the isolation and purification of proteins. Since the ideal crystal is formed by a three-dimensional repetition of identical molecules, purifications to a single homogeneous molecular species should in general help in obtaining crystals. Conditions that render a protein insoluble (pH, type of ions, ionic strength, temperature, protein concentration, etc.) are favorable for the nucleation and growth of crystals. A classical example is the crystallization by "salting out" of protein molecules in solution. Frequently, the same protein can be obtained in several different crystal forms by changing the conditions of crystallization. In the few cases in which these different crystalline forms of the same (or related) proteins were analyzed by X-ray diffraction, the same three-dimensional structure was found to be present in all, although the contact points between the molecules and the volume taken by the solvent vary from one crystal form to another. Most of the indirect evidence obtained suggests that the structure of a protein in the crystalline state is very similar to the structure of the protein in solution, since many reactions (for example, enzymatic activity) which take place in solution can also be shown to take place in the crystalline state. Detailed analysis of all the available evidence should perhaps be briefly summarized by saying that the structure in the crystalline form is at least one of several possible "ground states" of the molecule. Since X-ray diffraction measurements of proteins take place over extended periods of time (hours), only stable conformations can be studied by this method.

B. Experimental Diffraction Techniques

Protein crystals are mounted in sealed (thin) glass or quartz capillaries surrounded by their "mother liquor" (buffer or solution from which they were crystallized), carefully avoiding any drying during the crystal mounting operation. The ideal dimensions for such crystals are about $0.5 \times 0.5 \times 0.5$ mm (i.e., they are visible by eye). Crystals should measure at least 0.05 mm on each side before they can be used for single crystal X-ray diffraction experiments. Smaller crystals (which are frequently obtained with many proteins) do not diffract strongly enough to permit observation of their single crystal diffraction pattern.

X-rays are produced by water-cooled stationary- or rotating-anode tubes (both commercially available). A copper anode from which Cu K_a X-rays of wavelength $\lambda = 1.542$ Å are obtained is most frequently used in protein work. Photographic techniques are always used for preliminary studies such as the investigation of the crystallinity of the material, its unit cell dimensions, and its symmetry. Precession photographs provide a picture of the "reciprocal lattice" (i.e., the diffraction pattern) of a crystal and make the determination of its unit cell dimensions and symmetry a relatively simple operation. The unit cell dimensions, symmetry (the way in which molecules are packed in the crystal), and crystal density can be used to calculate the molecular weight contained in the "asymmetric unit" of the crystal. By allowing for the presence of solvent (which can be measured), the molecular weight of an individual molecule (or molecues) contained in the asymmetric unit can be determined.

As the size of the asymmetric unit of a crystal increases (with increasing molecular weight), so do the number of X-ray reflections that must be measured to determine the molecular structure. Furthermore, as the size of the asymmetric unit increases, the reflections generally become weaker and their measurement more difficult. Thus, the difficulty in obtaining diffraction data from larger macromolecules (such as immunoglobulins and crystalline viruses) necessitates special techniques for intensity measurements. Computer controlled X-ray diffractometers have been most widely used for the automatic measurement of X-ray intensities from protein crystals. In these instruments, the crystal and an X-ray counter (scintillation or proportional) are set to the appropriate angular values to measure a given reflection. The angular values are calculated by a computer which is connected "on-line" to the diffractometer. Since reflections have to be measured in a temporal sequence which extends over periods of several hours, a highly stabilized X-ray source is required. Photographic techniques, which were used in the early days of X-ray diffraction, are regaining an important role in protein crystallography by virtue of the fact (among others) that their use allows the recording of many reflections simultaneously. In this way, the speed of data collection is increased, providing an invaluable help when the crystalline material is damaged by radiation. The diffraction films may then be measured by film scanners which provide the output information in a form suitable for further computer processing (for example, on magnetic tape).

C. Isomorphous Replacement Method

As stated above, the intensities of the X-rays diffracted by a crystal can be measured by films or by radiation counters, but the relative phases of these reflections cannot be measured directly. To determine the relative phases, the method of isomorphous heavy atom substitution is used. This method consists of introducing one or a few atoms of high electron density (i.e., "heavy" atoms) into specific sites in the asymmetric unit of the crystal without altering the conformation of the protein molecule under study or the relative positions of the molecules in the crystal. If this condition is achieved, the native protein crystals and those in which solvent or other atoms have been replaced by the heavy atoms are said to be isomorphous. Intensity changes, which can be seen by comparing the diffraction pattern of the native protein crystals with that of isomorphous crystals containing heavy atoms, are an indication of a possible heavy atom substitution. The Fourier transform of the measured intensity changes (in the form of a two-dimensional or three-dimensional autocorrelation map called the Patterson function) can be analyzed to determine the location of the heavy atoms. If this analysis has been successfully completed for two or more different heavy atom substituents, the contribution of the heavy atom derivatives can be calculated, and the phases thus obtained can be used to determine the native protein phases. An example of a heavy atom substituion is the titration of a (cys-) SH group of a protein by a mercurial such as p-chloro-mercuribenzoic acid. In such a case the substitution can be performed before or after crystallization. In most cases, heavy atoms are introduced by diffusion into already grown crystals by "soaking" the crystals in a solution containing heavy atoms. Coordination of the substituent in a favorable environment of protein side chains accounts for their binding at the few specific sites that are required. A few rules can be mentioned here to summarize the preceding paragraphs: 1) It is important that the isomorphism be as perfect as possible so that distortions of the protein configuration will not interfere with the determination of its structure. This criterion becomes more exacting as the resolution of the analysis is increased. 2) The substitution should take place at a few sites in one molecule and in all or most molecules in the crystal leading to a few sites with high occupancy. A high occupancy is particularly desirable for a large protein so that the heavy atom scattering can be measured accurately over that of the large number of (lighter) atoms of the protein. 3) A minimum of two heavy atoms (at different sites) is necessary to solve the protein phases. A number in excess of two is desirable to increase and improve the phase information. If the number of reflections to be measured for the native protein crystals is N, the total number of reflections to be measured for all the derivatives will be $N(n + 1)$, where n is the number of heavy atom derivatives that are used in the process of phase determination. 4) Heavy atom attachment to crystalline proteins is, in most cases, a trial and error process. Fortunately, results can be analyzed by X-ray diffraction methods; visual inspection of photographs is enough to detect the intensity changes that occur if substitution has taken place. Because it is unpredictable, isomorphous heavy atom substitution remains one of the most difficult and elusive steps in the study of protein structures by X-ray crystallographic methods.

D. Resolution

Although in theory the resolution depends on the wavelength of the radiation used, in practice the intensity of the X-ray diffraction pattern of proteins decreases rapidly with increasing diffraction angle so that it is difficult to measure reflections beyond 2 Å which would be needed for atomic resolution. (A 2 Å reflection can be visualized as obtained from an imaginary set of parallel planes spaced 2 Å apart from each other following the condition known as Bragg's law, $\lambda = 2d \sin \theta$, where λ is the wavelength of X-rays, d is the 2 Å spacing of the set of planes, and θ is the angle made by both the incident and the diffracted beams and the planes.) Because of crystalline disorder, it is frequently observed that the diffraction pattern of proteins fades at much lower resolutions. In these cases only a gross structure of the molecule can be determined. Features of secondary structure such as polypeptide chains in a-helical configuration can be detected at a resolution of 6 Å, as has been demonstrated by the X-ray analyses of myoglobin and hemoglobin. When the helical content of a protein is small, it is mostly features of tertiary and quaternary structure that can be determined at a low resolution such as 6 Å.

The number of reflections to be measured increases sharply with increasing resolution. If the number of reflections to be measured for a resolution of 6 Å is N, the number of reflections will be (approximately) $2N$ for a resolution of 4 Å, $5N$ for a resolution of 3.3 Å, and $25N$ for a resolution of 2 Å. If one considers that N is of the order of 10^3 for a native protein crystal (and for each heavy atom derivative), the increasing amount of work with increasing resolution becomes clear. It is also clear that if 3–2 Å is the resolution limit that can be attained with a given protein crystal even if good phase information is available, it will be necessary to have access to the amino acid sequence for a complete interpretation of the Fourier map of the electron density.

E. Phase Refinement and Interpretation of Fourier Maps

Heavy atom parameters such as positional coordinates, relative occupancies, and a measure of their thermal vibrations in space can be refined by least squares techniques from the intensities of the diffraction pattern. Refinement of these parameters leads to more precise phase information. An index called the "figure of merit" is frequently used to express the average error in the phase angles for all the reflections that were calculated. The average figure of merit m is a measure of the cosine of the average angular error in the calculated phase angles. The range of m is, evidently, 0 to 1; a value above 0.7 is considered satisfactory, i.e., the average error in phase angle is less than $45°$. The value of m tends to decrease as the resolution increases, due to factors that were mentioned above such as poorer experimental data and lack of strict isomorphism.

Fourier maps of the electron density describe the structure under study. In low-resolution maps (for example, 6 Å) it is possible to define the shape of a molecule. However, in regions of the map where one molecule comes into contact with another, this task may be difficult and may require noncrystallographic information (such as a knowledge of the approximate molecular shape by light scattering or electron microscopy, etc.) or an arbitrary decision. An electron-dense "marker" such as the heme group in hemoglobin can be easily located and used as a reference point in the interpretation of low and high resolution maps. In spite of their higher electron density, disulfide bonds cannot be easily located in low resolution maps. In high-resolution maps (3 Å or smaller spacings), runs of continuous polypeptide chains can be seen, and if sequence information is available, amino acid side chains can be matched with the electron density map. Some side chains or the ends of a polypeptide chain may be freely rotating and thus they are difficult to locate in a map. Solid models of a material such as balsa wood are usually built from low-resolution maps. They represent features of electron density above the background due to the intermolecular solution of crystallization. Skeletal wire models of amino acids are used to interpret high-resolution maps in terms of polypeptide chains. A good fit of the amino acid sequence to the electron density map constitutes the ultimate test of the determination of a protein structure.

IV. X-RAY DIFFRACTION STUDIES OF IMMUNOGLOBULINS

A. IgG Immunoglobulins

The most advanced crystallographic analysis of a whole IgG molecule has been reported by Sarma *et al.* (1971*a,b*). These studies were carried on IgG Dob, a cryoglobulin that crystallizes spontaneously on cooling. One L chain and one H chain are contained in the asymmetric unit of the crystal and are related to the other H chain and L chain of the molecule by a twofold axis of symmetry which could run through the two inter-H-chain disulfide bonds ("parallel" polypeptide chains) or between them ("antiparallel" chains), assuming that IgG Dob has the typical IgG1 structure. Because of structual disorder, the X-ray diffraction pattern of IgG Dob does not extend to high resolutions, making it difficult to measure intensities with resolution greater than 6 Å. Also, irradiation of the IgG Dob crystals affects the intensity pattern after relatively short exposures, thus making the collection of intensity data a difficult problem even at low resolution. Four heavy atom derivatives were used for phase determination; three of which, $Hg(CN)_2$, p-chloromercuribenzene sulfonate, and 1,4-diacetoxymercuri-2,3-dimethoxybutane (Baker dimercurial), share one major binding site. The final figure of merit reported for 2010 reflections was $m = 0.800$ (Sarma *et al.*, 1971*b*). A Fourier map of the electron density at a nominal resolution of 6 Å was interpreted as showing two globular regions. One of these is located around a twofold axis of symmetry and must therefore constitute the Fc part of the molecule since the Fc consists of two (idential) C_H2 and C_H3 homology regions (Fig. 1). The other globular structure contained in the asymmetric unit must correspond to the Fab region of the molecule. Sarma *et al.* (1971*b*) found four possible ways of assembling a complete IgG Dob molecule from these two globular subunits (see Fig. 3). Although one model (IV, Fig. 3) was chosen among the four possibilities, this choice was present as a tentative structure. In this structure the IgG molecule is T-shaped. Its stem corresponds to the Fc region which measures 72 × 45 × 38 Å, agreeing with the dimensions reported by Valentine and Green (1967) from electron microscopy studies and by Goldstein *et al.* (1968) from X-ray diffraction studies. The Fab regions have dimensions of 70 × 50 × 40 Å, making the longer axis of the molecule

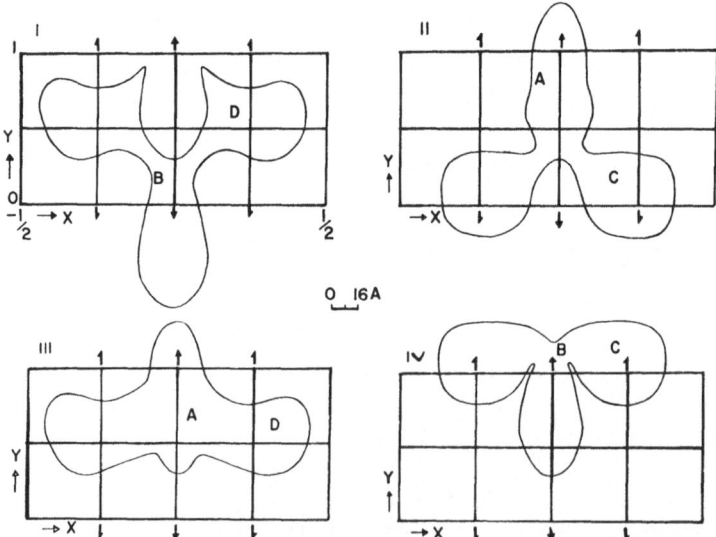

Figure 3. Schematic representation of four possible immunoglobulin structures from the 6 Å resolution Fourier map of IgG Dob. (Reproduced from Sarma *et al.*, 1971*a*, with permission of the American Society of Biological Chemists.)

approximately 140 Å long. In conclusion, the crystallographic analysis of IgG Dob has shown that there is an exact twofold axis of symmetry relating identical H and L chains to build the four-chain structure of IgG and has provided a tentative T-shaped model for human IgG. The first of these two conclusions confirms a result which had already been obtained by biochemical analysis. The determination of the shape of the molecule is of considerable importance as a test of hypotheses such as the "click open" proposal of Feinstein and Row (1965). A T-shaped molecule which becomes Y-shaped when reacting with antigen (Valentine and Green, 1967) is in disagreement with such a hypothesis. However, it should be emphasized that the result obtained by Sarma *et al.* (1971*a*) applies to the crystalline state of a molecule in which there may be a flexible (hinge) region (see for example Yguerabide *et al.*, 1970). A T-shaped model would be in agreement with the interpretation of small angle X-ray scattering data (Pilz *et al.*, 1970) although the molecular dimensions proposed to account for the small angle X-ray data are considerably larger (see below).

Edmundson *et al.* (1970) have reported a preliminary crystallographic study of IgG Mcg, a crystalline protein that gives a diffraction pattern extending to a resolution of 3.5 Å. The crystals are reasonably stable under the X-ray beam so that IgG Mcg appears to be a favorable specimen for X-ray diffraction studies on a whole IgG. As in IgG Dob, a twofold axis of symmetry relates two identical halves of the structure of IgG Mcg. However, study of allotypic markers and partial sequence data indicates that the hinge region of the H chains of this IgG is deleted and that the L chains are present as a covalently linked (S-S) dimmer, so that in this sense IgG Mcg is not a typical IgG molecule (Deutsch and Suzuki, 1971).

A rabbit anti-*p*-azobenzoate antibody has been crystallized by Nisonoff *et al.* (1967). The antibody was elicited by an antigen prepared by diazotizing *p*-aminobenzoic acid and coupling it to bovine γ-globulin carrier. Analysis of allotypic markers, binding experiments, and disc electrophoresis patterns have indicated that the antibody is a homogeneous (or nearly homogeneous) molecular species, a finding that helps to explain the fact that it crystallized spontaneously at 5°C. An X-ray crystallographic study was attempted (Nisonoff and Poljak, 1967, unpublished) but no X-ray pattern could be observed beyond a few relfections at very low resolution. Similar behavior has been observed in experiments with other crystalline IgG materials that were examined by X-ray diffraction (Edmundson *et al.*, 1971; Poljak, unpublished).

B. Light Chains, Bence-Jones Proteins, and Their Fragments

A crystalline Bence-Jones protein (Schiffer *et al.*, 1970) has recently been analyzed to 6 Å resolution by crystallographic methods (Edmundson *et al.*, 1971, 1972). This Bence-Jones L chain was obtained from the same patient from which their crystalline pathological IgG Mcg (see preceding section) was derived. The Mcg Bence-Jones protein was crystallized as a dimer consisting of two identical (λ) chains connected by a disulfide interchain bond at the penultimate C-terminal amino acid residue. Two crystal forms were obtained: an ortho-rhombic form crystallized by dialysis against deionized water and a trigonal form grown in 1.6–1.9 M ammonium sulfate, 0.1 M ammonium phosphate, pH 6.2. The trigonal crystals are of good size (approximately 0.5 × 0.5 × 1.0 mm), give an intense diffraction pattern to high resolutions, and are sufficiently stable under X-ray irradiation to constitute an excellent material for crystallographic analysis. Two heavy atom derivatives were prepared using mersalyl and o-chloro-mercuriphenol. The intensities of the diffraction patterns were measured by diffractometer techniques. After phase refinement, the average figure of merit was $m = 0.66$, a reasonable value considering that only two heavy atom derivatives were used. The Fourier map of the electron density showed a striking feature of the structure: the L-chain Mcg dimer consists of two structural units or "modules" separated by a crevice but still linked by features of electron density that run from one module to the other (see Fig. 4). The maximum length of this structure is 78 Å, close to the maximum length (75 Å) that has been obtained for low-angle X-ray scattering (Holasek et al., 1963). Edmundson and his colleagues found that the two globular regions (see Fig. 4) differ in size and structure so that they cannot each represent an L-chain monomer. Since the C-terminal regions are covalently linked by an S–S bond, one of the modules must approximately represent the constant homology region of both L chains $[(C_L)_2]$ and the other structural module must contain the variable regions of the L chains $[(V_L)_2]$. This result indicates that the homology regions C_L and V_L fold into separate globular structures which interact more closely with the homologous parts of a second chain than they do with each other. In this

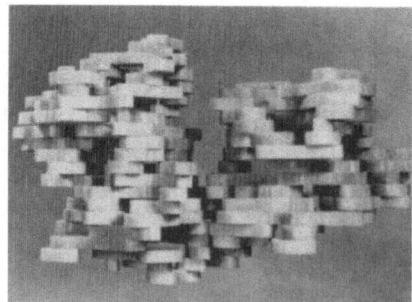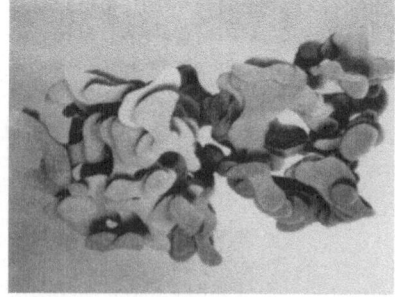

Figure 4. Two different views of the 6 Å resolution model of Bence-Jones protein Mcg. Two subunits of structure or modules can be clearly seen. (Reproduced from Edmundson et al., 1972; courtesy of Dr. A.E. Edmundson and with the permission of the American Chemical Society.)

respect, the results of this elegant study are very close to those obtained with Fab (see below) and confirm the notion that immunoglobulins contain globular subunits of structure which are formed by two different polypeptide cahins. This study also provides a model to explain several of the physicochemical properties of L-chain monomers and dimers which will be discussed below in the section dealing with Fab.

Immunoglobulin L chains from different sources have been obtained in crystalline form. L chains derived from a macroglobulin (IgM) have been crystallized (Suzuki and Deutsch, 1967) after separation from the parent IgM and subsequent purification. However, the crystals appeared to be too small for X-ray diffraction studies. L chains belonging to the κ antigenic class are under study (R. Huber, personal communication). V fragments obtained by controlled enzymatic digestion of L chains have also been obtained in crystalline form and are under study by crystallographic methods (Solomon *et al.,* 1970).

C. Fab Fragments

The Fab and Fab$'$ fragments of immunoglobulins retain the antibody activity and the antigen binding specificity of the parent molecule. Thus their structural study is of considerable interest. Three human myeloma IgG1 proteins have been reported to yield crystalline Fab fragments suitable for X-ray studies. Fab New and Fab$'$ New obtained from IgG New (λ, Gm 1^+, 3^-, 4^-, 5^-; Rossi and Nisonoff, 1968; Rossi *et al.,* 1969) are isomorphous, crystallize in space group C2 with one Fab or Fab$'$ molecule per asymmetric unit, and have unit cell dimensions $a = 111.43 \pm 0.10$ Å $b = 56.68 \pm 0.10$ Å, $c = 90.30 \pm 0.10$ Å, $\beta = 116.46 \pm 0.10°$ (Avey *et al.,* 1968; Poljak *et al.,* 1971). The crystals, grown in 1.7–1.9 M ammonium sulfate, pH 6.5, have prismatic shape and dimensions of the order of $1.0 \times 0.5 \times 0.2$ mm. X-ray precession photographs show reflections extending beyond 2.8 Å. Crystalline Fab New and Fab$'$ New can be irradiated for prolonged periods of time (over 24 hr) before the intensity of the overall diffraction pattern decreases below 90% of the original intensity. Thus, Fab New and Fab$'$ New are well suited for X-ray crystallographic studies. In spite of the fact that human Fab$'$ is longer by ten amino acid residues in its Fd$'$ polypeptide chain than Fab, no major intensity differences are observed between the diffraction patterns of Fab New and Fab$'$ New. For this reason, the terms Fab or Fab$'$ will be used indistinctively in the following description. A preliminary crystallographic study of Fab Hil and Fab Smo (Humphrey *et al.,* 1969) showed that these two fragments each have two molecules per asymmetric unit. The cell dimensions of Fab Hil are $a = 111.1$ Å, $b = 127.8$ Å, $c = 66.1$ Å (± 0.2 Å), orthorhombic, space group $P2_12_12_1$. Although Fab Hil [from cryoglobulin IgG1 Hil (λ, Gm 1^+, 3^-, 4^-, 5^-)] diffracts well, intensity measurements are considerably more difficult than in the case of Fab New because of the larger number of reflections to be measured (twice that of Fab New). Fab Smo [from IgG1 Smo, κ Inv(a^-), Gm(a^+; b^1, b^3, b^4, x, f, c^-)] gives a poorer diffraction pattern and appears unsuitable for detailed structural studies. Evidently, Fab New is the most suitable form for detailed crystallographic analysis. It should be emphasized here that the differences in morphology and diffraction patterns of different human myeloma Fab fragments do not imply that each will be found to have a different tertiary structure. Rather, they imply that the variation in amino acid sequence determines in each case a different set of intermolecular contacts or interactions, giving rise to unique crystalline lattices.

Although gram quantities of IgG New are available, crystallographic experiments on Fab New were carried out using a minimum amount of material in order to preserve most of the material for primary structure determination. Screening of heavy atom derivatives was performed by soaking one or two small crystals (0.05 × 0.1 × 0.5mm) in a solution of the heavy atom compound to be tested. The crystals were then mounted in sealed glass capillaries under a polarizing microscope and examined by recording, on precession photographs, the $h0l$ "centric" reflections (thus obtaining a section of the diffraction lattice corresponding to a projection of the structure down the unique axis of twofold symmetry). An extensive search for isomorphous heavy atom substitution could be conducted in this way using a minimum of crystalline material. X-ray intensities from the native and the heavy atom substituted Fab crystals were recorded by photographic techniques and also measured by a computer-controlled, four-circle diffractometer (Poljak *et al.*, 1971). The possibility of titrating the SH groups generated in the reduction step leading from F(ab')$_2$ to Fab' was explored. In the preparation of native Fab', after reduction of the inter-H-chain S—S bonds, the SH groups thus obtained were alkylated with iodoacetic acid and the resulting Fab' separated from unreduced F(ab')$_2$ by gel filtration on G-100 Sephadex columns. In different experiments, iodoacetic acid was replaced by mercurials such as methylmercuric nitrate (Poljak *et al.*, 1971) and the CH_3Hg-Fab' obtained in this was was set to crystallize. The crystals obtained by this method were of different external morphology than native Fab' and were too small to be useful in X-ray diffraction experiments. Similar trials with other mercurials proved unsuccessful. However, in the soaking experiments, different mercury compounds were bound to Fab crystals at several sites, some of which were common to all of the mercurials. By using as heavy atom substituents organic mercurials of varying molecular dimensions and stereochemistry, the number of binding sites was limited so that the difference in Patterson functions could be unambiguously interpreted. At least nine heavy atom substitutions were characterized and found to be useful in the phase determination procedure. These nine substituents are: phenylmercuric acetate, uranyl nitrate, *p*-chloromercuriphenylsulfonic acid, 1,4-diacetoxymercuri-2,3-dimethoxybutane (Baker dimercurial), diacetoxymercury dipropylenedioxide, mersalyl, mercuhydrin, and iodine. The use of a large number of heavy atom derivatives provided better phase information for the Fourier coefficients in the electron density map, thus enhancing the quality of the final electron density map of Fab New. The average figure of merit for 1225 reflections used to calculate the 6 Å resolution electron density map was 0.87, which means that the average phase angle error for the 1225 amplitudes was less than 30° (Poljak *et al.*, 1972).

At different stages during the course of the refinement process, electron density maps of Fab' were calculated. Preliminary study of these maps revealed several featureless regions of low electron density, in particular around the twofold axes of symmetry, which must be regions of intermolecular spacing since an Fab molecule does not have twofold symmetry in itself. Very few rodlike features of high electron density were seen, as was expected because of the low helical content of IgG molecules predicted by optical rotatory dispersion measurements (Jirgensons *et al.*, 1966). As refinement proceeded, successive balsa wood models were constructed representing features of electron density above the average value. The final Fourier map calculated at the end of the phase refinement process allowed an unequivocal definition of the molecular boundaries in most regions. A striking feature of all models that were built is the presence of two structural subunits of relatively compact globular shape and of nearly equal size, with approximate dimensions of 30 X 40 X 50 Å. These two

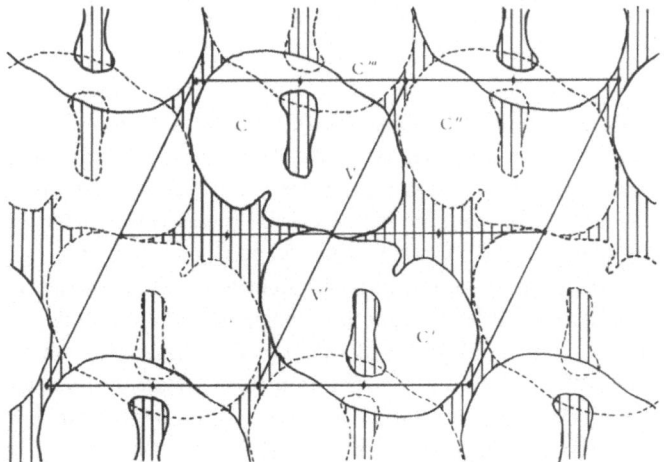

Figure 5. Schematic representation of the crystalline packing of Fab' New, viewed along the twofold axis (b) of the crystal. V and C are the two structural subunits of Fab'. The space between V and C and between neighboring molecules is shaded. (Reproduced from Poljak *et al.* (1972), with the permission of *Nature.*)

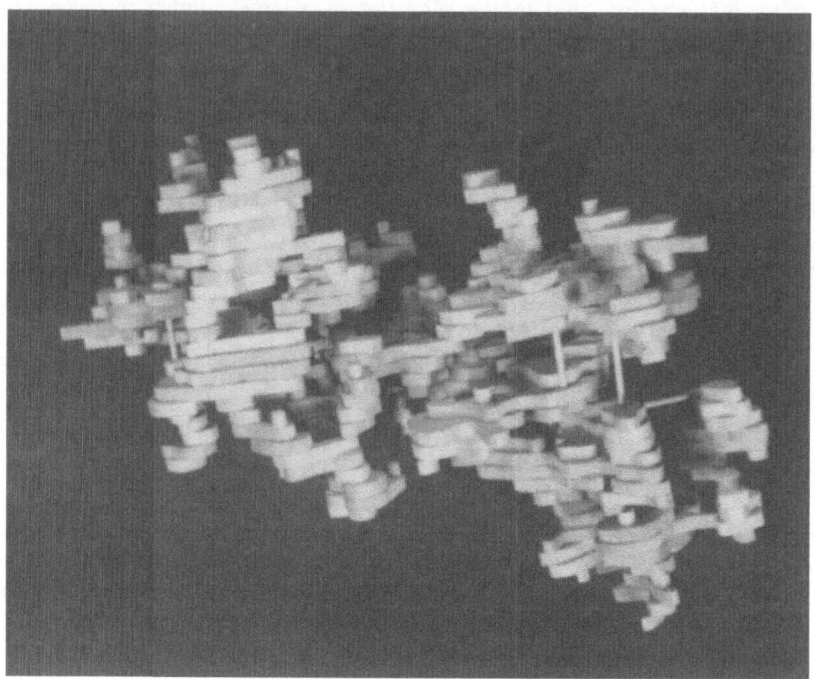

Figure 6. Balsa wood model of Fab' New at 6' Å resolution. Two globular subunits, corresponding to V and C of Fig. 5 are clearly seen.

subunits, although linked by features of positive electron density could be separated from each other as clearly as they could be separated from neighboring Fab molecules. This aspect of the structure is illustrated schematically in Fig. 5 in which the molecular packing in the crystal is described in terms of the two different globular subunits (V and C, Figs. 5 and 6).

With this preliminary description of Fab in terms of two structural subunits, it would appear reasonable that one of the subunits corresponds to the L chain and the other to the Fd fragment of the H chain. However, such an interpretation is not consistent with the results obtained by electron microscopy (Valentine and Green, 1967; Green et al., 1971) and X-ray diffraction (Edmundson et al., 1972). The combination of the structural subunits V and C (Figs. 5 and 6) gives an Fab molecule of approximate dimensions 40 X 50 X 80 Å, which is in good agreement with the dimensions obtained by electron microscopy (Valentine and Green, 1967). The electron microscopy studies have shown that the antigen binding site is at the end of the longer axis in the Fab region. If the long axis of Fab New is oriented parallel to the long axis of the Fab region of IgG

anti-DNP antibodies seen by electron microscopy (Fig. 2) then one must con-
clude that either the V subunit alone, or the C subunit alone contains the
antigen binding site. However, since it is known that the binding site is formed
by both L and H chains, the subunits V and C cannot correspond to the L and
Fd chains.

The structural model of a Bence-Jones λ-chain dimer obtained by Edmundson et al. (1972) also rules out the interpretation that the subunits V and C
correspond to the L and Fd chains. In the L-chain model of Edmundson et al.
(1972) discussed above, an L chain consists of two modules corresponding to the
homology regions V_L and C_L. Since it is expected that the structure of the L
chain in Fab New must be similar to that of the L chain described by Edmundson et al. (1972), it cannot correspond to one of the globular subunits (V or C)
of Fab New.

A closer study of the Fab' New Fourier map and of the 6 Å resolution
model built on the basis of the map provides a clearer answer to the meaning of
the V and C subunits and a more detailed picture of Fab. Starting at one end of
the molecular model (in the V subunit) two separate chains of electron density
can be traced. These two chains fold into several loops and determine the
globular structure of the V subunit, then continue independently into the C
subunit by way of two relatively linear bridges. However, the two chains do not
come into very close contact with each other in the V subunit. Inside the C
subunit both chains are compactly folded in a globular structure with closer
spatial relationship and several contact points. Since a 6 Å resolution map in
general cannot show the detailed folding of the polypeptide chain, no attempt
was made to correlate the electron density chains with the partially known
amino acid sequence of Fab New. However, it is most reasonable to believe that
these two continuous electron density chains correspond to the L and Fd
polypeptide chains. Figure 7 illustrates the model obtained for Fab in which the
continuous electron density chains are indicated with different colors. Both
chains appear to start in the V subunit with a short linear stretch, then go into a
more complex folding pattern including a loop, and emerge from the globular V
region to cross in a relatively linear fashion to the C subunit. Inside C they
resume a globular shape and become more interrelated than in the V subunit.
The overall arrangement of Fab, as illustrated in Fig. 7 is that of a distorted
tetrahedron. At the beginning of the V subunit the two chains jointly define a
cavitylike space which is easily accessible from the intermolecular spacing. This
cavity-shaped region has dimensions compatible with the requirements of an
antigen binding site, a feature that identifies the V subunit as one that includes
the variable regions of both L and H chains (V_L and V_H). The C subunit must
consist of the homology regions C_H1 and C_L.

From an electron microscopy study of an IgA murine myeloma protein
(MOPC 315) which binds dinitrophenyl groups, it has been concluded (Green et

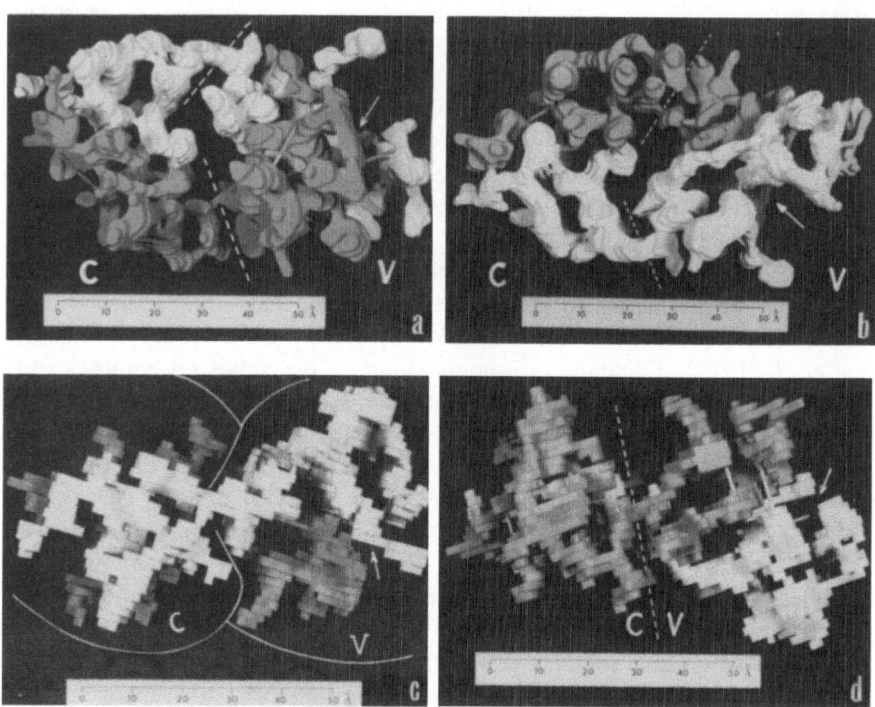

Figure 7. "Top" (a), "bottom" (b), and "side" (c,d) views of the 6 Å resolution model of Fab'. Dashed lines indicate the two connections between the V and C subunits; arrows on the right hand side of the figures point to the cavitylike area in the V subunit. The two continuous chains of electron density described in the text are shown as lighter and darker colored parts of the model. (Reproduced from Poljak *et al.* (1972), with the permission of *Nature.*)

al., 1971) that there are IgA subunits ("domains") which include parts of both the L and the H (*a*) chains. However, similar subunits could not be consistently observed in IgG proteins. The 6 Å model shown in Fig. 7 provides a plausible explanation for this apparent difference between IgG and IgA. Looking at the Fab region of IgG in the orientation shown in Figs. 6, 7c, and 7d, two structural subunits (V and C) are immediately evident. In this orientation they should be revealed by the negative staining technique used in electron microscopy. However, the "top" view (shown in Figs. 7a and 7b and along a nearly vertical line in Figs. 6, 7c, and 7d) will not necessarily display the subunit arrangement (it should also be considered that in Figs. 7a and 7b the model has been raised at its V end for photographic reproduction). It seems most likely that the way in which IgG molecules are deposited on electron microscope grids (providing the "top" view of Figs. 7a and 7b) prevents the detection of subunits, whereas the "side" view (Figs. 6, 7c, and 7d) which is probably obtained with MOPC 315 IgA (Green *et al.*, 1971) makes the subunits more evident.

The 6 Å Fab New structure provides a three-dimensional model to explain some of the physicochemical properties of immunoglobulin molecules. For example, fragments of light chains which appear to be of catabolic origin have been reported in human urine samples (Solomon and McLaughlin, 1969; Baglioni *et al.*, 1967). *In vitro* cleavage of human myeloma L chains by controlled enzymatic digestion has been shown (Solomon and McLaughlin, 1969; Karlsson *et al.*, 1972) to generate fragments having a more compact shape as judged by the radius of gyration and frictional coefficient than the parent L chain. Studies of allotypic and idiotypic markers (Solomon and McLaughlin, 1969), peptide mapping, and partial amino acid sequence data (Karlsson *et al.*, 1972) indicate that the fragments obtained by enzymatic action on L chains correspond to the V_L and C_L homology regions. Cleavage of the parent polypeptide chain occurs at the "switch" connecting the V_L and C_L homology regions, which is probably easily accessible to proteolytic attack by enzymes. In the Fab model, both L and Fd chains do indeed show easily accessible linear regions around the middle of their total length which connect the globular V and C subunits described above. Cleavage at the middle point of the L chain would generate two L-chain fragments of globular shape with a radius of about 15 to 20 Å, which compares well with the value of 16 Å obtained for the radius of gyration of several C_L and V_L fragments (Karlsson *et al.*, 1972). In fact the model of Fab New suggests that it should be possible to cleave Fab itself into two fragments of molecular weight 25,000 each; one of which should correspond to the V subunit and which could presumably retain antigen binding activity. It is interesting to note that a similar type of cleavage can be obtained in the Fc region (Turner and Bennich, 1968) leading to the appearance of an Fc′ fragment of molecular weight approximately 25,000. The overall similarity in tertiary structure between the L and Fd chains of Fab provides a structural model for the formation of dimers of L chains and dimers of H chains (Bjork and Tanford, 1971).

Studies of the conformational equilibria of the Fab fragment of a human myeloma IgG as a function of guanidine hydrochloride concentration (Rowe, 1971) have been interpreted in terms of a structural model consisting of a V and a C region. These regions are assumed to behave independently in the transition from the native conformation to a denatured state, giving rise to intermediate states in which one region is denatured while the other is still native. When the experimental data (optical rotatory dispersion measurements) were analyzed in terms of this model, one of the regions was found to be more stable than the other by two to four orders of magnitude. It was then proposed (Rowe, 1971) that the more stable region with stronger interactions consists of the constant homology regions $C_L + C_H 1$; the $C_L - C_H 1$ interactions would promote the assembly of H and L chains including the more weakly interacting $V_L - V_H$

domains. This proposal is consistent with the structure of Fab New in which the L and Fd chains appear less closely related in the V subunit than they are in the C subunit.

The X-ray crystallographic model of Fab New also shows a definite correlation between the internal homologies in amino acid sequence and the tertiary structures of immunoglobulins. In fact, it verifies that the homology regions fold into compact structures or domains linked by linear connecting regions. The striking structural feature of Fab is the presence of two globular subunits, V and C, each comprised of two distinct polypeptide chains. The hypothesis of a gene duplication process (Hill *et al.*, 1966) could be extended to say that gene duplication determined a structural duplication to build increasingly larger precursors of immunoglobulin molecules by the addition of globular subunits. The type of structure determined for Fab New can then be extended to the whole IgG molecule to provide the scheme shown in Fig. 8. In this schematic representation the V subunit consists of the homology regions V_L and V_H, C_1 consists of C_L and $C_H 1$, and C_2 and C_3 consist of $(C_H 2)_2$ and $(C_H 3)_2$, respectively. C_2 and C_3 constitute the Fc region in which an exact twofold axis of symmetry relates two $C_H 2$ and two $C_H 3$ domains (Goldstein *et al.*, 1968).

Affinity labeling experiments with rabbit anti-DNP antibodies have been interpreted (Singer *et al.*, 1967) to indicate that there is an approximate twofold axis of symmetry in the antigen binding region, very much like the one that relates the a to β chains in hemoglobin (Perutz *et al.*, 1960). This hypothesis appears consistent with the fact that the cavitylike region of the V subunit is delineated by both the H and the L chains. At 6 Å resolution the hypothesis appears plausible since there appear to be similarities in the structure of the two chains. A more definitive test will be provided by the high resolution studies.

The suggested "antigen binding site" of Fab New has dimensions of approximately 30 X 15 X 15 Å. These dimensions are close to those obtained from the geometry and dimensions of polypeptide and polysaccharide antigens mentioned above.

A preliminary 3.5 Å resolution Fourier map of Fab New has recently been calculated (Amzel *et al.*, 1972). Approximately 6000 native amplitudes were

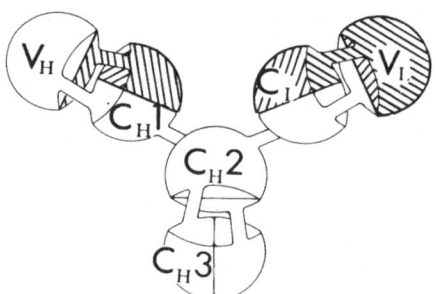

Figure 8. Schematic model of the structure of an IgG molecule incorporating the structural features determined for the Fab fragment and extrapolating these structural features to the Fc region. (Reproduced from Poljak *et al.* (1972) with the permission of *Nature.*)

measured using a computer-controlled diffractometer. Six heavy atom derivatives were included in the phase refinement process. The average figure of merit was 0.80. The definition of the molecular boundaries and of the subunits confirms the results obtained in the 6 Å resolution analysis. The C subunit includes regions of very compact folding in which it is difficult to distinguish the "backbone" polypeptide from the amino acid side chains; L and Fd chains are closely related. In the V subunit the two chains make much looser contact and appear to have similar tertiary structures, further supporting the notion of a local twofold axis of symmetry. Several stretches of extended polypeptide chain can be seen in both subunits, and in many places bulky side chains are clearly visible. The complete interpretation of this Fourier map and of the 3 Å resolution map to be calculated next will require a detailed correlation of the three dimensional structure with the amino acid sequence.

D. Fc Fragments

The Fc fragments from rabbit IgG and from human myeloma IgG were the first immunoglobulin materials to be analyzed by crystallographic methods (Poljak and Dintzis, 1966; Poljak et al., 1967; Humphrey, 1967; Goldstein et al., 1968). Crystals of the rabbit Fc fraction obtained from animals of different genetic constitution (allotypes) gave diffraction patterns which are identical in unit cell dimensions and intensity distribution. Although these observations were limited to some of the X-ray reflections having resolution less than 3.5 Å, they are enough to indicate virtual identity in the main features of polypeptide folding in the rabbit Fc. This result was in agreement with those obtained by Small, Reisfeld, and Dray (1966), who compared tryptic peptide maps and concluded that the Fc piece is constant or nearly constant in IgG molecules obtained from rabbits of different allotypic constitutions.

Human Fc crystals from several IgG1 myeloma proteins of different allotype have been examined by X-ray diffraction (Humphrey et al., 1969; Poljak, unpublished observations). The diffraction pattern of human Fc crystals extends to reflections of spacings d = 3 Å. The relatively large size and favorable symmetry of these crystals make them suitable for structural work. However, a major difficulty encountered in the determination of the structure of Fc has been that of obtaining suitable heavy atom derivatives.

The work of Goldstein et al. (1968) has shown that there is a twofold axis of symmetry relating the two identical halves of the Fc and that the molecule can be enclosed in a parallelepiped of 50 × 40 × 70 Å. These dimensions are in agreement with those determined by Valentine and Green (1967) by electron microscopy. Reduction of the S—S interchain bonds of human Fc and titration with Hg atoms of the SH groups thus created has been successfully attempted by Steiner and Blumberg (1971). Unfortunately, the Hg-Fc crystals obtained by this procedure diffract poorly and have not provided a useful heavy atom derivative of Fc (Steiner and Blumberg, 1971). Thus, because of the difficulty in obtaining suitable heavy atom substitutions no major progress has yet been made in the crystallographic study of the structure of the Fc fragment of human IgG.

E. Future Prospects

The detailed three-dimensional structure of immunoglobulin fragments (Fab) and L chains will be worked out in the not too distant future. These studies will provide a three-dimensional model of immunoglobulins and a correlation between amino acid sequence and structure. Since several different immunoglobulins are being investigated, the studies will also show the effects of variable amino acid sequences on the conformation of the molecules. In addition, the studies will give an indication of the geometry and stereochemistry of possible binding sites. However, unless antibody function or specificity for these myeloma proteins is found, these studies will not provide a system for the study of the chemical interactions between antigen and antibody. Therefore, it will be desirable to screen these human myeloma proteins to detect any possible antibodylike binding of haptens. It is even more desirable to obtain crystals of several induced antibodies of different specificity. The crystallographic analysis of a hapten–antibody complex would then give a model of a biologically significant interaction. Recent progress in obtaining induced antibodies of restricted heterogeneity in high yields indicates that the crystallographic study of induced antibodies may be a feasible project.

ACKNOWLEDGMENT

I am grateful to Dr. L. M. Amzel and Mr. Frederick Saul for reviewing the manuscript. The author's work cited in this review was supported by research grants AI 08202 (National Institutes of Health), E 638 (American Cancer Society) and by Research Career Development Award AI 70091 from the U.S. Public Health Service.

REFERENCES

Amzel, L.M., Avey, H.P., and Poljak, R.J. (1972). (in preparation)
Avey, H.P., Poljak, R.J., Rossi, G., and Nisonoff A. (1968). *Nature* **200**: 1248.
Baglioni, C., Cioli, D., Gorini, G., Ruffilli, A., and Alescio-Zonta, L. (1967). *Cold Spring Harbor Symp. Quant. Biol.* **32**: 147.
Bjork, I., and Tanford, C. (1971). *Biochemistry* **10**: 1271.
Cebra, J.J., Ray, A., Benjamin, D., and Birshtein, B. (1971). In Amos, B. (ed.), *Progress in Immunology*, Academic Press, New York, p. 269.
Deutsch, H.F., and Suzuki, T. (1971). *Ann. N.Y. Acad. Sci.* **190**: 472.
Dickerson, R.E. (1964). In Nevrath, H. (ed.), *The Proteins*, Vol. II, Academic Press, New York, p. 603.

Edelman, G.M., and Gall, W.E. (1969). *Ann. Rev. Biochem.* **38**: 415.
Edelman, G.M., Cunningham, B.A., Gall, W.E., Gottlieb, P.D., Rutishauser, V., and Waxdal, M.J. (1969). *Proc. Natl. Acad. Sci. U.S.* **63**: 78.
Edmundson, A.B., Wood, M.K., Schiffer, M., Hardman, K.D., Ainsworth, C.F., Ely, K.R., and Deutsch, H.F. (1970). *J. Biol. Chem.* **245**: 2763.
Edmundson, A.B., Schiffer, M., Wood, M.K., Hardman, K.D., Ely, K.R., and Ainsworth, C.F. (1971). *Cold Spring Harbor Symp. Quant. Biol.* **36**: 427.
Edmundson, A.B., Schiffer, M., Ely, K.R., and Wood, M.K. (1972). *Biochemistry* **11**: 1822.
Feinstein, A., and Rowe, A.J. (1965). *Nature* **205**: 147.
Goldstein, D.J., Humphrey, R.L., and Poljak, R.J. (1968). *J. Mol. Biol.* **35**: 247.
Green, N.M., Dourmashkin, R.R., and Parkhouse, R.M.E. (1971). *J. Mol. Biol.* **56**: 203.
Haber, E., Richards, F.F., Spragg, J., Austen, K.F., Vallotton, M., and Page, L.B. (1967). *Cold Spring Harbor Symp. Quant. Biol.* **32**: 299.
Haimovich, J., Givol, D., and Eisen, H.N. (1970). *Proc. Natl. Acad. Sci. U.S.* **67**: 1656.
Hill, R.L., Delaney, R., Fellows, Jr., R.E., and Lebowitz, H.E. (1966). *Proc. Nat. Acad. Sci. U.S.* **56**: 1762.
Holasek, A. Kratkey, O., Mittlebach, P., and Wawra, H. (1963). *J. Mol. Biol.* **7**: 321.
Holmes, K.C. and Blow, D.M. (1966). *The Use of X-ray Diffraction in the Study of Protein and Nucleic Acid Structure*, Interscience, New York.
Humphrey, R.L. (1967). *J. Mol. Biol.* **29**: 525.
Humphrey, R.L. and Owens, A.H. Jr. (1972). In Harvey, A.M., Johns, R.J., Owens, A.H. Jr., and Ross, R.S. (eds.), *The Principles and Practice of Medicine*, Appleton Century Crofts, New York, p. 1206.
Humphrey, R.L., Avey, H.P., Becka, L.N., Poljak, R.J., Rossi, G., Choi, T.K., and Nisonoff, A. (1969). *J. Mol. Biol.* **43**: 223.
Jirgensons, B., Saine, S., and Ross, D.L. (1966). *J. Biol. Chem.* **241**: 2314.
Kabat, E.A. (1966). *J. Immunol.* **97**: 1.
Kabat, E.A. (1968). *Structural Concepts in Immunology and Immunochemistry*, Holt, Rinehart and Winston, New York.
Karlsson, F.A., Peterson, P.A., and Berggord, I. (1972). *J. Biol. Chem.* **247**: 1065.
Maurer, P.H. (1964). *Progr. Allergy* **8**: 1.
Milstein, C., and Pink, J.R.L. (1970). In Butler, J.V.A. and Noble, D. (eds.), *Progress in Biophysics and Molecular Biology*, Vol. 21, Pergamon Press, New York, p. 209.
Nisonoff, A., Wissler, F.C., Lippman, L.N., and Woer, D.L. (1960). *Arch. Biochem. Biophys.* **89**: 230.
Nisonoff, A., Zappacosta, S., and Jureziz, R. (1967). *Cold Spring Harbor Symp. Quant. Biol.* **32**: 89.
Perutz, M.F., Rossman, M.G., Cullis, A.F., Muirhead, H., Will, G., and North, A.C.T. (1960). *Nature* **185**: 416.
Pilz, I., Puchwein, G., Kratky, O., Herbst, M., Naager, O., Gall, W.E., and Edelman, G.M. (1970). *Biochemistry* **9**: 211.
Poljak, R.J., and Dintzis, H.M. (1966). *J. Mol. Biol.* **17**: 546.
Poljak, R.J., Goldstein, D.J., Humphrey, R.L., and Dintzis, H.M. (1967). *Cold Spring Harbor Symp. Quant. Biol.* **32**: 95.
Poljak, R.J., Amzel, L.M., Avey, H.P., Becka, L.N., Goldstein, D.J., and Humphrey, R.L. (1971). *Cold Spring Harbor Symp. Quant. Biol.* **36**: 421.
Poljak, R.J., Amzel, L.M., Avey, H.P., Becka, L.N., and Nisonoff, A. (1972). *Nature New Biology* **235**: 137.
Porter, R.R. (1959). *Biochem. J.* **73**: 119.
Putnam, F.W., Titani, K., Wikler, M., and Shinoda, T. (1967). *Cold Spring Harbor Symp. Quant. Biol.* **32**: 9.
Rossi, G., and Nisonoff, A. (1968). *Biochem. Biophys. Res. Commun.* **31**: 914.
Rossi, G., Choi, T.K., and Nisonoff, A. (1969). *Nature* **233**: 837.
Rowe, E.S. (1971). Ph.D. Thesis, Department of Biochemistry, Duke University.
Sage, H.J., Deutsch, H.F., Fasman, G., and Levine, L. (1964). *Immunochemistry* **1**: 133.

Sarma, V.R., Silverton, E.W., Davies, D.R., and Terry, W.D. (1971a). *J. Biol. Chem.* **246:** 3753.

Sarma, V.R., Davies, D.R., Labaw, L.W., Silverton, E.W., and Terry, W.D. (1971b). *Cold Spring Harbor Symp. Quant. Biol.* **36:** 413.

Schechter, I. (1971). *Ann. N.Y. Acad. Sci.* **190:** 394.

Schiffer, M., Hardman, K.D., Wood, M.K., Edmundson, A.B., Hook, M.E., and Ely, K.R. (1970). *J. Biol. Chem.* **245:** 728.

Sela, M. (1969). *Science* **166:** 1365.

Singer, S.J., Slobin, L.I., Thorpe, N.O., and Fenton, J.W. (1967). *Cold Spring Harbor Symp. Quant. Biol.* **32:** 99.

Small, P.A., Reisfeld, R.A., and Dray, S. (1966). *J. Mol. Biol.* **16:** 328.

Solomon, A., and McLaughlin, C.L. (1969). *J. Biol. Chem.* **244:** 3393.

Solomon, A., McLaughlin, C.L., Wei, C.H., and Einstein, J.R. (1970). *J. Biol. Chem.* **245:** 5289.

Steiner, L.A., and Blumberg, P.M. (1971). *Biochemistry* **26:** 4725.

Suzuki, T., and Deutsch, H.F. (1967). *J. Biol. Chem.* **242:** 2725.

Turner, M.W., and Bennich, H. (1968). *Biochem. J.* **107:** 171.

Valentine, R.C., and Green, N.M. (1967). *J. Mol. Biol.* **27:** 615.

Welscher, H.D. (1969). *Int. J. Protein Research* **1:** 267.

Wu, T.T., and Kabat, E.A. (1970). *J. Exp. Med.* **132:** 211.

Yguerabide, J., Epstein, H.F., and Stryer, L. (1970). *J. Mol. Biol.* **51:** 573.

Chapter 2

Structural Analysis of the Antibody Combining Site

David Givol

Department of Chemical Immunology
The Weizmann Institute of Science
Rehovot, Israel

I. INTRODUCTION

The central problem of immunochemistry is to find the structural basis for antibody specificity. In view of the very wide range of different antigenic determinants and the overall similar basic structure of all antibodies the task seems formidable, and this problem has invited some paradoxical solutions in the past. However, it is now becoming increasingly apparent that the general architecture of antibody sites will not be different in principle from that of the active sites of enzymes. With the help of statistical analysis of amino acid sequences from myeloma proteins, affinity labeling of antibodies, and X-ray crystallographic analyses of crystals of antibody–hapten complexes, it seems that in the near future we will resolve the three-dimensional structure of an antibody site. It is already possible to speculate that in all antibodies the parts contributing to form the specific site are derived from similar sections of the variable region. I shall summarize here our studies which have had a role in the formation of this speculation and I shall discuss them in view of similar studies by others. In these studies we used both induced anti-DNP antibodies and mouse myeloma proteins with anti-DNP activity. The myeloma proteins are generally considered as representatives of homogeneous antibodies since in their reaction with DNP ligands they exhibit all the characteristics of binding sites of conventionally induced antibodies (Eisen *et al.*, 1968).

II. LOCALIZATION OF THE ANTIBODY COMBINING SITE

The antibody combining site is contained within the Fab fragment (Porter, 1959) which is composed of a light (L) chain and the N-terminal half (Fd) of the

27

heavy (H) chain (Fleischman *et al.*, 1963). It is generally agreed that antibody specificity results from different amino acid sequences and this is strongly supported by experiments on refolding of completely unfolded Fab or peptide chains (Haber, 1964; Whitney and Tanford, 1965; Freedman and Sela, 1966; Jaton *et al.*, 1968). However, only the N-terminal half of L (105–109 residues) or Fd (115–120 residues) contain sequences which vary from one IgG molecule to another, whereas the C-terminal halves of the polypeptides of the Fab fragment have constant sequences within the subclass. Theoretically, it is not impossible for the binding site to be in the constant region and modulated by different sequences in the variable region. It is also possible that the constant region of the Fab fragment is necessary for the maintenance of the combining site. Although affinity-labeling experiments have tugged residues only within the variable region of the H and L chains (Thorpe and Singer, 1969; Goetzl and Metzger, 1970; Givol *et al.*, 1971; Haimovich *et al.*, 1972; Franek, 1971; Cebra *et al.*, 1971; Ray and Cebra, 1972), it will be preferable to obtain a more direct evidence for the localization of the site.

The Fab fragment (molecular weight $\sim$50,000) can be obtained by a variety of methods (for positions of various splits see Givol and DeLorenzo, 1968). An early report (Kulberg and Tarkhanova, 1962) on the production of a smaller

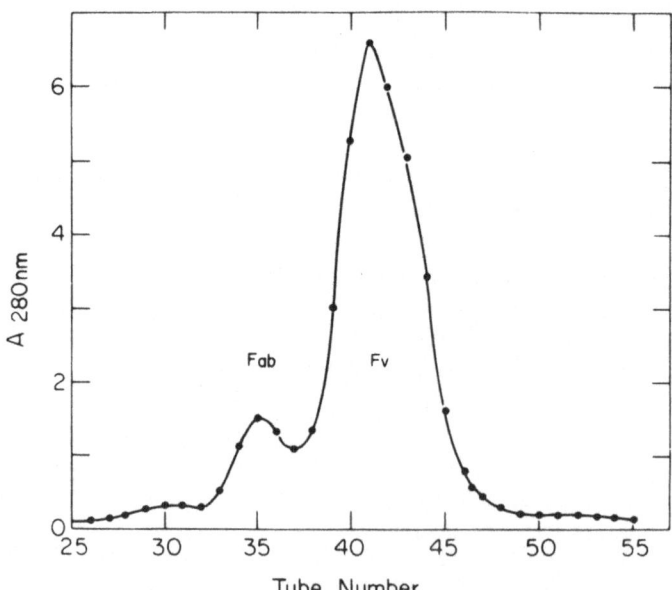

Figure 1. Fractionation on Sephadex G-75 of the fraction from pepsin-digested Fab' that binds to DNP-lysine-Sepharose. Column size was 2.7 X 140 cm and fractions of 5 ml were collected.

fragment (molecular weight $\sim$13,000) by digestion of Fab with papain in 6M urea was not followed up and other attempts to produce an active fragment with molecular weight smaller than 46,000 have been unsuccessful (Haber and Stone, 1967).

Direct evidence for the localization of the antibody combining site in the variable region of both the H and L chains was provided by studies with Fv, a fragment which is approximately the N-terminal half of the Fab fragment and which retains the complete antigen-binding activity. Our approach (Inbar et al., 1972) was based partly on the observation of Solomon and McLaughlin (1969) that under acidic conditions L can be split with pepsin into the variable and constant fragments. The mouse myeloma protein MOPC 315, an IgA which has anti-DNP activity (Eisen et al., 1968), was chosen for this purpose. The Fab' of MOPC 315 (Inbar et al., 1971) was digested with pepsin at pH 3.6 for 4 hr and fractionated by affinity chromatography on a DNP-lysine-Sepharose column. The material which bound to the immunoadsorbent (60% of the absorbance at 280nm) was eluted by DNP-glycine and further fractionated on a Sephadex G-75 column (Fig. 1). A comparison of various physical, chemical, and biological properties of Fab' and the peptic fragment Fv derived from it (Fig. 1) is given in Table I. The sequence of the first 7 residues of the Fv fragment (Asp–Val–Glx–Leu–Glx–Glx–Ser) is identical with the N-terminal sequence of the MOPC 315 H chain (Eisen, personal communication) and the N-terminal residue of L is PCA: These data also indicate that there are no internal peptide splits in the Fv. The molecular weights of Fv in aqueous solution and in SDS (Table I) imply that it is composed of two peptide chains of similar size (molecular weight $\sim$12,500), thus suggesting that Fv is composed of V_L and V_H. The very similar binding data of Fab and Fv indicate that the antibody site in MOPC 315 resides entirely in the variable domain and is independent of the constant portion of Fab.

These results provide also some support for the "domain hypothesis" (Edelman et al., 1969). On the basis of the repetitive homologous regions and periodic arrangement of disulfide bonds, it was suggested that each homologous region is a separately-folded globular domain stabilized by a single intrachain

Table I. Characteristics of Fab' and Fv

Property	Fab'	Fv
$S_{20,w}$	3.7S	2.6S
Molecular weight	59,000	25,000
Molecular weight in SDS	22,000	12,500
N-terminal residues	Asp–Val–Glx	Asp–Val–Glx
Isolectric point	4.7	5.4
K_a (M^{-1})	2.4×10^7	2.8×10^7
Binding sites per molecule	1.02	1.04

disulfide bond. The domains are linked by less tightly folded stretches of the peptide chain which are more susceptible to enzymic digestion. Our results indicate that in the intact Fab, the corresponding "domains" from the L and H chains are intercalated as one globular unit. This is particularly consistent with the recent X-ray analysis data of human Fab crystals (Poljak *et al.*, 1972).

III. CRYSTALS OF ANTIBODY–HAPTEN COMPLEX

Obviously, as with active sites of enzymes, the definitive structure of the antibody combining site will come from comparative X-ray crystallographic analysis of several antibody–hapten complexes. Crystals of human Ig or their Fab fragments are being analyzed in several laboratories. However, no known binding activities have been assigned to these proteins. Consequently, we attempted to crystallize MOPC 315 with its hapten. The Fab' of MOPC 315 can be crystallized near its isoelectric point (*p*H 4.6) at low salt concentration (Inbar *et al.*, 1971). The crystals formed were needlelike (Fig. 2), comprising at least 85% of the protein.

Crystallization of the Fab' fragment in the presence of the hapten Nϵ-DNP-lysine or Nϵ-DNP-amino caproate was performed under similar conditions except that the hapten was present at a concentration of 10^{-3}M. The Fab'–hapten complex formed yellow crystals. To test the molar ratio of Fab' to hapten in the crystals, crystallization was performed with ^{14}C-labeled Nϵ-DNP-lysine. The

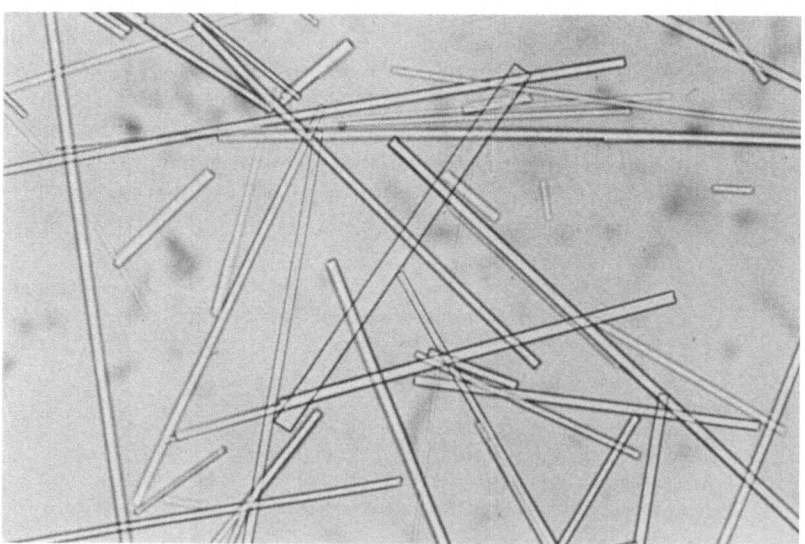

Figure 2. Crystals of Fab' in 0.002 M sodium acetate, *p*H 4.7, photographed on a 35 mm film X 78. (Reduced 35% for reproduction.)

ratio of hapten to protein in the dissolved crystals was 1.05, indicating that the combining sites of all the Fab' molecules in the crystals were occupied by the ligand. The difference spectrum between this solution and that of Nε-DNP-lysine with identical concentration showed two maxima at 470 and 383 nm, respectively, which was similar to the results of Eisen *et al.* (1968). This finding provides some evidence that the hapten is present in the combining site of the crystallized Fab'. No difference was observed in the general shape of the Fab' crystals obtained either in the absence or presence of hapten. Moreover, when crystalline Fab' was dialyzed against 0.002 M sodium propionate, 0.001 M, Nε-DNP-lysine at pH 4.7, the crystals became yellow. These crystals, however, are still unsuitable for X-ray analysis. Nevertheless, it is an important step in initiating similar attempts with other mouse or human myeloma proteins or with homogeneous antibodies which show anti-hapten activity. Such studies are under way in some laboratories and it seems likely that a complete picture of the antibody combining site will soon be available. However, as was the case with enzymes, chemical data on the active site can be obtained before the three-dimensional picture is available.

IV. AFFINITY LABELING OF ANTIBODIES

Undoubtedly the method of choice for obtaining data on the structure of the antibody combining site is affinity-labeling, a technique which was pioneered by Singer and his colleagues (Wofsy *et al.*, 1962). This method requires the preparation of hapten analogs which are modified to include a chemically reactive group capable of forming a covalent bond with certain amino acid residues. Due to the high local concentration of the modified hapten in the site, chemical reaction will take place predominantly there. It is clear that this method will become more versatile as different types of reagents are developed. Singer and his colleagues used the diazonium group as the chemical reactive moiety, whereas Porter and his colleagues introduced a photosensitive aromatic azide which upon exposure to light decomposed to give a highly reactive nitrene (Fleet *et al.*, 1969). In order to prepare affinity-labeling reagents with different chemical properties, we introduced the bromoacetyl derivatives of haptens (Weinstein *et al.*, 1969). Some characteristics of these reagents are given in Table II.

The main features of the bromoacetyl reagents are their high specificity, ease of identification of the labeled residues, and the possibility of mapping the site by a homologous series of reagents (Fig. 3) in which the chemically reactive group is situated at increasing distance from the haptenic group (Strausbauch *et al.*, 1971). As in other studies on affinity labeling of antibodies (Wofsy *et al.*, 1962; Singer, 1967) special care was taken to insure that each reagent in the series was indeed site specific (Strausbauch *et al.*, 1971). This was demonstrated

Table II. Comparison of Affinity Labeling Reagents

Property	Reagent type		
	Diazonium	Aromatic azide	Bromoacetyl
Reactive group is part of the antigenic determinant	No	Yes	No
Specificity to residue	Tyr, His, Lys	Any C-H bond	Tyr, His, Lys, Cys, Met, Asp, Glu
Rate of reaction	Fast	Very fast	Slow
Number of sites labeled	0.3	1.2	1–1.6
Possibility of preparing homologous series of reagents	No	No	Yes
Identification of labeled residue	By spectral analysis	By sequence of peptides	As CM-amino acid

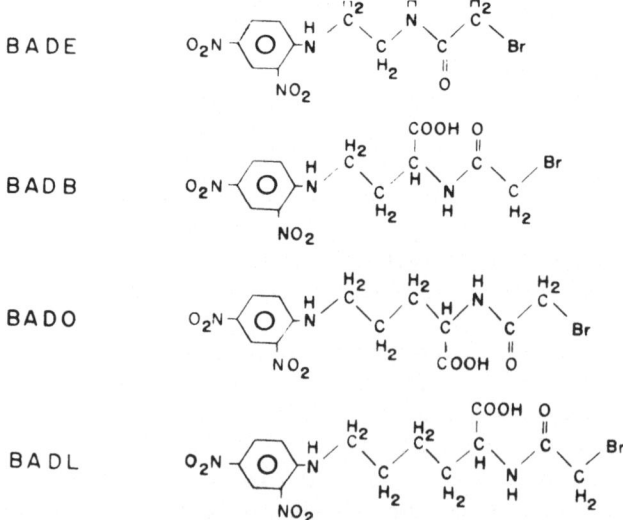

Figure 3. Homologous series of bromoacetyl reagents.

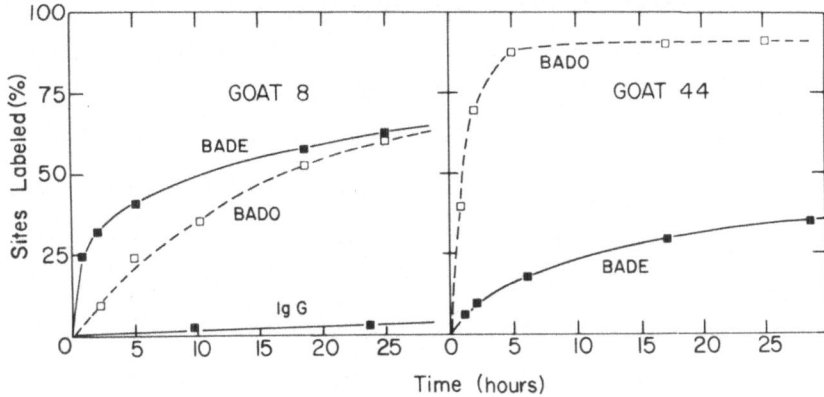

Figure 4. Reaction of BADE (■) and BADO (□) with purified anti-DNP antibodies from individual goats, and reaction of BADE (■) with normal goat immunoglobulin. Reaction conditions: antibody (10^{-6} M) and reagent (4×10^{-6} M) were incubated at 37° in 0.1 M $NaHCO_3$, pH 9.0.

by the following findings: 1) The reactions were stoichiometric, restricted to specific antibodies, and negligible with normal immunoglobulins. 2) The rate and extent of the reaction were not enhanced by increasing the excess of labeling reagent, indicating that covalent binding takes place within the specific complexes that are formed between the antibodies and their reagents. 3) Specific haptens protect the antibodies from labeling by competing with the labeling reagents for the vacant sites of the antibody. 4) After covalent attachment of the labeling reagent, there is no dislocation of the haptenic group and the red shift in the absorption spectrum (which is characteristic of DNP haptens bound to anti-DNP antobidies) is preserved. These data, together with the fact that upon covalent binding there is a loss of free antibody sites proportional to the extent of labeling (Weinstein *et al.*, 1969), strongly indicate that the labeling occurs either at or near the binding site.

The most interesting finding of the study with induced anti-DNP antibodies was the difference in kinetics and specificity of labeling with different reagents and with antibodies from different animals. For example, antibodies from goat 8 reacted more rapidly and to a larger extent with BADE* than with BADO, while reciprocal results were obtained with goat 44 (Fig. 4). Further details about the behavior of antibodies with the various reagents are given in Table III. With goat 8, the rate of reaction is maximal with BADE and decreases with increasing of

* Abbreviations used: BADE, N-bromoacetyl, N'-DNP-ethylene diamine; BADL, Nα-bromo-acetyl, Nε-DNP-lysine; BADB, N-bromoacetyl, Nγ-DNP-diamino-L-butyric acid; BADO, Nα-bromoacetyl, Nδ-DNP-L-ornithine; MNBD, *m*-nitro-benzenediazonium fluoroborate; NAP, nitroazidephenyl, CM, carboxymethyl.

Table III. Labeling of Goat Anti-DNP Antibodies with Affinity-Labeling Reagents[a]

Antibody preparation	Reagent	Extent of reaction[b]	Half-life time of reaction (hr)[c]
Goat 44	BADE	0.64	58.0
	BADE	0.84	41.0
	BADO	1.81	1.5
	L-BADL	0.96	25.5
	D-BADL	1.30	9.0
Goat 8	BADE	1.20	6.5
	BADE	1.60	7.0
	BADO	1.17	15.5
	L-BADL	0.96	26.0
	D-BADL	1.30	15.0
Goat 36	BADE	0.61	45.0
	L-BADL	0.62	30.0

[a] Reaction conditions: 1 mμmole/ml of antibody in 0.1 M NaHCO$_3$, pH 9.5, were reacted at 37° with 4 mμmoles/ml affinity-labeling reagent.

[b] Extent of reaction is given as moles of radioactive reagent covalently bound per 2 moles of hapten combining sites after 24 hr reaction. Number of combining sites was determined by fluorescence quenching.

[c] Time required for covalent labeling of 50% of the available sites.

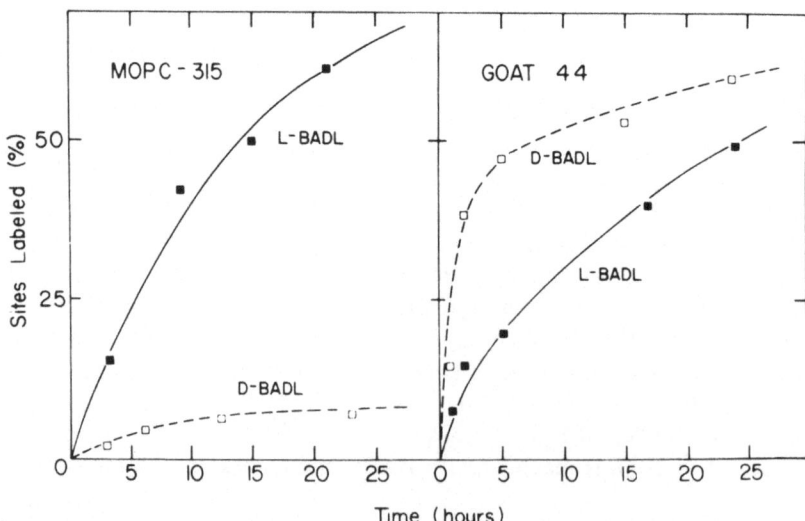

Figure 5. Stereospecificity in the labeling of myeloma protein MOPC 3.5 and anti-DNP antibodies from goat 44. Both proteins were reacted with either the D (□) or L (■) isomers of BADL under the conditions described in Fig. 4.

the reagent's size. On the other hand, with antibodies from goat 44, the rate increases with increasing size until the size of BADO is reached. Further increase in the size of the reagent results in a decrease in the rate of reaction. Another manifestation of the variability in behavior of various antibodies is reflected in the differences observed with two diastereoisomers of the same reagent (L- and D-BADL). For example, the antibodies from goat 44 react with the D isomer faster than with the L isomer (Fig. 5). Stereospecificity was even more accentuated in the case of the myeloma protein MOPC 315 (Fig. 5) which dramatically differentiates between the two diastereoisomeric reagents and essentially reacts only with the L isomer (Givol *et al.*, 1971; Strausbauch *et al.*, 1971).

In contrast to pooled rabbit antibodies, in which 95% of the label was on tyrosyl residues (Weinstein *et al.*, 1969), goat antibodies were labeled on both tyrosine and lysine. However, the distribution of the label between these two amino acids varied markedly in antibodies from different animals (Strausbauch *et al.*, 1971). The antibodies obtained from goat 8 were labeled mostly on tyrosine while in goat 44 most of the label was found on lysine. Moreover, antibodies from bleedings made at various times over a period of 18 months showed a fairly consistent distribution of the label between tyrosine and lysine characteristic for each animal (Fig. 6). This trait was preserved even after additional immunization. Since the difference in specificity of labeling probably reflects differences in amino acid sequences in the variable region, the labeled

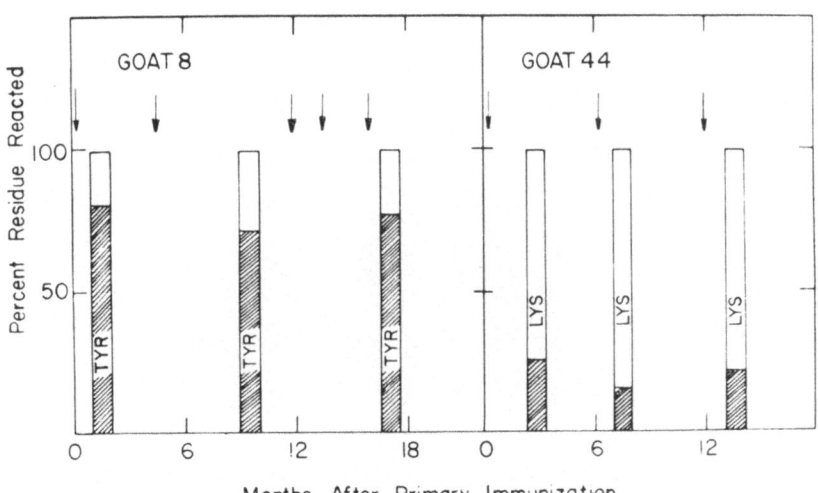

Figure 6. Affinity labeling of goat anti-DNP antibodies isolated at different times following immunization. Bar graphs indicate the percentage of lysyl (unshaded) and tyrosyl (shaded) residues labeled by BADE. Initial immunization was made at time zero. Arrows mark booster injections.

residue may serve as a genetic marker for this region. This possibility is further supported by affinity-labeling of anti-DNP antibodies from different strains of mice (Weinstein *et al.*, 1972). The results (Fig. 7) clearly show strain-related differences in the ratio of Tyr to Lys which was labeled in their anti-DNP antibodies. It is hoped that genetic crosses between strains showing high and low Tyr:Lys affinity-label ratios will reveal whether this can be used as a genetic marker in the hypervariable region of antibodies.

These results further demonstrate the potential of affinity labels for the study of variations in the combining sites and their biological significance. It is clear that in such a study it is important to select appropriate reagents which label specific amino acid residues and to try to analyze the biological background of the differences observed. The bromacetyl reagents are particularly suitable for this type of study because they label more than one type of amino acid and since the label can be identified easily.

In the case of affinity labeling with diazonium-type reagents, the remarkable result was the confinement of labeling to only one residue. With three different

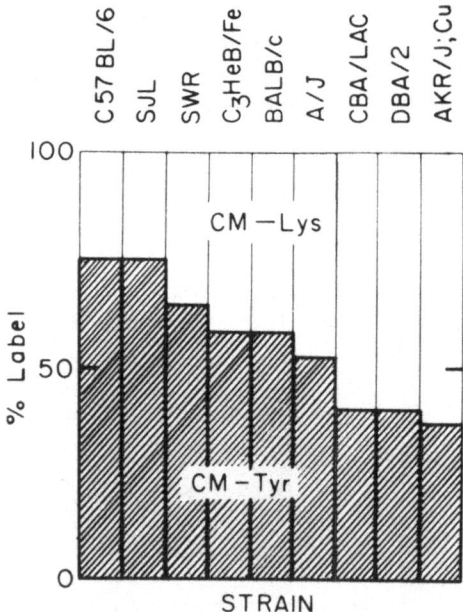

Figure 7. The distribution of affinity-labeled Tyr and Lys in anti-DNP from various mice strains. Antibodies were obtained from pooled sera of 20 mice and also from individual mice. Labeling was performed with BADL under the conditions specified in Fig. 4. The labeled CM-amino acids were quantified by high voltage paper electrophoresis or on the amino acid analyzer.

antibenzenoid antibodies, anti-*p*-azobenzenearsonate (Wofsy *et al.*, 1962), anti-DNP (Good *et al.*, 1968), and anti-*p*-azophenyltrimethylammonium (Fenton and Singer, 1965), only tyrosine residues were labeled. However, Wofsy *et al.*, (1967*a,b*) reported that with anti-carbohydrate antibodies some residues other than tyrosine were labeled. In rabbit anti-β-lactoside or anti-β-galactoside, the H chain was labeled at a tyrosine residue, but the labels on the L chains had a spectrum which could not be identified with either azotyrosine or azohistidine. Equine anti-lactoside antibodies were labeled primarily on histidine residues (Wofsy and Parker, 1967*c*).

Similar studies in different mice strains (Wofsy *et al.*, 1970) showed that there are indeed some strain differences. These differences are predominantly in the amount of affinity label attached to the antibodies. Pressman and his colleagues (Koyama *et al.*, 1968*a*) analyzed variability among rabbit anti-*p*-azobenzenearsonate by affinity labeling with the diazonium reagent and found remarkable quantitative and qualitative differences between antibodies from individual rabbits. Antibodies from one rabbit were labeled exclusively (0.5 residue/mole) on tyrosine. Antibodies from another rabbit were not significantly labeled, and antibodies from a third rabbit were labeled on both tyrosine and histidine. There were also striking differences in the kinetics of antibody labeling in the different rabbits. The observed differences which could not be correlated with the binding constants of the antibodies were probably due to different orientations of the reagent in the active site (Koyama *et al.*, 1968*a*). This theory was supported by experiments which combined chemical modification and affinity labeling (Koyama *et al.*, 1968*b*). Antibodies which are iodinated, in the presence of hapten were labeled at rates, degrees, and residues different from the noniodinated antibodies. For example, the antibody which was not susceptible to affinity labeling (see above) could be labeled extensively following iodination; the residue labeled was histidine. These authors further demonstrated that iodination in the presence of haptene did not change the binding constant of the antibody. They concluded, therefore, that the iodination caused conformational changes in the vicinity of the haptene-binding site making the histidine available for affinity labeling.

These results again demonstrate the ability of affinity labels to distinguish variability within the combining sites of different antibody populations. It will be of particular value to apply affinity labeling to antibodies of restricted heterogeneity, to antibodies of different classes or subclasses, and to antibodies obtained from animals with different genetic make-up of the immune response such as high and low responders from inbred guinea pigs or mice.

V. AFFINITY LABELING AND TOPOLOGY OF THE ANTIBODY SITE

In an extensive series of studies Singer and his colleagues analyzed many of the structural features of antibody sites by affinity labeling. With a variety of antibodies of different hapten specificities and with anti-DNP antibodies from several species, affinity labeling with diazonnium reagents labeled tyrosine residues on both L and H chains with a remarkable similarity in the distribution of label between the chains (H/L ratio of label was between 2 and 4). This led to 1) the hypothesis that all antibody sites are more or less uniform, having both H and L chains in close proximity in the combining site, and 2) the recognition of the evolutionary homology between H and L chains (Singer and Doolittle, 1966). Further studies suggested that a pseudodyad axis may relate the homologous L chain and Fd piece of the Fab fragment and the regions contributed by these to the antibody active site (Singer and Thorpe, 1968). This was indeed confirmed by X-ray analysis of Fab' crystals (Poljak et al., 1972).

The localization of the labeled tyrosine in the amino acid sequence met with difficulties due to the heterogeneity of antibodies. However, isolation of a labeled dipeptide, Asp–Tyr, from mouse anti-DNP light chain established that the labeled tyrosine must be in the variable portion since there is no such sequence in the constant part of mouse light chain (Thorpe and Singer, 1969). The same argument was applied for labeled dipeptide (Thr–Tyr from rabbit anti-DNP heavy chain. Moreover by comparison with the available sequences of myeloma proteins, Singer and Thorpe (1968) came to the conclusion that the labeled tyrosine in mouse and rabbit was tyrosine 86 in L chain and tyrosine 96, its homolog, in H chain. Since then, a sequence Thr–Tyr was indeed found by Porter and his colleagues in that position in rabbit heavy chain. It is interesting that these tyrosines, although very close to the third hypervariable region (Kabat and Wu, 1971), are extremely constant residues in both mouse and man Ig. It was suggested by Singer and Doolittle (1966) that antibody sites will be composed of a specificity region differing from one antibody to another and a conservative region which is shared by all antibody sites.

The studies on induced antibodies showed how complicated the analysis of the site labeled on each chain in heterogeneous antibody population can be. Hence, we turned to homogeneous myeloma proteins with anti-DNP activity. Figure 8 illustrates the results of affinity labeling of MOPC 315 with different reagents. BADE, and to a great extent BADB, labeled only Tyr on L chains whereas BADL labeled only Lys on H chains (Haimovich et al., 1970; Givol et al., 1971). A difference of only 3 Å in length (between BADB and BADL) resulted in a marked change in specificity in both the residue modified and the chain labeled. These observations strongly support the view that labeling reactions are sterically directed in the reversible complex of protein and reagent. Further support for this contention is provided by the result with D- and L-BADL (Fig. 5). L-BADL labeled a heavy chain lysine but D-BADL was not reactive even though MOPC 315 has the same intrinsic affinity for each reagent (Givol et al., 1971).

Reagent		Labeled residue and chain	
		%Tyr (L)	%Lys (H)
BADE	DNP-NH-CH$_2$-CH$_2$-NH-X	96	4
BADB	DNP-NH-CH$_2$-CH$_2$-CH-NH-X COOH	87	13
BADO	DNP-NH-CH$_2$- CH$_2$-CH$_2$-CH-NH-X COOH	66	34
BADL	DNP-NH-CH$_2$-CH$_2$-CH$_2$-CH$_2$-CH-NH-X COOH	5	95

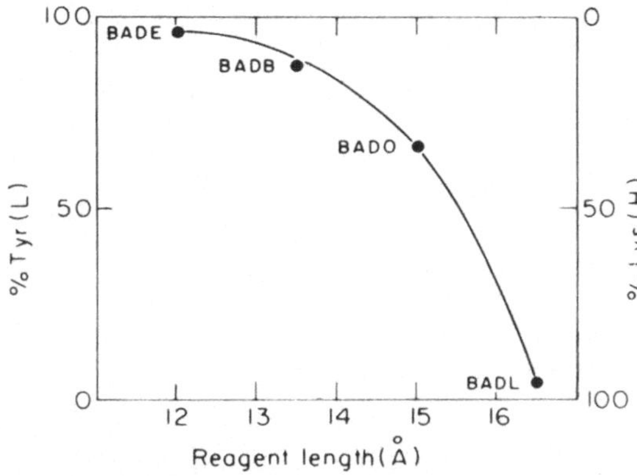

Figure 8. The specificity of affinity labeling of MOPC 315 by different reagents. The upper part of the figure gives the proportion of peptide chain and amino acid residue labeled by the different reagents. This was determined from heavy and light chains isolated on SDS-polyacrylamide gels. The lower part gives a schematic representation of the relation between the above specificity and the size of reagents (X = COCH$_2$Br).

If indeed the specificity of the chemical reaction is a function of the positioning of the bromoacetyl group, the foregoing results indicate that the distance between the labeled lysine on the H chain and the labeled tyrosine on L chain is approximately equal to the difference in the length of BADE and BADL (about 5 Å). Hence, a bifunctional reagent with two bromoacetyl groups separated by a distance equal to the difference in length between BADE and BADL would react simultaneously with both lysine and tyrosine and thus would cross-link the heavy and light chains. The data depicted in Fig. 9 show that the bifunctional reagent DNPHN–(CH$_2$)$_2$CH–(–HNCOCH$_2$Br)CO(NH)$_2$COCH$_2$Br (DIBAB) covalently cross-linked the H and the L chains to yield a molecule with

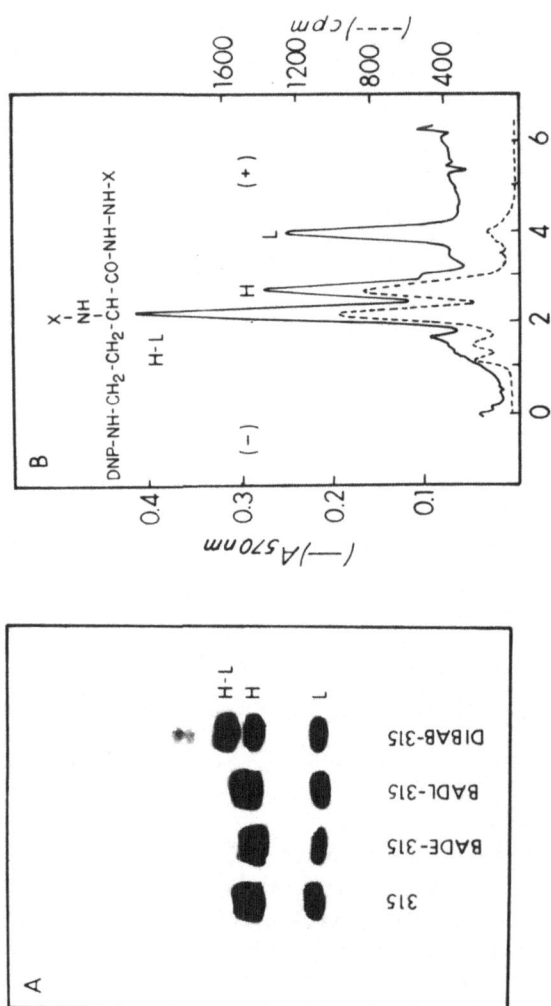

Figure 9. SDS-polyacrylamide gel electrophoresis of DIBAB-, BADL-, and BADE-labeled MOPC 315. 100 μg of protein in 100 μl were applied to the gel. After the run, the gel was stained and either scanned at 570 nm or sliced into 50 slices (1.3 mm) which were then dissolved in Soluene and counted in toluene scintillant. A) Electrophoretic pattern of affinity-labeled MOPC 315, protein migration from top to bottom. B) Distribution of protein and radioactivity in the gel of DIBAB-labeled protein. H, heavy chain; L, light chain; H–L, cross-linked chains.

a molecular weight of 72,000 (Givol *et al.*, 1971). The H-L band contained labeled Tyr and Lys in a ratio of 1:1 indicating that Tyr (on L) and Lys (on H) were involved in the cross-linking. This affinity-directed cross-linking of two peptide chains demonstrates the close spatial arrangement of H and L chains in the construction of the antigen-binding site. A schematic representation of this view is given in Fig. 10. In a slightly different manner, Hadler and Metzger (1971) succeeded in cross-linking H and L chains on the basis of affinity labeling. They labeled protein MOPC 315 with MNBD followed by reduction of the diazo bond with dithionite. The NH_2 tyrosine was then used, due to the low pK of its amino group, as the "first hook" for the bifunctional reagent 1,5-difluoro-2,4-dinitrobenzene. Subsequently the pH of the solution was raised and the second fluorine of the reagent reacted with neighboring residue on the heavy chain. This site-directed cross-linking is consistent with a distance of 3–4 Å between Tyr 34 (the affinity-labeled residue) on the L chain and an as yet unidentified residue on the H chain.

These results support the view that the antibody site is quite rigid and that the hapten has very little motility in the site. Thus the chemical reaction of the bound hapten depends on an exact positioning of the reactive bromoacetyl group in the vicinity of the residue to be labeled. Therefore, use of such a homologous series of reagents would facilitate an approach to mapping the structure of the site. In order to accomplish this, it is necessary to locate the labeled residues in the primary sequence of the peptide chains. It is also of

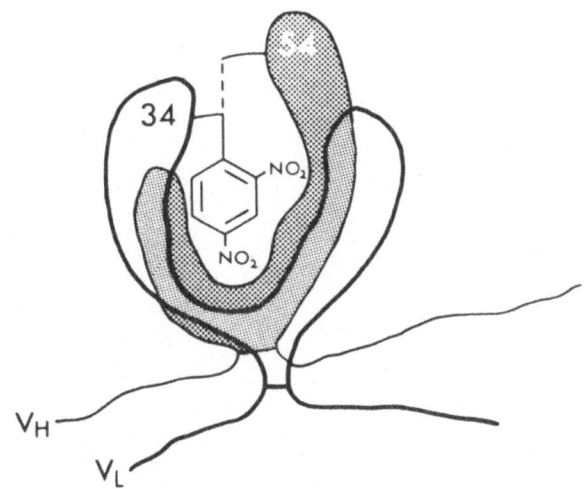

Figure 10. A schematic representation of the involvement of both V_H and V_L in the antibody site as revealed by affinity labeling. The numbers designate the affinity-labeled and the affinity-cross linked residues in L and H (see text).

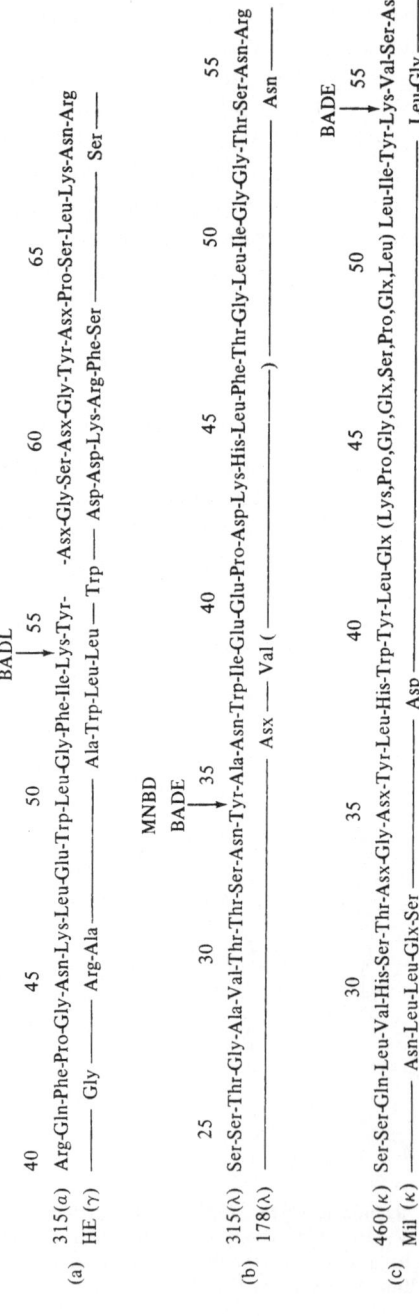

Figure 11. Combining site peptides. The sequences of affinity-labeled peptides isolated by affinity chromatography on anti-DNP-Sepharose. The sequences are given with homologous sequences from known heavy and light chains of myeloma proteins. (a) BADL-labeled peptide from H of MOPC 315 (Haimovich *et al.*, 1972). The sequence is compared with that of human protein HE (Cunningham *et al.* 1969). (b) BADE- or MNBD-labeled peptide from L of MOPC 315 (Goetzel and Metzger, 1970; Haimovich *et al.*, 1972). The sequence is compared with that of mouse protein 178 (Weigert, cited in Goetzel and Metzger, 1970; see also Schulenberg *et al.*, 1971) (c) BADE-labeled peptide from L of protein 460 (Haimovich *et al.*, 1972). The sequence is compared with that of human Bence-Jones protein Mil (Dreyer *et al.* 1967).

particular interest to extend this study to other DNP-binding myeloma proteins in order to establish whether differences in affinity and specificity can be reflected by differences in the susceptibility to affinity-labeling by these rea gents. Protein 460, a mouse IgA myeloma protein (Jaffe *et al.*, 1971), was selected for this purpose. In this protein, BADL labeled only 0.3 sites per molecule of protein whereas BADE labeled 1.2 sites per molecule. Contrary to the results with protein MOPC 315, BADE labeled predominantly lysine on light chains of protein 460.

The isolation of the labeled tryptic peptides from the peptide chains of proteins MOPC 315 and 460 (65–90% yield) was accomplished by affinity chromatography on anti-DNP-Sepharose columns (Givol *et al.*, 1970; Wilchek *et al.*, 1971). The labeled residues were localized largely on the basis of sequence homology with other Ig (Haimovich *et al.*, 1972). The sequences of the combining site peptides are given in Fig. 11. BADE labeled Tyr 34 on the light chain of MOPC 315 and Lys 54 on the light chain of protein 460, whereas BADL labeled Lys 54 on the heavy chain of MOPC 315 (Haimovich *et al.*, 1972).

A tryptophan residue was present in each of the affinity-labeled tryptic peptides. The DNP moiety of the peptides from MOPC 315 showed a red shift in absorption spectrum, resembling that observed when DNP ligands are specifically bound noncovalently in the combining sites of the intact protein. An illustration of the BADL-modified peptide showing BADL bound to Lys 54 and interacting with Trp 49 is given in Fig. 12. As expected, this red shift disappears after cleaving the peptide with thermolysin (Fig. 12). The results suggest that in the isolated peptides (and perhaps in the intact protein as well) the DNP group makes contact with Trp 49 or Trp 37 of the heavy and light chain, respectively, of MOPC 315, or possibly with both of these tryptophan residues. The results

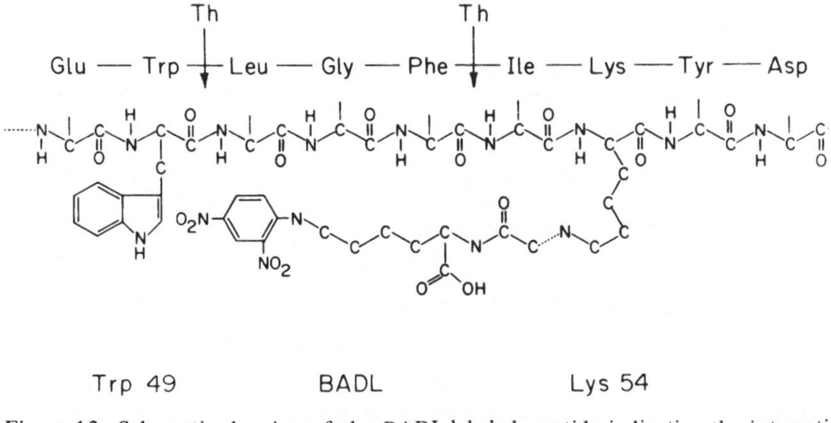

Figure 12. Schematic drawing of the BADL-labeled peptide indicating the interaction between DNP (bound to Lys 54) and Trp 49. The red shift of DNP absorption due to this interaction disappears upon thermolysin (Th) digestion.

from other similar studies and the positions of the labeled residues are summarized in Table IV.

It is notable that Tyr 34 in the light chain of MOPC 315 was labeled by *m*-nitrobenzenediazonium (Goetzl and Metzger, 1970) and also by BADE, which in its extended configuration is about 6 Å longer than the diazonium reagent. The BADE probably assumes a coiled configuration when bound to the combining site, allowing the bromacetyl moiety to approach the same residue as the diazonium group of the diazonium reagent. This suggests that the BADL, with an extended length of about 17 Å, might also be bound in a coiled configuration since it labels residues that are close to the site associated with DNP binding.

In each of the four affinity-labeling experiments, the two myeloma proteins, and practically all conventionally raised anti-DNP antibodies (Table IV), residues are labeled at positions found within one or another of the restricted hypervariable segments of the variable light or heavy chain domains. (Franek, 1971; Milstein, 1967; Wu and Kabat, 1970; Kabat and Wu, 1971; Kehoe and Capra, 1971.) The hypervariable segments which occupy positions 24–34, 50–56, and 89–97 of light chains and positions 31–35, 50–65, 81–87, and 95–102 of heavy chains (Kabat and Wu, 1971) comprise approximately 30% of the residues in the variable regions. If affinity-labeling reagents are free to combine with residues anywhere in the variable segments (V_L or V_H), then it seems unlikely that in four out of four experiments (with two myeloma proteins and three different reagents) all labeled residues were found only in the hypervariable region. It would seem rather likely that residues in these restricted segments of light and heavy chains actually constitute the specific combining sites, and are thus available for consistent labeling. Other indications that the hypervariable segments form the specific combining sites are provided by the remarkable similarity of sequences in these sections in diverse immunoglobulins with similar

Table IV. Affinity-Labeled Residues in Various Anti-DNP Immunoglobulins

Protein	Reagent	Labeled residue	Reference
315	BADL	Lys 54 on H chain	Haimovich *et al.* (1972)
315	BADE	Tyr 34 on L chain	Haimovich *et al.* (1972)
460	BADE	Lys 54 on L chain	Haimovich *et al.* (1972)
315	MNBD	Tyr 34 on L chain	Goetzl and Metzger (1970)
Pig anti-DNP	MNBD	Tyr 33 and Tyr 93 on L chain	Franek (1971)
Rabbit anti-DNP	MNBD	Tyr 96 on H chain	Singer and Thorpe (1968)
Mouse anti-DNP	MNBD	Tyr 86 on L chain	Thorpe and Singer (1969)
Guinea pig anti-DNP	MNBD	Tyr 33, Tyr 60, and positions between 99–119 on H chain	Cebra *et al.* (1971)
Rabbit anti-NAP	NAP	Cys 98 and Ala 99 on H chain	Porter (1971), Press *et al.* (1971)

binding specificies (Capra and Kunkel, 1970; Capra *et al.,* 1972). These authors compared the sequences of the 40 amino terminal residues of five L chains and two H chains from human myeloma proteins with anti-IgG specificity. They found striking differences between the sequences of these proteins and other non-anti-IgG myeloma proteins. The anti-IgG proteins however, showed marked sequence similarities, particularly in the first hypervariable region of both H and L chains (Capra *et al.,* 1971) and in the third hypervariable region of the H chains (Capra and Kehoe, personal communication). Some unusual replacements in the hypervariable region of L chains (e.g., Asn 30 and Ser 31) appear in most of these anti-IgG proteins (and not in other myeloma proteins) and may be related to antibody specificity.

Weigert *et al.* (1970) analyzed 10 mouse myeloma λ chains. Six of the proteins were identical, two proteins differed by one amino acid substitution, and two differed by two and/or three amino acid substitutions. All the substitutions were located in the hypervariable regions (positions 25, 32, 50, 52, 97). It has been suggested that the diversity within the variable region is by antigen-selected, single-step mutations. The fact that the first mutants to be selected are those which occur in hypervariable positions, strongly reinforces the theory that these regions are responsible for specificity. Another striking piece of evidence for this theory was obtained from the results of Cebra and his colleagues who identified the same hypervariable regions by comparative sequencing of "normal" Ig and anti-DNP antibodies from guinea pig (Birshtein and Cebra, 1971). The labeled residues in these anti-DNP antibodies (Cebra *et al.,* 1971; Ray and Cebra, 1972) fell in the hypervariable region of the H chain. (Table IV.) In addition, the amino acid sequence in these hypervariable segments of these anti-DNP antibodies was much simpler than that of pooled Ig (Ray and Cebra, 1972).

It may be of significance that BADL and BADE labeled only the first and second hypervariable segments, whereas MNBD and NAP labeled also the third hypervariable segments which is toward the end of the V fragment. This may be due to the fact that in NAP and MNBD the chemical reactive group is attached to the benzene ring and in NAP it is also a part of the haptenic determinant. If so, it may indicate that either the third or the third and fourth hypervariable segments in L or H, respectively, provide residues which are more in contact with the benzene ring of the determinant.

The lysyl residues that were labeled in the heavy chain of MOPC 315 and in light chain of protein 460 are replaced by other residues in the sequences of many other light and heavy chains (Milstein and Pink, 1970, also Fig. 11A and C). Hence these residues might not only be present in the combining site but they might also help to determine its specificity. The labeled tyrosine (Tyr 34) in MOPC 315 is homologous to Tyr 32 in most human light chains (Milstein and Pink, 1970). Of 20 human L chains analyzed, 10 have Tyr, 5 have Phe, and the remaining 5 each have a different residue at position 32 (Wu and Kabat, 1970). It has not yet been established whether this position is considered to be in a hypervariable region. It is, however, possible that this residue can assume different orientations in three dimensions and thus contribute to the specificity of the site. Another possibility is that Tyr 34 and Tyr 32 are part of the limited conservative region of the combining site of antibodies, regardless of specificity (Singer and Doolittle, 1966).

It is of interest that while BADL labeled Lys 54 in the heavy chain of MOPC 315, it did not label the neighboring Tyr 55 (Fig. 11A) whose hydroxyl group is probably not vicinal to the ε-amino of Lys 54 in the combining site of the intact protein. In addition to emphasizing the extraordinary dependency of the covalent labeling reaction on steric factors, these findings imply that the DNP reagent is highly immobilized when bound specifically (noncovalently) in the active site and that the amino acid residues that make up the site are also fixed in a relatively rigid configuration. If the polypeptide chains were flexible in this region, or if the bound ligand had some freedom in mobility, then labeling of Tyr 55 (on the heavy chain of MOPC 315) would have been expected (Haimovich *et al.*, 1972).

The absorption spectra of the labeled peptides isolated from MOPC 315 provide additional information on the protein's combining site. The red shift in the absorbance of the DNP group implies interaction with the indole ring of a tryptophanyl residue in each of these peptides (Little and Eisen, 1967). Though not proven, it is likely that Trp 49 in the peptide isolated from the heavy chain (Fig. 12) forms an intramolecular charge—transfer complex with the DNP moiety covalently bound to Lys 54. Trp 37 in the light chain of MOPC 315 probably forms a similar complex with the DNP group attached to Tyr 34 of this chain, since the corresponding peptide also exhibits the red shift. It is possible, therefore, that in the combining site of the intact immunoglobulin, either Trp 34 of the light chain or Trp 49 of the heavy chain, or possibly both of these Trp residues, interact with the bound DNP ligand in the combining site. This would account for the red shift observed when DNP is bound by the intact protein (Eisen *et al.*, 1968; Givol *et al.*, 1971). If both of these tryptophan residues interacted with the same molecule of specifically bound DNP, then the relevant heavy and light chain residues should be within 3–5 Å of each other. This possibility is supported by affinity-labeling studies with the bifunctional reagent that covalently links the H and L chains of MOPC 315, presumably at Tyr 34 of L chains and at Lys 54 of H chains. (Givol *et al.*, 1971).

VI. CONCLUDING REMARKS

The foregoing results clearly give some insight into the general architecture of the antigen-binding sites of antibodies. In fact, these results are at the same level of sophistication as those obtained from affinity-labeling and chemical modification studies of enzymes. The main conclusions can be summarized as follows: 1) The antibody site occupies only the V region. 2) There are close spatial associations between V_H and V_L in the site with possible distances of the order of 3–5 Å. 3) Spatial relationships can be suggested between several residues (e.g., Lys 54 and Tyr 55 on H chains, Trp 49 on H and Trp 37 on L chains, and Lys 54 on H and Tyr 34 on L chains. 4) Three main segments in L chains and probably four segments in H chains contribute contact residues to the antibody site. These segments superimpose the hypervariable segments identified by statistical analysis of sequences. 5) These segments appear in relatively similar positions in both V_H and V_L, indicating "symmetrical" contribution by both. Although most of the studies were conducted with anti-DNP antibodies, the good agreement with data on hypervariable regions obtained by comparing all known sequences of myeloma Ig strongly suggests that the general conclusion on the involvement of three segments of the V region in specific sites may hold for all antibodies. A schematic drawing of the model of the site which attempts to bring together all the labeled positions is given in Fig. 13.

It is of interest to compare the present results with those of substrate-binding by lysozyme. This enzyme is quite similar in size to V_H or V_L. Its

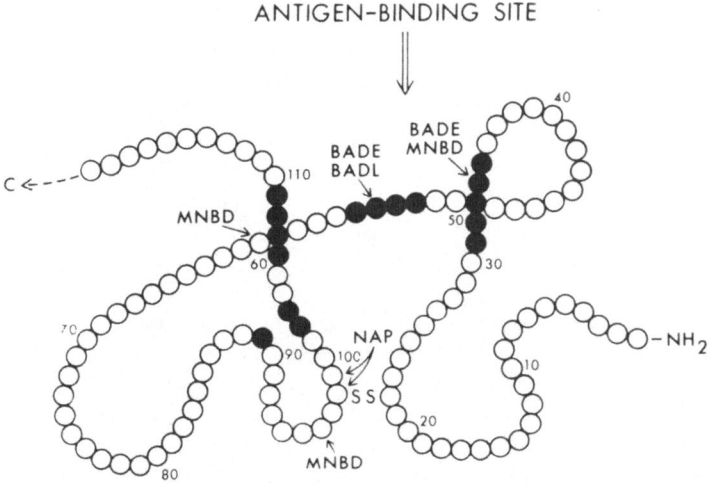

Figure 13. Schematic model of the antibody combining site of a variable fragment. The model mainly illustrates how the three affinity-labeled (hypervariable) segments are being brought together to the cleft of the site. It is assumed that variable fragments from the other chains complements this variable fragment. Numbering is as in V_H. Positions of labels on either V_H or V_L are according to Table IV. Black circles are hypervariable positions.

substrate or inhibitor is similar in size to that of saccharide antigenic determinants and the enzyme–inhibitor complex was fully analyzed crystallographically. The lysozyme site is proposed as a cleft of about 20 residue in the enzyme molecule which accommodates the ligand by noncovalent interactions. The positions of the residues which line the lysozyme cleft are shown in Fig. 14. There is a striking similarity between the three main segments which contribute contact residues and their position in lysozyme, and the hypervariable segments in the variable regions of antibody chains (compare with Fig. 13 and with Wu and Kabat, 1970; Kabat and Wu, 1971). It is therefore possible, as suggested by Porter (1971), that the antigen-binding site is constructed as a similar type cleft lined by about 20 residues contributed from the three hypervariable segments of each chain. As in enzymes, a change in one or two of these contact residues may lead to a big change in the specificity of binding (Hartley, 1970) without necessitating changes elsewhere in the molecule (i.e., in the nonhypervariable segments of the V region).

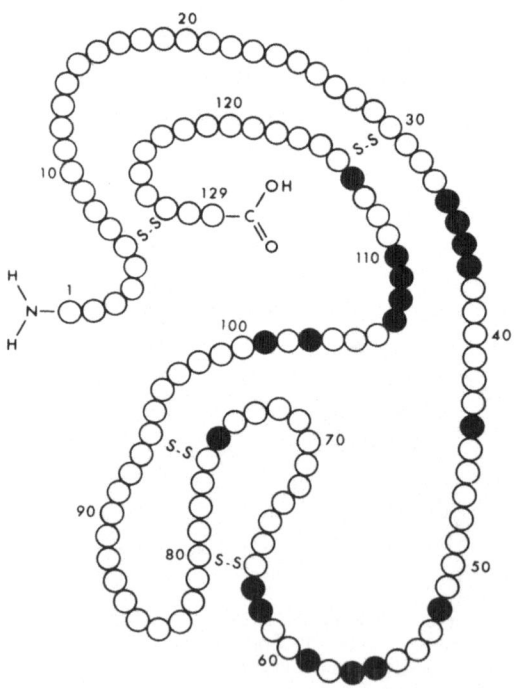

Figure 14. The primary sequence of lysozyme. The black circles represent residues which line the cleft (Phillips, 1966).

Table V. Some General Properties of Antibodies and Enzymes

Property	Enzymes	Antibodies
Range of specificity	Very broad	Very broad
Protein structure	Very different	Very similar
Active site	Binding and catalysis	Binding
Active site	One chain	Two chains (H and L)
Gene–protein relationship	One gene–one chain	Two genes (V and C)–one chain
Selection pressure	Against mutations at the active site	Favors mutations at the combining site

Although the basic architecture of the active sites of antibodies and enzymes may be similar in principle, it may be of interest to compare some of the general properties of enzymes and antibodies (Table V). It is evident that these two classes of proteins demonstrate basic differences in the biological background of the origin of their structure. The complementation of two different peptide chains in forming a binding site is a unique feature of immunoglobulins. However, the most fundamental problem of antibody structure is the origin of its diversity, and it is very likely that this problem will not be solved by our understanding of the structure of the site.

ACKNOWLEDGMENT

This work was supported in part by the Jane Coffin Child Memorial Fund for Medical Research and by United States Public Health Service Project (HD-05894).

REFERENCES

Birshtein, B.K., and Cebra, J.J. (1971). *Biochemistry* 10: 4930.
Capra, J.D., and Kunkel, H.J. (1970). *Proc. Natl. Acad. Sci. U.S.*
Capra, J.D., Kehoe, J.M., Winchester, R.J., and Kunkel, H.J. (1971). *Ann. N.Y. Acad. Sci.* 190: 371.
Cebra, J.J., Ray, A., Benjamin, D., and Birshtein, B. (1971). In Amos, B. (ed.), *Progress in Immunology*, p. 269, Academic Press, New York.
Dryer, W.J., Gray, W.R., and Hood, L. (1967). *Cold Spring Harbor Symp. on Quant. Biol.* 32: 353.
Edelman, G.M., Cunningham, B.A., Gall, W.E., Rutishauser, U., and Waxdal, M.J. (1969). *Proc. Natl. Acad. Sci. U.S.* 63: 78.
Eisen, H.N., Simms, E.S., and Potter, M. (1968). *Biochemistry* 7: 4126.
Fenton, J.W., and Singer, S.J. (1965). *Biochem. Biophys. Res. Commun.* 20: 315.
Fleet, G.W.J., Porter, R.R., and Knowles, J.R. (1969). *Nature* 224: 511.
Fleischman, J.B., Porter, R. R., and Press, E.M. (1963). *Biochem. J.* 88: 220.
Franek, F. (1971). *European J. Biochem.* 19: 176.
Freedman, M.H., and Sela, M. (1966). *J. Biol. Chem.* 241: 5225.
Givol, D., and DeLorenzo, F. (1968). *J. Biol. Chem.* 243: 1886.
Givol, D., Weinstein, Y., Gorecki, M., and Wilchek M. (1970). *Biochem. Biophys. Res. Commun.* 38: 825.

Givol, D., Strausbauch, P.H., Hurwitz, E., Wilchek, M., Haimovich, J., and Eisen, H.N. (1971). *Biochemistry* **10**: 3461.
Goetzl, E.J., and Metzger, H. (1970). *Biochemistry* **9**: 3862.
Good, A.H., Ovary, Z., and Singer, S.J. (1968). *Biochemistry* **7**: 1304.
Haber, E. (1964). *Proc. Natl. Acad. Sci. U.S.* **52**: 1099.
Haber, E., and Stone, M. (1967). *Biochemistry* **6**: 1974.
Hadler, N., and Metzger, H. (1971). *Proc. Natl. Acad. Sci. U.S.* **68**: 1421.
Haimovich, J., Givol, D., and Eisen, H.N. (1970). *Proc. Natl. Acad. Sci. U.S.* **67**: 1656.
Haimovich, J., Eisen, H.N., Hurwitz, E., and Givol, D. (1972). *Biochemistry* **11**: 2389.
Hartley, B.S. (1970). *Phil. Trans. Roy. Soc. London, Ser. B:* **257**: 77.
Inbar, D., Rotman, M., and Givol, D. (1971). *J. Biol. Chem.*, **246**: 6272.
Inbar, D., Hochman, Y., and Givol, D. (1972). *Proc. Natl. Acad. Sci. U.S.* **69**: 2659.
Jaffe, B.M., Simms, E.S., and Eisen, H.N. (1971). *Biochemistry* **10**: 1693.
Jaton, J.C., Klinman, N.R., Givol, D., and Sela, M. (1968). *Biochemistry* **7**: 4185.
Kabat, E.A., and Wu, T.T. (1971). *Ann. N.Y. Acad. Sci.* **190**: 382.
Kehoe, J.H., and Capra, J.D. (1971). *Proc. Nat. Acad. Sci. U.S.* **68**: 2019.
Koyama, J., Grossberg, A.L., and Pressman, D. (1968*a*). *Biochemistry* **7**: 1935.
Koyama, J., Grossberg, A.L., and Pressman, D. (1968*b*). *Biochemistry* **7**: 2369.
Kulberg, A.Y., and Tarkhanova, I.W. (1962). *Folia Biol. (Prague)* **8**: 147.
Little, J.R., and Eisen, H.N. (1967). *Biochemistry* **6**: 3119.
Metzger, H., Wofsy, L., and Singer, S.J. (1963). *Biochemistry* **2**: 979.
Milstein, C. (1967). *Nature* **216**: 330.
Milstein, C., and Pink, J.R.L. (1970). *Prog. Biophys. Mol. Biol.* **21**: 211.
Phillips, D.C. (1966). *Scientific American* **215**: 78.
Poljak, R.J., Amzel, L.M., Avery, H.P., Becka, L.N., and Nisonoff, A. (1972). *Nature New Biology* **235**: 137.
Porter, R.R. (1959). *Biochem. J.* **73**: 119.
Porter, R.R. (1971). *Harvey Lectures Ser.* **65**: 157.
Press, E.M., Fleet, G.W.J., and Fisher, C.E. (1971). In Amos, B. (ed.), *Progress in Immunology,* Academic Press, New York, p. 234.
Ray, A., and Cebra, J.J. (1972). *Biochemistry* **11**: 3647.
Schulenberg, E.P., Lynch, R.G., Bradshaw, R.A., and Eisen, H.N. (1971). *Proc. Natl. Acad. Sci. U.S.* **68**: 2623.
Singer, S.J. (1967). *Adv. Protein Chem.* **22**: 1.
Singer, S.J., and Doolittle, R.F. (1966). *Science* **153**: 13.
Singer, S.J., and Thorpe, N.O. (1968). *Proc. Natl. Acad. Sci. U.S.* **60**: 1371.
Solomon, A., and McLaughlin, C.L. (1969). *J. Biol. Chem.* **244**: 3393.
Strausbauch, P.H., Weinstein, Y., Wilchek, M., Shaltiel, S., and Givol, D. (1971). *Biochemistry* **10**: 4342.
Thorpe, N.O., and Singer, S.J. (1969). *Biochemistry* **8**: 4523.
Weigert, M.G., Cesari, I.M., Yonkovick, S.J., and Cohn, M. (1970). *Nature* **228**: 1045.
Weinstein, Y., Wilchek, M., and Givol, D. (1969). *Biochem. Biophys. Res. Commun.* **35**: 694.
Weinstein, Y., Givol, D., and Strausbauch, P.H. (1972). *European J. Immol.* **2**: 186.
Whitney, P.L., and Tanford, C. (1965). *Proc. Natl. Acad. Sci. U.S.* **53**: 524.
Wilchek, M., Bocchini, V., Becker, M., and Givol, D. (1971). *Biochemistry* **10**: 2828.
Wofsy, L., Metzger, H., and Singer, S.J. (1962). *Biochemistry* **1**: 1031.
Wofsy, L., Kimura, J., Bing, D.H., and Parker, D.C. (1967*a*). *Biochemistry* **6**: 1981.
Wofsy, L., Klinman, N.R., and Karush, F. (1967*b*). *Biochemistry* **6**: 1988.
Wofsy, L., and Parker, D.C. (1967*c*). *Cold Spring Harbor Symp. Quant. Biol.* **32**: 111.
Wofsy, L., Parker, D.C., Corneil, I., and Burr, B. (1970). In Sterzl, J., and Riha, I. (eds.), *Developmental Aspects of Antibody Formation and Structure,* II, Academic Press, New York, p. 425.
Wu, T.T., and Kabat, E.A. (1970). *J. Exp. Med.* **132**: 211.

Chapter 3

The Primary Structure of Rabbit and Mouse Immunoglobulin Light Chains: Structural Correlates of Allotypy

Ettore Appella and John K. Inman

Laboratory of Cell Biology
National Cancer Institute
and Laboratory of Immunology
National Institute of Allergy and Infectious Diseases
National Institutes of Health
Bethesda, Maryland

I. INTRODUCTION

Studies of immunoglobulin structure have been advancing at a considerable rate in the last few years. In spite of the obstacles of heterogeneity, information has become available concerning the overall structure of antibody molecules. A number of laboratories, particularly those of Porter (Porter, 1959; Fleischman *et al.*, 1963) and Edelman (Edelman and Gally, 1966), have contributed to the elucidation of the general structure of immunoglobulins. Immunoglobulins are multichain proteins made up of light and heavy chains linked by noncovalent interactions (Edelman and Poulik, 1961) and by disulfide bonds. A number of immunoglobulin classes have been defined according to serologically recognized determinants located in their heavy chains. Within a given class of heavy chains, subclasses have been distinguished by further antigenic determinants. Two major classes of light chains, κ and λ, are found associated with all classes of immuno-globulins. Although the immunoglobulins share the same overall structure, within a single class or subclass they are a heterogeneous mixture of chemically different molecules. Chemically homogeneous immunoglobulins are however available in large amounts as the protein secreted by cells of multiple myeloma tumors in men and mice. These proteins, considered earlier as "paraproteins" or abnormal products of tumor metabolism, have been clearly shown to have the same structure as normal immunoglobulins, and they appear to be made up of one or another of the many different molecules present in normal heterogeneous immunoglobulins (Edelman and Gally, 1962; Kunkel, 1965). Results of work over the past several years in amino acid sequence analysis of myeloma proteins, particularly Bence-Jones proteins (light chains) and more recently heavy chains, have established that the carboxyl-terminal portions of these peptide chains have essentially invariant sequences within each class or subclass. Limited variability occurs which is heritable in accordance with simple Mendelian principles (Terry *et al.,* 1969). The amino-terminal portions of immunoglobulin peptide chains, on the other hand, possess a high degree of variability in amino acid sequence. To account for this unusual structural arrangement, it has been suggested that two separate genes may specify the sequence of each variant and invariant region, and that sequence variation in antibodies may arise as a result of processes in addition to natural selection during evolution (Dreyer and Bennett, 1965). A debate has been generated, but a clear solution to the problem of the genetic origin of antibody variability and its relationship to specificity and to the biology of the selective immune response has not yet been provided.

Amino acid sequences of a large number of human light chains have been determined (Edelman and Gall, 1969; Milstein and Pink, 1970; Smith *et al.,* 1971). However, most of the existing sequence data on light chains of mouse and rabbit origin have been reported only recently or have not as yet been published. In this review we wish to summarize all the available sequence data on the light chains from these two species and to discuss the problem of allotype-associated residues.

II. RABBIT LIGHT CHAINS

Early studies on antigenic specificities giving rise to the concept of allotypy in rabbits were published by Oudin (1956). He arrived at a definition of allotypic specificity as being any serological specificity that is not shared by all members of a given animal species. The expression of these specificities was found to be controlled by different alleles (Oudin, 1956). These observations were subsequently confirmed by both Dray and Young (1958) and Dubiski *et al.* (1959). An early list and classification of six allotypic specificities associated with rabbit immunoglobulins was presented by Oudin (1960). At the present time, seven specificities including the above six are clearly recognized as being under the control of two unlinked genetic loci, *a* and *b*. The specificities are designated accordingly, a1, a2, a3 and b4, b5, b6, b9.

Dray, Young, and Gerald (1963) reported another specificity which they first called "P" and later renamed c7. It appears to be determined by molecules which comprise less than 10% of the total immunoglobulins. Recently, a new allotype, c21, has been identified and found to be genetically related to the c7 allotype (Vice *et al.*, 1969). These new allotypes segregate as if controlled by allelic genes. However, progenic data of a few families suggest that the genes may be closely linked, i.e., pseudoalleles (Gilman-Sachs *et al.*, 1969).

The discovery of two kinds of polypeptide chains in the immunoglobulin molecule (Edelman and Benacerraf, 1962; Fleischman *et al.*, 1962) led to the first insight into the possible chain localization of rabbit allotypic specificities. From many subsequent studies, it has become clear that the *a*-locus specificities are carried on the heavy chains, and that specificities controlled by genes at the *b* and *c* loci are expressed on the light chains (Kelus, 1963; Mage *et al.*, 1968).

The problem of the relationship between the allotypic specificities and the primary structure of immunoglobulin light chains has been approached in many different ways. Reisfeld, Dray, and Nisonoff (1965) were the first to compare the amino acid composition of light chains from rabbits homozygous for allotypes b4 and b5. They found differences, of 25 residues per light chain, involving 7 different amino acids. Reisfeld and Inman (1968) compared the

Table I. Amino Acid Composition of Rabbit IgG Light Chains with Different Allotypic Specificities[a]

Amino acid	b4[b]	b4[c]	b5[c]	b6[d]	b9[e]
Lys	8.7	8.8	9.6	7.6	7.5
His	1.2	1.3	1.4	1.3	2.3
Arg	3.1	3.1	3.1	4.0	4.7
Cys	(7.0)[f]	(7.0)[f]	(7.0)[f]	6.9	6.8
Asp	18.7	18.5	17.9	17.8	19.7
Thr	28.2	29.8	25.3	23.1	22.4
Ser	20.6	21.5	23.1	29.0	23.0
Glu	20.1	19.8	19.8	18.8	22.1
Pro	11.2	11.8	13.4	12.8	14.7
Gly	19.5	18.0	18.1	17.5	15.7
Ala	16.0	15.6	16.4	17.3	14.4
Val	21.2	21.0	18.5	17.5	16.2
Met	0.9	0.7	0.7	0.8	1.0
Ile	7.4	7.3	7.3	8.1	10.5
Leu	10.5	10.7	13.5	12.2	13.9
Tyr	10.2	9.8	9.6	10.1	9.3
Phe	6.5	6.3	6.3	6.1	6.7

[a]Calculated as residues on the basis of 204 residues for all amino acids except tryptophan, half-cystine and derivatives of the latter. (Data herein used with the permission of the publishers.)
[b]From data of Reisfeld *et al.* (1965).
[c]Calculated from data of Reisfeld *et al.* (1965).
[d]Data from Reisfeld and Inman (1968).
[e]From data of Appella *et al.* (1970).
[f]Assumed correct value from data of Reisfeld *et al.* (1965).

above compositions with the amino acid analysis of light chains from homozygous b6 rabbits. The average difference in composition between b4 and b6 chains involved 28 residues. The difference between b5 and b6 chains was 17 residues. The composition of light chains pooled from a group of b9 rabbits was reported by Appella *et al.* (1970). A comparison of the compositions of light chains bearing the four allotypes is presented in Table I. Differences in composition are given in Table II. The large compositional difference between the b9 and b4 chains is noteworthy. These reported compositions of light chains from serum pools of unimmunized individuals homozygous for a given allotype have been shown to be reproducible (Appella, unpublished observations). The observed compositional differences are compatible with the assumption that some of the amino acid positions are involved in determining the special antigenic properties associated with allotypy. The assumption that considerable differ-

**Table II. Differences in Amino Acid Composition[a]
Among Rabbit IgG Light Chains
with Different Allotypic Specificities[b]**

Amino acid	Allotypes			
	b6–b4[c]	b6–b5	b5–b4[c]	b9–b4[c]
Lys	−1.1	−2.0	+0.9	−1.2
His	0.0	−0.1	+0.1	+1.1
Arg	+0.9	+0.9	0.0	+1.6
Asp	−0.8	−0.1	−0.7	+1.1
Thr	−5.9	−2.2	−3.7	−6.7
Ser	+8.0	+5.9	+2.1	+2.0
Glu	−1.2	−1.0	−0.2	+2.1
Pro	+1.3	−0.6	+1.9	+3.2
Gly	−1.2	−0.6	−0.6	−3.1
Ala	+1.5	+0.9	+0.6	−1.4
Val	−3.6	−1.0	−2.6	−4.9
Met	0.0	+0.1	−0.1	+0.2
Ile	+0.7	+0.8	−0.1	+3.2
Leu	+1.6	−1.3	+2.9	+3.3
Tyr	+0.1	+0.5	−0.4	−0.7
Phe	−0.3	−0.2	−0.1	+0.3

[a] Italic numerals indicate differences considered significant in this study since they exceed 0.4 residues of individual amino acids or ten times the standard error, whichever is greater.
[b] Differences are expressed in residues per light chain and are taken directly from data presented in Table I.
[c] An average of the two b4 compositions reported in Table I is used here.

ences in observed composition may be involved in allotype expression is further supported by the observation that a minimum of two or three regions along the light polypeptide chain bear allotypic determinants (Mage *et al.*, 1966). An additional step in studying the relationship of allotypy and primary structure was provided by peptide map analysis of rabbit light chains as reported by Small, Reisfeld, and Dray (1965) and by Frangione, Franklin, and Kelus (1968). The maps from these two studies show about 7 peptides (out of about 30) that are characteristic for each allotype.

Human immunoglobulin light chains were the first to be recognized as falling into two distinct structural classes currently designated κ and λ (Mannik and Kunkel, 1962). Studies of amino acid sequences showed that chains of either class possessed a half-cystine residue at or near the carboxyl terminus which participated in the formation of the interchain disulfide bond joining light and heavy chains (Hilschmann and Craig, 1965; Milstein, 1965). Doolittle and Astrin (1967) were able to isolate from light chains of allotype b4 a peptide containing this half-cystine residue. When its sequence was compared with known C-terminal sequences of human and mouse light chains, 6 out of 7 positions were identical with the human κ chain, and 5 out of 7 positions were the same as the mouse κ chain. This strong homology suggested that the majority of rabbit light chains are of the κ type. These studies were extended to chains of allotypes b5 and b6 (Appella *et al.*, 1969). Characteristic amino acid interchanges were found between any two C-terminal sequences from chains of the three allotypes (Table III). These results established a clear sequence correlation with *b*-locus allotypy.

Studies on the amino-terminal residues of normal rabbit immunoglobulin and of several specific antibodies were initially carried out by Porter (1950) and by McFadden and Smith (1955). Their results indicated an average of 1.0 residue of alanine, 0.4 residue of aspartic acid and small amounts of leucylvaline per 7S immunoglobulin molecule at the N-terminal position. After the demonstration that 7S immunoglobulin could be separated into light and heavy polypeptide chains (Edelman and Benacerraf, 1962), these N-terminal amino acids were found to be associated with light chains. The heavy chains were shown to have no reactive N-terminal residues (Fleischmann *et al.*, 1962). The above N-terminal analyses were carried out exclusively with the Sanger dinitrophenylation method (Sanger, 1945). Doolittle (1966), using the Edman degradation, reexamined the amino-terminal portions of b4 light chains from normal rabbit immunoglobulin and from antibody specific for dinitrophenyl groups. In the course of 6 Edman cycles, the two types of preparation were qualitatively similar but quantitatively different. In normal pooled light chains, alanine was the major amino acid found at position 1, but a significant amount of isoleucine occurred there also (Table IV). When anti-dinitrophenyl light chains were examined, the ratio of alanine to isoleucine at position 1 decreased appreciably. Comparison of these mixed

Table III. Amino Acid Composition and Sequence of Tryptic and Chymotryptic Peptides from Partially Sulfitolyzed Rabbit b5, b6, and b4 κ-L$_{II}$ Chains[a]

Peptides	Amino acid composition							Sequence
	CySO$_3$H	Asp	Ser	Gly	Phe	Arg	Lys	
K(L$_{II}$) b5 T1 (40%)[b]	1.0	1.0					1.0	Lys-Asn-Cys
K(L$_{II}$) b5 C1 (20%)	0.9	1.0				1.0	1.0	Ser-Arg-Lys-Asn-Cys
K(L$_{II}$) b5 T2 (10%)	1.0		1.0		0.8	1.0	1.0	Phe-Ser-Arg-Lys
K(L$_{II}$) b6 T1 (30%)	1.0		1.0				1.0	Lys-Ser-Cys
K(L$_{II}$) b6 C1 (25%)	1.0		1.6			1.0	1.0	Ser-Arg- Lys-Ser-Cys
K(L$_{II}$) b6 T2 (15%)			1.0		0.6	1.0		Phe-Ser-Arg
K(L$_{II}$) b4 T1 (25%)	1.0	0.8		1.0				Gly-Asn-Cys
K(L$_{II}$) b4 C1 (40%)	1.0	2.0		1.0		1.0		Asp-Arg-Gly-Asn-Cys
K(L$_{II}$) b4 T2 (10%)	1.0	1.0	1.0		1.0	1.0		Ser-Phe-Asp-Arg

[a] Appella et al., 1970. (With the permission of the publisher.)
[b] Yields of the purified peptide as the percent recovery from the isolated whole light chain.

Table IV. PTH-Amino Acids Identified at Amino-Terminal End of Immunoglobulin Light Chains[a]

Light-chain source	Position in peptide chain[b]					
	1	2	3	4	5	6
Rabbit γ-globulin	Ala (Ile, Asp, Glu)	Val (Leu)	Val Leu (Gln/Glu)	Val (Gln/Glu)	Gln	Gln (Thr, Ala)
Rabbit anti-DNP	Ala Ile (Asp, Glu)	Val	Val Leu (Gln/Glu)	Val (Gln/Glu)	Gln Ala	Gln Ala (Thr)
Mouse and human[c]	Asp Glu	Ile	Val Gln	Val Leu Met	Thr	Gln

[a] Doolittle (1966). (With the permission of the publisher.)
[b] Positions numbered from amino-terminal end. PTH-amino acids shown in parentheses occurred in small amounts.
[c] Summarized from Hood et al. (1966) and Perham et al. (1966).

sequences with human and mouse κ chains showed that positions 1 and 2 of rabbit light chains did not show homology. However, positions 3 and 6 were essentially identical in all three species (Doolittle, 1966). Fraser and Edman (1970) successfully applied the automated sequential degradation method to b4 rabbit light chains from normal immunoglobulin and anti-p-azobenzenearsonate antibodies. A high degree of heterogeneity was found in the first 10 positions of normal light chains, but fewer amino acid substitutions were seen at corresponding positions in the antibody chains. An interesting feature of their findings is that a given amino acid can be recovered at successive steps of the degradation indicating that chains of different length were present in the sample. Severe limitations to further characterization of amino acid sequence was imposed by the heterogeneity of these preparations. Antibodies of highly restricted heterogeneity, as judged from binding studies and electrophoretic separations, have been obtained from rabbits immunized with streptococcal vaccines (Krause, 1970), pneumococcal vaccines (Pincus et al., 1970), p-azobenzoate conjugates of bovine γ-globulin (Roholt et al., 1970), and with p-azobenzenearsonate-coupled edestin (Mage et al., 1973). It became apparent from partial sequence studies of light chains from these antibodies that the restricted heterogeneity applied also to the primary structure. Examination of all the data from these studies (Table V) indicated that at least three or four distinct populations of rabbit antibody light chains could be discerned on the basis of specific deletion or substitution

Appella and Inman

Table V. Summary of Amino-Terminal

Antibody to	Rabbit light chain	Subgroup	0	1	2	3	4	5
Strep. Grp. C	2711^a	V_{KI}	Ala	Asp	Val	Val	Met	Thr
Pneu. Type VIII	1305^c			Asp	Val	Val	Met	Thr
Pneu. Type III	$G222-2^d$			Asp	Val	Val	Met	Thr
Pneu. Type III	268		Ala	Asp Val	Ile	Val	Met	Thr
Strep. Grp. C	2436^a	V_{KII}		Ala	Phe	Glx	Leu Met	Thr
Strep. Grp. C	2690^a	V_{KIII}			Ile	Val	Met	Thr
p-Azobenzoate	2717^e	V_{KIV}		Val	Glu	Val	Leu	Thr
p-Azobenzene-arsonate	$DD8^f$			Ala	Val	Val	Leu	Thr

[a] Hood et al. (1970a).
[b] Glx = Glu or Gln.
[c] Jaton et al. (1970).

patterns that occurred among certain positions (Hood et al., 1970a). In view of the sequence data on restricted light chains, it was interesting to reexamine by automated methods the sequences of normal rabbit light chains bearing each of the four allotypic specificities. Results so far obtained show that chains of each allotype are apparent mixtures of the three or four above-mentioned sequence classes found from the studies of restricted antibodies. But, the relative abundances of chains of these classes were found to vary in a characteristic pattern from one allotype to another (Hood et al., 1971; Chersi et al., 1971). It is not known yet whether any appreciable number of individual variable region genes are uniquely associated with any one allotype.

Skarova, Rejnek, and Kotynek (1968) separated rabbit light and heavy chains by means of gel filtration on Sephadex G-100 in 6 M urea, 0.05 M formic acid following partial oxidative sulfitolysis. They observed that light chains were distributed between two distinct fractions which they designated L_I and L_{II} in the order of elution. Both L_I and L_{II} material possessed the b4 allotypic

Sequences of Rabbit Light Chains

					Residue number									
6	7	8	9	10	11	12	13	14	15	16	17	18	19
Glx[b]	Thr	Pro	Ala	Ser	Val	(Ser)	Glu	Pro	Val	Gly	Gly		
Glx	Thr	Pro	Ala	Ser	Val	Ser	Glx	Pro	Val	Gly	Gly		
Glx	Thr	Pro	Ala	Ser	Val	Glx	Ala	Ala	Val	Gly	Gly		
Glx	Thr	Pro	Ala	Ser	Val Thr	Glx	Glx Ala	Val Ala	Val	Gly	Gly		
Glx	Thr	Pro	Ser Ala	Ser	Val	Glx Thr	Ala	Ala	Val	Gly	Gly		
Glx	Thr	Pro	Ser	Ser	( )	Ser	Val	Pro	Val	Gly	Gly		
Glx	Thr	Pro	Ser	Pro	Val	Ser	Ala	Ala	Val	Gly	Gly		
Glx	Thr	Ala	Ser	Pro	Val	Ser	Ala	Pro	Val	Gly	Gly		

[1] Appella et al., unpublished.
[2] Appella et al. (1971).
[f] Mage et al. (1973).

specificity of the original immunoglobulin and showed the molecular weight of undegraded light chain. Rejnek et al. (1969a) extended these observations to light chains prepared from normal immunoglobulins of rabbits homozygous for each of the four allotypes. In all cases L_I and L_{II} fractions were obtained and the respective allotypic specificity was expressed in both fractions. Significant differences in relative amounts of L_I and L_{II} fractions were found to be associated with allotype.

The L_{II} fractions from any of the 4 allotypes contained only κ-type chains as determined by chemical and immunological studies (Rejnek et al., 1969a), whereas the L_I fraction was in each case a mixture of κ light chains and molecules bearing no κ or b-locus allotypic determinants. The latter subgroup of L_I was identified with the "b" chains which carry an antigenic determinant, c7, which appeared to be controlled by a distinct locus, c (Mage et al., 1968).

The L_{II} κ fractions from b4 and b5 rabbits were found by careful amino acid analysis to contain 7 half-cystine residues per chain (Rejnek et al., 1969a;

Appella, unpublished observations). This number of half-cystines is apparently a unique feature of rabbit light chains. Half-cystine-containing peptides from b4 and b5 κ chains found in L_{II} fractions were isolated and sequenced by Frangione and Lamm (1970) and by Appella *et al.* (1971) (Table VI). It was feasible to place these peptides into about 7 groups on the basis of sequence homology; only 4 of the peptide groups were recovered in good yield, and these showed a single sequence for a given allotype (Table VI). One of these 4 peptides was the C-terminal segment with the allotype-associated interchanges noted above. Only one other half-cystine peptide showed any amino acid interchange that was related to allotypic specificity involving a position (169) with Ala from b4 and Asp from b5. Studies on the amino acid sequence of large, half-cystine-containing tryptic peptides from b4 light chains from two highly restricted rabbit antibodies have been reported recently (Appella *et al.*, 1972; Fraser *et al.*, 1972) (Table VII). From these data, the half-cystine residues of 6 of the 7 peptides have been located at positions homologous with those numbered 23, 88, 134, 171, 194, and 214 in the human κ protein Ag (Putnam *et al.*, 1967). The remaining peptide cannot be placed according to any obvious homology as yet. But, since this peptide is heterogeneous in both b4 and b5 light chains, it is thought to be part of the variable region. Poulsen and Haber (1972) have recently shown that one intrachain disulfide bond links a position in the variable region with a position in the constant region. Lamm and Frangione (1972) have shown, furthermore, that constant-region half-cystine 171 is linked to a half-cystine in the variable region, but the position of the latter has not yet been assigned. In previous work on normal light chains of b4 and b5 allotypes, Frangione and Lamm (1970) reported that a constant-region Ala–Asp interchange occurs at position 169 with Ala associated with b4 and Asp with b5. Fraser *et al.* (1972) also found Ala at position 169 in a highly restricted anti-pneumococcal antibody of allotype b4. However, Appella *et al.* (1971) found Asp at the same position in a peptide isolated from a highly restricted anti-*p*-azobenzoate antibody that was also of the b4 allotype. Thus, the relationship between b4 and b5 allotypy and the interchange occurring at position 169 is presently unclear.

Another interesting situation arose in connection with position 174 in normal pooled L_{II} κ chains from homozygous b4 and b5 rabbits. Three different amino acids (Leu, Val, and Asx) were found in this constant-region position. Leu alone was found at position 174 in highly restricted anti-*p*-azobenzoate b4 light chain (Appella *et al.*, 1971), and Val alone was found at the same position in restricted b4 anti-pneumococcal antibody (Fraser *et al.*, 1972) (Table VII). These data raised the question of whether these two constant-region sequences associated with a single allotype represent isotypic forms or two subgroups of the allotype. Decision on this matter must await analysis of the pertinent peptide isolated from light chains of a single individual.

Table VI. Half-Cystine-Containing Peptides Isolated from Rabbit Light Chains of Allotypes b4 and b5*

Suggested position of Cys residue	Allotype	Sequence
23	b4	Ser Ile-Asn-Cys
23	b5	Ser Ile-Asn-Cys
88	b4	Tyr-Tyr-Cys-Gln-Gln-Gly-Ser-Tyr
		Ser Tyr-Tyr-Cys-Gln-Gly-Ala
		Asn Tyr-Tyr-Cys-Gln-Gln-Ser-Gly
88	b5	Tyr-Tyr(Cys,Gln,Gln,Gly)Ser-Tyr
		Tyr-Tyr(Cys,Gln,Gln,Gly,Ser,Asp,Ala)
V region	b4	Leu Asx† Val-Glu-Cys-Ala-Asp-Ala-Ala-Thr
	b5	Leu Asx Val-Glu-Cys-Ala-Asp-Ala-Ala-Thr
171	b4	Thr-Pro-Glx-Asx-Ser-Ala-Asx-Cys-Thr
171	b5	Thr-Pro-Gln-Asn-Ser-Asp-Asp-Cys-Thr
134	b4	Ile-Val-Cys-Val-Ala-Asn-Lys
134	b5	Ile-Val-Cys-Val-Ala-Asn-Lys
194	b4	Glu-Tyr-Thr-Cys-Lys
194	b5	Glu-Tyr-Thr-Cys-Lys
214	b4	Ser-Phe-Asn-Arg-Gly-Asn-Cys
214	b5	Phe-Ser-Arg-Lys-Asn-Cys

* Frangione and Lamm (1970), Appella *et al.*, (1971), Lamm and Frangione (1972).
† Asx = either Asp or Asn.

Table VII. Partial Amino Acid Sequence* of Rabbit Light Chains of b4 Allotypes from Pools and Anti-*p*-Azobenzoate-Restricted Antibody 2717†

Block 1 (positions 1–19)

Pos	b4 Pool	2717
1	Ala / Asp	Val
2	Val / Asp / Ile / Leu / Tyr	Glu
3	Val / Ile / Asp	Val
4	Thr / Val / Met	Leu
5	Thr / Met / Glx / Ser	Thr
6	Glx / Thr / Gly / Val	Glx
7	Gly / Val / Pro / Glx	Thr
8	Pro / Val / Gly / Ser	Pro
9	Gly / Pro / Val / Ser	Ser
10	Val / Ala / Ser / Pro / Leu	Pro
11	Val / Ser / Leu / Pro	Val
12	Glx / Ala / Ser / Val	Ser
13	Ala / Val / Glx	Ala
14	Asp / Ala / Val	Ala
15	Val / Gly	Val
16	Gly / Val	Gly
17	Gly / Val / Ser	Gly
18	Val / Thr / Thr	Thr
19	Val / Thr	Val

Block 2 (from position 20)

- b4 Pool: 20 Thr / Gly · Ser / Ile · Ile · … · 27 …
- 2717: Thr · Ser · Glx · Cys · Ile · Ser · Thr · Lys · …

Block 3 (positions ~78–100)

- b4 Pool: Leu / Val · Glu · 80 Cys · Asx [Asp / Ala] · Ala · Ala · 85 Thr · … Glx · 90 Gln / Gly · (Ser / Ala / Gly) · … Gly · 100 Gly · Gly · Thr
- 2717: Tyr · Tyr · Cys · (Gly, Gly, Ala) · Asx · Tyr · …

(table rotated 90° on the printed page; residues given N→C, b4 Pool compared with mouse 2717)

						110										120		
b4 Pool	Glx	Val	Val	Lys	Gly	Asp	Pro	Val	Ala	Pro	Thr	Val	Leu	Ile	Phe	Pro	Pro	Ala	Ala
2717	┊	—	—	┊	Gly	———	———	———	———	———	———	———	———	———	———	———	———	———	———

							130											
b4 Pool	Asx	Gln	Val	Ala	Thr	Gly	Thr	Val	Ile	Val	Cys							
2717	———	———	———	———	———	———	———	———	———	———	Cys							

	162								170									
b4 Pool	Ser	Lys	Thr	Pro	Glu	Asp	Ser	Ala	Asp	Cys	Thr	Tyr	Leu/Val/Asn	Leu	Ser	Ser	Thr	Leu
2717	———	———	———	———	Ile	Ser	———	———	Asp	———	———	———	Leu	———	———	———	———	┊

	180								190										
b4 Pool	Thr	Leu	Thr	Ser	Tyr	Asp	Ser	His	Lys	Glu	Tyr	Leu	Ile	Thr	Cys	Lys	Gly	Thr	Val
2717	┊	┊	┊	———	———	———	———	———	———	———	———	———	———	———	———	———	———	———	Val

		210			214	
b4 Pool	Phe	Asn	Arg	Gly	Asp	Cys
2717	┊	┊	┊	———	———	Cys

* ———— sequences not determined.
——— sequences identical to the b4 pool.
† Appella *et al.* (1971, 1972).

Table VIII. Comparison of Sequences of Half-Cystine-Containing Peptides of Rabbit (b^-) Light Chains and Human, Mouse, Avian, and Pig Chains

Residue No.	20	21	22	64	65	66	67	68	69	70	71	72	73	74	75	76	77
Rabbit	Leu	Thr	Cys	Phe	Ser	Gly	Ser	Thr	Asp	Gly	Tyr	Thr	Ala	Ser	Leu	Thr	Ile
Mouse 104[a]	Leu	Thr	Cys	Phe	Ser	Gly	Ser	Leu	Ile	Gly	Asn	Lys	Ala	Ala	Leu	Thr	Ile
Mouse 315[b]	Leu	Thr	Cys	Phe	Ser	Gly	Ser	Leu	Ile	Gly	Asx	Lys	Ala	Ala	Leu	Thr	Ile
Human[c]	Ile	Thr / Ser	Cys	Phe / Ile	Ser	Gly	Ser	Ser / Lys	Ser	Gly / Asn	His / Thr / Asp	Thr / Ser	Ala / Ala	Ser / Thr	Leu	Thr / Gly / Ala	Ile / Val
Pig[d]	Leu	Thr	Cys										Ala	Thr / Ala	Ala	Thr / Leu / Gly	Ile
Avian[e]	Ile	Thr	Cys														

Residue No.	78	79	80	81	82	83	84	85	86	87	88	89	90	132	133	134	135
Rabbit	Thr	Gly	Ala	Glx	(Gly)	Val	Asp	Glx	Ala	Asx)	Tyr	Tyr	Cys	Ala	Thr	Leu	Val
Mouse 104[a]	Thr	Gly	Ala	Glu	Thr	Glu	Asp	Glu	Ala	Ile	Tyr	Phe	Cys	Ala	Thr	Leu	Val
Mouse 315[b]	Thr	Gly	Ala	Glx	Thr	Glx	Asx	Glx	Ala	Met	Tyr	Phe	Cys	Ala	Thr	Leu	Val

Residue No.	136	189	190	191	192	193	194	195	206	207	208	209	210	211	212	213	214
Human[c]	Thr Ser	Gly	Ala Leu Thr	Glu Arg	Ala Thr Ser	Glu Glx Gly Val	Asp Asx	Glu Glx	Ala	Asp His	Tyr	Tyr His Phe	Cys	Ala	Thr	Leu	Val
Pig[d]	Thr	Gly	Ala	Gln	Ala	Glu Asn	Asp	Glu	Ala	Asp	Tyr	Phe	Cys				Val
Avian[e]														Ala	Thr	Leu	Val
Rabbit	Cys	Ser	Tyr	Gln	Val	Ser	Thr	Cys		Ser	Leu	Ala	Pro	Ala	Glu	Cys	Ser
Mouse 104[a]	Cys	Ser	His	Ser	Tyr	Ser	Ser	Cys	Lys	Ser	Leu	Ser	Arg	Ala	Asp	Cys	Ser
Mouse 315[b]	Cys	Ser	His	Asp	Phe	Ser	Thr	Cys		Ser	Leu	Ser	Pro	Ala	Glu	Cys	Leu
Human[c]	Cys	Ser	His	Arg Lys	Ser	Tyr	Ser	Cys	Lys	Thr	Val	Ala	Pro	Thr	Glu	Cys	Ser
Pig[d]	Cys					Phe	Thr	Cys		Thr	Val	Thr	Pro	Ser	Glu	Cys	Ala
Avian[e]	Cys	(Ser	His	Thr	Ser	Tyr	Ser	(Cys)		Thr	Leu	Lys	Arg	Ser	Glu	Cys	

[a] Data from Appella (1971).
[b] Data from Schulenburg et al. (1971).
[c] Data from Milstein (1966); Titani et al. (1967); Langer et al. (1968); Milstein et al. (1967).
[d] Data from Franek (1967).
[e] Data from Grant et al. (1971).

The L_I fraction, as described above, contained a mixture of both κ and b^- light chains. In the course of further investigation of the L_I fraction, these two forms were separated (Rejnek *et al.*, 1969*b*) by the use of an immunoadsorbent to which was coupled anti-b5 antibody (reacting with the κ chains only). The b^- chains obtained in this way not only lacked *b*-locus determinants, but shared determinants with a distinct type of light chain isolated from the immunoglobulin of rabbits immunologically suppressed with respect to the expression of *b*-locus allotypes (Dubiski, 1967). The b^- light chain isolated from the suppressed rabbit was also shown by amino acid and partial sequence analysis to be strictly homologous with the λ-type chain of man and mouse (Appella *et al.*, 1968). The b^- or λ chains occur in all individuals regardless of their *b*-locus allotype (Rejnek *et al.*, 1969*a*), and have been shown to contain (for b5-suppressed b^- chain) 5 half-cystine residues (Appella *et al.*, 1973). The amino acid sequence of the isolated 5 half-cystine containing peptides is shown in Table VIII.

The κ portion of the L_I fraction was shown to be very similar in amino acid composition to the κ portion of the L_{II} fraction. A notable exception was that the former contained the more normal 5 rather than 7 half-cystine residues per chain (Rejnek *et al.*, 1969*a*). Since one of the extra half-cystines of the κ portion of the L_{II} fraction has been located at position 171 of the constant region, another interchange in this region would have to occur. Also, since immunoglobulins from individual rabbits have both L_I and L_{II} fractions, there must be at least two isotypes of the κ-chain constant-region sequence.

III. MOUSE LIGHT CHAINS

Murine myeloma tumors have been induced in the inbred BALB/c strain by intraperitoneal injections of mineral oil or some of its chemical components (Potter and Boyce, 1962; Anderson and Potter, 1969). Among the secreted products of these tumors are found a variety of immunoglobulin types. Except in rare instances, individual myeloma (plasma cell) tumors will secrete immunoglobulin having a single type of light chain and a single type of heavy chain. Often, a tumor-bearing mouse excretes in its urine an intact light chain, or Bence-Jones protein, which has been shown to have the same amino acid composition and sequence as the light chain from the whole immunoglobulin secreted by the tumor cells. Two serological types of Bence-Jones proteins from mouse urine have been recognized. Partial amino acid sequence analysis demonstrated that these two types of light λ chain were strictly homologous with the κ and λ types of human light chains (Appella and Perham, 1967). Moreover, the first complete sequence of two mouse κ chains (MOPC 41 and MOPC 70E) showed a high degree of homology with human κ chains (Gray *et al.*, 1967). In addition, the MOPC 70E protein has 4 amino acid residues inserted between positions 27 and 28* (Gray *et al.*, 1967). Early studies on the primary structure of κ chains from different BALB/c tumors revealed striking differences in peptide maps which involved at least 10 different peptides (Potter *et al.*, 1964). Five of these κ chains were examined with regard to their N-terminal sequences by the use of subtilisin degradation along with the Sanger N-terminal analysis method (Perham *et al.*, 1966) or by manual Edman degradation (Hood *et al.*, 1966). Amino acid sequence differences were clearly detected, and the patterns of variation were specific for each individual tumor protein. With one notable exception, all κ chains in these studies possessed aspartic or glutamic acids as N-terminal residues. Protein Adj-PC-9 did not have a reactive N-terminal amino group owing to the fact that the N-terminal residue was pyrrolidone-carboxylic acid (Glp).

By the use of the automatic sequence method of Edman and Begg (1967) 18 more amino-terminal sequences (up to position 23) have been published for mouse myeloma κ chains (Hood *et al.*, 1970b). Twenty-six more κ sequences have been determined for residues 1–22 by this method (Appella, unpublished data). A composite presentation of all the κ-sequence data appears in Table IX. A large degree of variability can be noted. The only completely invariant positions are 6 and 23 which bear glutamine and half-cystine residues, respectively. From 2 to 7 different amino acids have been found at all the other positions in the partial sequences. This large variability and the absence of any extensive linkage pattern among the substitutions point to the existence of a large number of variable κ ($V_κ$) subgroups. Furthermore, examinations of 4 of the 6 presently available complete mouse κ-chain sequences (McKean *et al.*, 1973; Gray *et al.*, 1967; Svasti and Milstein, 1972) show considerable variability throughout the entire amino-terminal half of the chains (Table X). No two chains share any extensive linkage pattern. Thus, the 4 chains may be regarded as members of different subgroups. Recently, McKean *et al.* (1973) have reported three complete and very similar $V_κ$ sequences from selected BALB/c tumors. Two of these differ only in three positions (Table XI). The third one differs from either of the other two in 8 positions. These 3 light chains were selected from 18 κ-type myelomas on the basis of identity in the first 22 positions. However, comparisons of any one of the 3 sequences with that of MOPC 70E, also identical with these in the first 22 positions, revealed differences at many positions (Table X). Thus, it can be seen that subgrouping of sequences on the basis of the first 22 positions entails the hazard of arbitrary selection.

Edelman and Gottlieb (1970) have studied a half-cystine-containing peptide separated from tryptic digests of mouse κ chains following full reduction and alkylation. The chains were obtained from 17 different strains of mice. A unique peptide which included the half-cystine at position 23 was found in only 3 strains, AKR/J, C58/J, and RF/J. This peptide occurred in about 10% of the κ chains of the above 3 strains, and was a member of a family of peptides of

---

* Throughout the discussion, all residue positions in κ chains refer to the numbering system applied to the human myeloma κ chain Ag by Putnam *et al.* (1967).

Table IX. Amino Terminal Sequences of Inbred BALB/c Mouse κ Chains*

	Residue number																						
	1	2	3	4	5	6	7	8	9	10	11	12	13	14	15	16	17	18	19	20	21	22	23
603†,384†,870†	D	I	V	M	T	Z	S	P	S	S	L	S	V	S	A	G	Z	K	V	T	M	S	C
HOPC 8†,TEPC 15†	D	I	V	M	T	Q	S	P	T	F	L	A	V	T	A	S	K	K	V	T	I	S	C
LPC 1†	D	I	V	M	T	Q	S	P	S	S	M	Q	A	S	I	G	E	K	V	T	I	S	C
265†,773†	E	T	T	V	T	Q	S	P	A	S	L	S	M	A	I	G	Z	K	V	T	V	S	C
157	D	I	V	M	T	Z	S	Z	S	F	M	S	T	S	V	G	D	R	V	S	V	T	C
641	D	I	V	M	T	N	S	X	X	F	M	S	T	S	V	G	D	R	V	S	I	T	C
843†	D	V	V	M	T	Z	T	P	L	T	L	S	V	T	I	G	E	P	A	X	I	S	C
674†	D	V	V	M	T	N	T	P	L	T	SL	S	V	T	I	G	Z	P	A	S	L	S	C
467†	D	V	V	M	T	Q	T	P	L	S	L	P	V	S	L	G	D	E	A	X	I	S	C
47†	N	V	V	M	T	N	T	P	L	S	L	A	V	S	L	G	X	Z	A	S	M	S	C
37†	D	V	L	M	T	Z	T	P	L	X	L	P	V	X	L	G	D	E	A	T	I	S	C
70E†,321†	D	I	V	M	T	Q	S	P	A	S	L	A	V	S	L	G	Q	R	A	T	I	S	C
613,124	D	I	V	M	L	Q	S	A	S	S	L	A	V	S	L	G							C

Protein	Sequence (single-letter code)
TEPC 29	E V V L T Q S P A I M S A S L G Q R V S M S C
172,46B,S23	D I V L T Q S P A T L S V T P G D S V S L S C
511	D I V I T Q D N L S K P V V S G N S V S I S C
167†	D I I S Q D S P — D L — — — — — — — — — — — C
MOPC 21	N V V L T Q S P A I M S A S P G Q R V T S M T C
3129,3434	D V V L T Q T G L S V S M G D R V S I S C
31B,31C,178	D I Q M T Q S P A S L S V S P G T T V T I T C
41†	D I Q M T Q S P S S L S A S L G D R V S L T C
173†	D I Q M T Q S P Y S S L S A S P G D X V X T C
23†	D I Q M T Q S P A S L S V S P G N N V T N T C
149	D I Q M T Q S P L Y D S L L G T V V N T C
3082,J606	D V Q M T Q S P A S L F M S V S D T V T M T C
600	D I Q M T Q S P E S E S S S I D N Z V S S T C
47A,47B	D I Q M T Q S P E S L A E X V R G G V T T C
611	D I Q M T Q S P A S L A X L S A V R R V T T C
SAPC 10,T191	E I V L T Q S P A I T A S A S L E R R V T S T C
21	N I V M T Q S P K S M S A K M A V G E R V S L T C

* The amino residues are expressed according to the single letter code: A = Ala, R = Arg, B = Asx, N = Asn, D = Asp, C = Cys, Q = Gln, E = Glu, G = Gly, H = His, I = Ile, Z = Glx, L = Leu, K = Lys, M = Met, F = Phe, P = Pro, S = Ser, T = Thr, W = Trp, Y = Tyr, V = Val, X = undetermined.
† Hood *et al.* (1970*b*). Other light chains were sequenced by Appella (unpublished data).

Table X. Partial Amino Acid Sequences of Four Mouse V$_K$ Polypeptides

Residues 1–25

										10										20					
321	D	I	V	L	T	Q	S	P	A	S	L	A	V	S	L	G	Q	R	A	T	I	S	C	R	A
70	D	I	V	L	T	Q	S	P	A	S	L	A	V	S	L	G	Q	R	A	T	I	S	C	R	A
41	D	I	Q	M	T	Q	S	P	S	S	L	S	A	S	L	G	E	R	V	S	L	T	C	R	A
21	N	I	V	M	T	Q	S	P	K	S	M	S	M	S	V	G	E	R	V	T	L	T	C	K	A

Residues 26–49 (30, 40)

										30										40					
321	S	K	S	V	B	T	Y	G	B	S	F	M	Q	W	Y	Z	Z	K	P	G	T	S	P	P	K	L
70	S	Q	S	V	B	B	S	G	I	S	F	M	N	W	F	Z	Z	K	P	G	T	I	S	P	P	K	L
41	S	Q	Q			B	B	B	I	G	S	L	B	W	L	Z	N	Z	G	B	B	Z	I	Z	K	R
21	S	Q	Q			N		N	V	T	Y	T	V	S	Y	Y	Q	Q	K	P	E	Q	S	P	K	L

Residues 50–72 (50, 60, 70)

										50										60				70
321	L	I	Y	R	A	A	S	N	L	Z	G	I	P	A	R	F	S	G	S	G	S	R	T	B	F
70	L	I	Y	A	A	S	N	Q	G	V	G	G	P	A	R	F	S	R	G	S	G	T	D	F
41	L	I	Y	A	T	S	S	L	B	S	G	V	P	K	R	F	S	G	S	G	S	G	D	Y
21	L	I	Y	G	A	A	S	N	R	Y	T	G	V	D	P	R	F	T	G	S	G	A	T	D	F

Residues 73–100 (80, 90, 100*)

								80										90								100*
321	T	L	T	I	B	P	V	Z	A	B	B	V	A	T	Y	F	C	F	Z	Z	N	B	Z	S	B	P	W	//S
70	S	L	N	I	H	P	M	Z	Z	B	B	T	A	M	Y	F	C	F	Z	Z	S	K	E	V	P	P	W	//G
41	S	L	T	S	S	L	E	S	E	D	F	V	D	Y	?	C	L	Q	L	Q	A	Y	S	P	S	//G
21	T	L	T	I	S	V	Q	A	E	D	L	A	D	Y	H	C	G	Q	G	Q	G	Y	S	Y	P	Y	//G

*The sequences of the constant regions of the four chains are identical and have been reported by the following investigators: 321, McKean et al. (1973); 70, 41, Gray et al. (1967); 21, Svasti and Milstein (1972).

Table XI. Summary of V_κ Mouse Sequence Variants*

Tumor	1	27	27d	50	58	83	91	94	100
M321	Asp	Lys	Thr	Arg	Ile	Val	Ser	Asx	Ser
T124	Asp	Gln	Trp	Arg	Ile	Val	Ser	Ala	Ser
M63	Asp	Gln	Ser	Leu	Val	Ala	Asx	Asx	Gly

* McKean *et al.* (1973).

similar length containing half-cystine 23. Breeding experiments demonstrated that genetic factors controlling the structure of the peptide were heritable in Mendelian fashion. These observations could suggest that only a small number of germ-line V_κ genes can exist in mice since it seems improbable that allelic variants can be maintained for long times when they are expressed in a large number of genes, but multiple subgroups, and thus multiple genes, can be inferred from sequence data.

In contrast, the half-cystine peptides of the constant region showed no variation. Complete amino acid analysis of tryptic peptides derived from the constant regions of a number of BALB/c myeloma κ chains indicates that only one gene controls the sequence of this region. An attempt to find allotypic determinants on mouse κ chains has so far failed (Lieberman, unpublished observations), whereas at least 4 allotypic markers are recognized in rabbit κ chains.

Mouse λ chains have been completely sequenced for two different myeloma proteins, one from the inbred BALB/c strain (MOPC 104E) and another from a cross between BALB/c and C57BL/ks (MOPC 315) (Appella, 1971; Schulenburg *et al.*, 1971). Even though both chains can be assigned to the λ class on the basis of serological specificity and sequence homology with human λ chain, they differ in their constant regions at 28 positions and in their variable regions only at 11 positions (Table XII). The variability in the constant region clearly establishes that there are two distinct types of λ chain, but it is not clear as yet whether these represent allotypes or isotypes. The latter interpretation is favored by the high probability that MOPC 315 is of BALB/c origin (as is 104E). This probability derives from the fact that MOPC 315 arose in a mouse from the seventh generation of backcrossings to BALB/c mice starting with an F_1 from a BALB/c $\times$ C57B1/ka mating. The progeny for backcrossing at each generation were selected on the basis of the presence of C57 heavy-chain markers. However, it can be reasonably assumed that heavy- and light-chain genes are unlinked in the mouse. Therefore, after 7 backcross generations, the probability that the MOPC 315 light chain was derived from the C57 genome is about 1/256 (Schulenburg *et al.*, 1971).

Table XII. The Amino Acid Sequence of Mouse Chain MOPC 104E and 315

	1									10								
MOPC 104E[a]	Glp	Ala	Val	Val	Thr	Gln	Gln	Ser	Ala	Leu	Thr	Thr	Thr	Ser	Pro	Gly	Glu	Thr
315[b]	Glp																Gly	

			20										30					
MOPC 104E[a]	Val	Thr	Leu	Thr	Cys	Arg	Ser	Ser	Thr	Gly	Ala	Val	Thr	Ser	Thr	Ser	Asn	Tyr
315[b]	Thr	Val										Ile		Ser				

						40						50					
MOPC 104E[a]	Ala	Asn	Trp	Val	Gln	Gln	Lys	Pro	Asp	His	Leu	Phe	Thr	Gly	Leu	Ile	Gly
315[b]																Ile	

								60									
MOPC 104E[a]	Gly	Thr	Asn	Arg	Ala	Pro	Gly	Val	Pro	Ala	Arg	Phe	Ser	Gly	Ser	Leu	
315[b]		Ser						Val									

		70									80						
MOPC 104E[a]	Ile	Gly	Asn	Lys	Ala	Ala	Leu	Thr	Ile	Thr	Gly	Ala	Gln	Thr	Glu	Asp	Glu
315[b]										Val							

				90									100				
MOPC 104E[a]	Ala	Ile	Tyr	Phe	Cys	Ala	Leu	Trp	Tyr	Ser	Asn	His	Trp	Val	Phe	Gly	Gly
315[b]	Met			Arg								Phe					

						110										
MOPC 104E[a]	Gly	Thr	Lys	Leu	Thr	Val	Leu	Gln	Pro	Lys	Ser	Ser	Pro	Ser	Val	Thr
315[b]				Val											Thr	Leu

Comparison of MOPC 104E[a] and 315[b] light-chain sequences (residues of MOPC 104E are given in full; for 315 only residues differing from MOPC 104E are shown).

	120										130						
MOPC 104E[a]	Leu	Phe	Pro	Pro	Ser	Ser	Glu	Glu	Leu	Thr	Glu	Asn	Lys	Ala	Thr	Leu	Val
315[b]	Val									Lys							

				140									150				
MOPC 104E[a]	Cys	Thr	Ile	Thr	Asp	Phe	Tyr	Pro	Gly	Val	Val	Thr	Asp	Trp	Lys	Val	
315[b]			Leu	Ser	Ser		Ser						Ala			Ala	

							160							170			
MOPC 104E[a]	Asp	Gly	Thr	Pro	Val	Thr	Gln	Gly	Met	Thr	Thr	Thr	Glu	Pro	Ser	Lys	Gln
315[b]					Ile				Val	Asp							

										180							
MOPC 104E[a]	Ser	Asn	Asn	Lys	Tyr	Met	Ala	Ser	Ser	Tyr	Leu	Thr	Leu	Thr	Arg	Ala	Trp
315[b]	Gly									Phe		His			Asp	Ser	

			190									200					
MOPC 104E[a]	Glu	Arg	Ser	His	Ser	Tyr	Arg	Ser	Cys	Gln	Val	Thr	(His)	Glx	Gly	His	(Thr)
315[b]					Asp	Phe	Pro	Thr					Asp				

					210					
MOPC 104E[a]	Val	Gln	Lys	Ser	Leu	Ser	Arg	Ala	Asp	Cys	Ser
315[b]	Leu			Pro					Glu		Leu

[a] Appella (1971). (With the permission of the publisher.)
[b] Schulenburg et al. (1971). (With the permission of the publisher.)

In an early study (Appella *et al.*, 1967; Appella and Perham, 1968), two mouse myeloma λ chains, MOPC 104E and RPC 20, were compared by tryptic peptide mapping. The maps were indistinguishable. The complete primary structure of these two chains has been shown to be identical (Appella, 1971). Weigert *et al.* (1970) partially sequenced the variable regions of 12 λ chains (including MOPC 104E). Eight of these sequences (V_λ) appeared to be identical. The other 4 chains varied in only one to four V_λ positions (Table XIII). MOPC 315, on the other hand, differed in about 11 positions throughout the N-terminal half of the chain when compared with MOPC 104E. These interchanges occur in the three hypervariable regions identified in the analysis by Wu and Kabat (1970). It is also interesting to note that the limited sequence variation in the selected chains studied by McKean *et al.* (1973) was confined to interchanges in the same hypervariable regions in two of the four chains studied, but not in the other two chains.

IV. CONCLUDING REMARKS

From results of studies on the relationship of primary structure with allotypy in rabbit immunoglobulin light chains, correlations have been defined both in the N-terminal and C-terminal sequences. However, these correlations have not solved the problem of the molecular basis of allotypic specificities. If one bears in mind that an allotypic site is that portion of the immunoglobulin structure with which the anti-allotype antibody molecule combines, then only the isolation of that segment of the entire immunoglobulin structure bearing all features necessary for maintaining the native site structure can define the

Table XIII. Summary of V_λ Mouse Sequence Variants*

Number of examples	Position					
	1	25	32	50	52	97
8	Glp†	Ser	Ser	Ile	Gly	His
1	Glp	*Asn*	Ser	Ile	Gly	His
1	Glp	Ser	Ser	*Leu*	Gly	His
1	Glp	*Thr*	*Gly*	Ile	Gly	His
1	Glp	*Asn*	Ser	Ile	*Asn*	*Arg*

* Weigert *et al.* (1970). (With the permission of the publisher.)
† Glp = pyrrolidone carboxylic acid.

structural basis of the specificity. This latter goal has not been achieved as yet for the *b*- or *c*-locus specificities.

Another consideration from the above studies is the relationship of the two-gene, one-polypeptide chain concept to the problem of antibody diversity. As has been argued many times, the disparity between the numbers of constant- and variable-region sequences points to a two-gene, one-chain mechanism for the specification of light-chain structure. The finding that constant regions of rabbit κ chains occur as two or possibly more isotypes raises the question of whether or not, in the long run, we will find as many constant-region sequences as there are variable-region subgroups. The implication for the two-gene, one-chain hypothesis is clear if one regards a subgroup as being encoded by a single germ-line gene and modulated in the "hot spot" positions by somatic mutations. Indeed, at present we see an obligatory association between that C-region isotype defined by the presence of half-cystine at position 171 (involved in the inter-regional disulfide bond) and a subgroup of variable sequences carrying the extra half-cystine which is bonded to position 171.

The allotype-associated distribution of rabbit V_κ subgroups can be interpreted in several ways in terms of strict germ-line concepts: The constant-region allele defined by a given allotype 1) controls the selection or expression of certain portions of a large pool of V_κ genes carried by the individual, or 2) is closely linked to a distinct set (in pseudoallelic fashion) of V_κ genes, and this set is different in subgroup distribution for each allotype.

Examination of the 44 partial N-terminal sequences (positions 1–22) of mouse κ chains (Table IX) soon reveals that an extensive and complex pattern of variability exists. As a first approximation, it appears that the number of possible V_κ subgroups is indeed large. This conclusion is based on data from a stretch of sequence outside of the hypervariable regions. In contrast, all the variant positions found in mouse λ chains occur in the hypervariable regions, indicating that the mouse can express only one indisputable variable-region subgroup of λ chain.

The variation in V_λ sequences that occur only in the hypervariable positions can be explained either by germ-line or somatic hypermutation models. With respect to the latter, Cohn (1971) has pointed out that this observed variability may be explained adequately by a process of stepwise antigen selection of somatic mutants.

REFERENCES

Anderson, P.N., and Potter, M. (1969). *Nature* **222**: 994.

Appella, E. (1971). *Proc. Natl. Acad. Sci. U.S.* **68**: 590.

Appella, E., and Perham, R.N. (1967). *Cold Spring Harbor Symp. Quant. Biol.* **32**: 37.

Appella, E., and Perham, R.N. (1968). *J. Molec. Biol.* **33**: 963.

Appella, E., McIntire, K.R., and Perham, R.N. (1967). *J. Molec. Biol.* **27**: 391.

Appella, E., Mage, R.G., Dubiski, S., and Reisfeld, R.A. (1968). *Proc. Natl. Acad. Sci. U.S.* **60**: 975.

Appella, E., Rejnek, J., and Reisfeld, R.A. (1969). *J. Molec. Biol.* **41**: 473.
Appella, E., Chersi, A., Rejnek, J., and Reisfeld, R.A. (1970). In Sterzl, J., and Riha, I. (eds.), *Developmental Aspects of Antibody Formation and Structure,* I, Academic Press, New York, p. 327.
Appella, E., Chersi, A., Roholt, O.A., and Pressman, D. (1971). *Proc. Natl. Acad. Sci. U.S.* **68**: 2569.
Appella, E., Chersi, A., Roholt, O.A., and Pressman, D. (1972). *Federation Proc.* **31**: 1296.
Appella, E., Chersi, A., Rejnek, J., Mage, R.G., and Reisfeld, R.A. (1973). (in preparation)
Chersi, A., Mage, R.G., and Appella, E. (1971). *Federation Proc.* **30**: 1307.
Cohn, M. (1971). *Ann. N.Y. Acad. Sci.* **190**: 529.
Doolittle, R.F. (1966). *Proc. Natl. Acad. Sci. U.S.* **55**: 1195.
Doolittle, R.F., and Astrin, K.H. (1967). *Science* **156**: 1755.
Dray, S., and Young, G.O. (1958). *J. Immunol.* **81**: 142.
Dray, S., Young, G.O., and Gerald, L. (1963). *J. Immunol.* **91**: 403.
Dreyer, W.J., and Bennett, J.C. (1965). *Proc. Natl. Acad. Sci. U.S.* **54**: 864.
Dubiski, S. (1967). *Nature* **214**: 1365.
Dubiski, S., Dudziak, Z., and Skalba, D. (1959). *Immunology* **2**: 84.
Edelman, G.M., and Benacerraf, B. (1962). *Proc. Natl. Acad. Sci. U.S.* **48**: 1035.
Edelman, G.M., and Gall, W.E. (1969). *Ann. Rev. Biochem.* **38**: 415.
Edelman, G.M., and Gally, J.A. (1962). *J. Exp. Med.* **116**: 207.
Edelman, G.M., and Gally, J.A. (1966). *Proc. Natl. Acad. Sci. U.S.* **51**: 846.
Edelman, G.M., and Gottlieb, P.D. (1970). *Proc. Natl. Acad. Sci. U.S.* **67**: 1192.
Edelman, G.M., and Poulik, M.D. (1961). *J. Exp. Med.* **113**: 861.
Edman, P., and Begg, G. (1967). *European J. Biochem.* **1**: 80.
Fleischman, J.B., Pain, R.H., and Porter, R.R. (1962). *Arch. Biochem. Biophys. Suppl.* **1**: 174.
Fleischman, J.B., Porter, R.R., and Press, E.M. (1963). *Biochem. J.* **88**: 220.
Franek, F. (1967). In *Nobel Symposium 3,* "Gamma Globulins, Structure, and Control of Biosynthesis," p. 221.
Frangione, B., and Lamm, M.E. (1970). *FEBS Letters* **11**: 339.
Frangione, B., Franklin, E.C., and Kelus, A.S. (1968). *Immunology* **15**: 599.
Fraser, K., and Edman, P. (1970). *FEBS Letters* **7**: 19.
Fraser, K., Strosberg, A.D., Margolies, M.N., Perry, D. and Haber, E. (1972). *Federation Proc.* **31**: 2968.
Gilman-Sachs, A., Mage, R.G., Young, G.O., Alexander, C., and Dray, S. (1969). *J. Immunol.* **103**: 1159.
Grant, J.A., Sander, B., and Hood, L.E. (1971). *Biochemistry* **10**: 3123.
Gray, W.R., Dreyer, W.J., and Hood, L.E. (1967). *Science* **155**: 465.
Hilschmann, N., and Craig, L.C. (1965). *Proc. Natl. Acad. Sci. U.S.* **53**: 1403.
Hood, L.E., Gray, W.R., and Dreyer, W.J. (1966). *Proc. Natl. Acad. Sci. U.S.* **55**: 826.
Hood, L.E., Eichmann, K., Lackland, H., Krause, R.M., and Ohms, J.J. (1970a). *Nature* **228**: 1040.
Hood, L.E., Potter, M., and McKean, D.J. (1970b). *Science* **170**: 1207.
Hood, L.E., Waterfield, M.D., Morris, J., and Todd, C.W. (1971). *Ann. N.Y. Acad. Sci.* **190**: 26.
Jaton, J.C., Waterfield, M.D., Margolies, M.N., and Haber, E. (1970). *Proc. Natl. Acad. Sci. U.S.* **66**: 959.
Kelus, A.S. (1963). *Biochem. J.* **88**: 49.
Krause, R.M. (1970). *Federation Proc.* **29**: 59.
Kunkel, H.G. (1965). *Harvey Lectures Ser.* **59**: 219.
Lamm, M.E., and Frangione, B. (1972). *Biochem. J.* **128**: 1357.
Langer, B., Steinmetz-Kayne, M., and Hilschmann, N. (1968). *Hoppe-Seyler's Z. Physiol. Chem.* **345**: 945.
Mage, R.G., Reisfeld, R.A. and Dray, S. (1966). *Immunochemistry* **3**: 299.
Mage, R.G., Young, G.O., and Reisfeld, R.A. (1968). *J. Immunol.* **101**: 617.

Mage, R.G., Appella, E., Young-Cooper, G.O., Winfield, J.B., Pincus, J.H., and Chersi, A.J. (1973). *J. Immunol.* (in press).
Mannik, M., and Kunkel, H.G. (1962). *J. Exp. Med.* **116**: 859.
McFadden, J.L., and Smith, E.C. (1955). *J. Biol. Chem.* **214**: 185.
McKean, D.J., Potter, M., and Hood, L.E. (1973). *Biochemistry* (in press).
Milstein, C. (1965). *Nature* **205**: 1171.
Milstein, C. (1966). *Proc. Roy. Soc. B* **166**: 113.
Milstein, C., and Pink, J.R.L. (1970). *Progr. Biophys. Mol. Biol.* **21**: 209.
Milstein, C., Clegg, J.B., and Jarvis, J.M. (1967). *Nature* **214**: 270.
Oudin, J. (1956). *Compt. Rend.* **242**: 2606.
Oudin, J. (1960). *J. Exp. Med.* **112**: 107.
Perham, R.N., Appella, E., and Potter, M. (1966). *Science* **154**: 391.
Pincus, J.H., Jaton, J.C., Bloch, K.J., and Haber, E. (1970). *J. Immunol.* **104**: 1143.
Porter, R.R. (1950). *Biochem. J.* **46**: 473.
Porter, R.R. (1959). *Biochem. J.* **73**: 119.
Potter, M., and Boyce, C. (1962). *Nature* **193**: 1086.
Potter, M., Dreyer, W.J., Kuff, E.L., and McIntire, K.R. (1964). *J. Molec. Biol.* **8**: 814.
Poulsen, K., and Haber, E. (1972). *Federation Proc.* **31**: 3131.
Putman, F.W., Titani, K., Wikler, M., and Shinoda, T. (1967). *Cold Spring Harbor Symp. Quant. Biol.* **32**: 9.
Reisfeld, R.A., and Inman, J.K. (1968). *J. Immunochemistry* **5**: 503.
Reisfeld, R.A., Dray, S., and Nisonoff, A. (1965). *J. Immunochemistry* **2**: 155.
Rejnek, J., Appella, E., Mage, R.G., and Reisfeld, R.A. (1969*a*). *Biochemistry* **8**: 2712.
Rejnek, J., Mage, R.G., and Reisfeld, R.A. (1969*b*). *J. Immunol.* **102**: 638.
Roholt, O.A., Seon, B.K., and Pressman, D. (1970). *Immunochemistry* **7**: 329.
Sanger, F. (1945). *Biochem. J.* **39**: 507.
Schulenburg, E.P., Lynch, R.G., Simms, E.S., Bradshaw, R.A., and Eisen, H.N. (1971). *Proc. Natl. Acad. Sci. U.S.* **68**: 2623.
Skarova, B., Rejnek, J., and Kotynek, O. (1968). *Folia Microbiol.* (*Prague*) **12**: 162.
Small, P.A., Reisfeld, R.A., and Dray, S. (1965). *J. Molec. Biol.* **16**: 328.
Smith, G.P., Hood, L.E., and Fitch, W.M. (1971). *Ann. Rev. Biochem.* **40**: 969.
Svasti, J., and Milstein, C. (1972). *Biochem. J.* **128**: 427.
Terry, W.D., Hood, L.E., and Steinberg, A.G. (1969). *Proc. Natl. Acad. Sci. U.S.* **63**: 71.
Titani, K., Wikler, M., and Putman, F.W. (1967). *Science* **155**: 828.
Vice, J., Hunt, W., and Dray, S. (1969). *Proc. Soc. Exp. Biol. Med.* **130**: 730.
Weigert, M.G., Cesari, I.M., Yonkovich, S.J., and Cohn, M. (1970). *Nature* **228**: 1045.
Wu, T.T., and Kabat, E.A. (1970). *J. Exp. Med.* **132**: 211.

Chapter 4

Studies of Rabbit Allotypes
by Cross-Linked Antisera

Roberto Tosi and Simonetta Landucci-Tosi

Laboratorio di Biologia Cellulare del C. N. R.
Rome, Italy
and
Osservatorio di Genetica Animale
Turin, Italy

I. INTRODUCTION

Immunoglobulin allotypes are genetic markers detected by serological reactions. It has become obvious that the genetics of antibody formation can hardly be understood without these genetic markers.

The rabbit allotype system is of special interest. Markers are known for most of the immunoglobulin chains. In addition, serological specificities are known for the variable region of the heavy chains. Most rabbit allotypes, unlike the markers available in other species, have the advantage of being detected by isoantisera, giving strong precipitation reactions. This makes it possible to use agar immunodiffusion (Ouchterlony) tests for typing, in addition to other classical immunological methods based on precipitation.

In rabbits, several groups or segregating series of allotypes have been detected. Light-chain allotypes of *b* group (4, 5, 6, 9) are located on κ chains; those of *c* group (7, 21) are located on λ chains. Heavy-chain allotypes of *a* group (1, 2, 3) are located in the V_H region, and are common to all heavy-chain classes, while the *e* group (14 and 15), *d* group (11 and 12), and allotypes 8 and 10 are exclusively $C\gamma$ markers. Heavy-chain allotypes of *f* group are exclusively located on IgA and those of the *Ms* group are exclusively located on IgM. Several review articles are available for further details (Kelus and Gell, 1967; Mage, 1967; Baglioni, 1970; Smith *et al.*, 1971; Mage, 1971; Dubiski, 1972).

When a quantitative immunochemical analysis of the different allotypic specificities present in a given immunoglobulin preparation is required, the precipitation reaction by specific antisera can be utilized. Precipitation curves can also be effected on a microscale by the use of radioiodinated antigens (Dray and Nisonoff, 1963). However, many anti-allotype sera do not completely precipitate the corresponding antigens, resulting in a variable proportion of soluble antigen—antibody complexes. Particularly the antisera directed against the *a*-group specificities precipitate poorly. This problem can be circumvented either by applying sequential precipitation steps to the same antigenic preparation, each time adding "carrier" antigen and antiserum (Dray *et al.*, 1963), or by using an "indirect" precipitation method (Chersi *et al.*, 1970; Hopper *et al.*, 1970). However, such procedures introduce additional complications. Moreover, the antisera directed against some of the γ-chain Fc markers such as 14 and 15 are usually nonprecipitating antisera. These allotypes are currently detected by passive hemagglutination-inhibition reactions with sheep red blood cells coated with Ig carrying the relevant allotype. This method, however, does not lend itself to precise quantitative analysis.

The disadvantage of nonprecipitating or poorly-precipitating antisera could be eliminated by a method measuring the primary antigen—antibody interaction instead of the secondary manifestations such as precipitation or hemagglutination. We attempted to establish such a method by using anti-allotype sera rendered insoluble and Ig labeled with [125]I. We will first give a detailed description of the methods involved, and then give a short review of the results obtained by their application.

II. EXPERIMENTAL PROCEDURES

A. Insolubilization of Antisera

Several techniques are available to insolubilize immunological reagents, i.e., antigens or antibodies. These can be divided into three categories (Centeno and Sehon, 1971): (1) covalent coupling to insoluble supporting media such as cellulose derivatives or synthetic polymers, (2) noncovalent adsorption onto insoluble particles such as glass beads or polyethylene tubes, and (3) polymerization or intramolecular condensation by cross-linking reagents such as ethyl chloroformate, glutaraldehyde, bisdiazotized benzidine, ethylene maleic anhydride, and others.

We adopted the method of cross-linking the antiserum proteins by using ethyl chloroformate as described by Avrameas and Ternynck (1967). The procedure routinely followed in our laboratory is as follows: 5–10 ml of antiserum is dialyzed overnight against 0.2 M sodium acetate buffer, *p*H 4.5, and then centrifuged for 2 hours at 2000 X *g* at 4°C. Ethyl chloroformate (British Drug House) is added to the supernatant in the proportion of 60 μl per ml of antiserum. The addition is performed dropwise with constant stirring in order to keep the drops of ethyl chloroformate in suspension throughout the solution. The pH is kept at 4.5 by continuous addition of 1 N NaOH. The whole procedure is performed at room temperature under an aspirating hood to avoid contact with the toxic ethyl chloroformate vapors. After 30 minutes, the insolubilization is essentially complete. The material is left without stirring for 60 minutes more, and is then suspended in 100 ml of PBS* in a Teflon homogenizer (Thomas, Catalog No. 4288 B). The suspension is centrifuged for 30 minutes at 2000 × g at 4°C, and the supernatant is removed. Then the sediment is washed by homogenization and centrifugation, first with a 0.1% sodium carbonate solution and then three times with PBS. If the cross-linked antiserum is required for absorption–elution experiments, the suspension is washed (before the last three washings with PBS) several times, with the eluting solution until the OD_{280} of the supernatant becomes negligible. The final pellet is resuspended in a volume of borate-buffered saline† corresponding to five times the initial antiserum volume. After thorough homogenization, this suspension can be easily pipetted, without clogging, with Lang–Levy-type or with Eppendorf-type micropipets. Care must be taken in order to avoid sedimentation of the cross-linked material during pipetting. After addition of 0.1% sodium azide, the suspension is stored at 4° C. Freezing produces heavy clumping and is therefore generally avoided.

B. Binding Reaction of Cross-Linked Anti-Allotype Sera With ^{125}I-Labeled Immunoglobulin

The proportion of molecules carrying the different allotypic determinants in an immunoglobulin preparation is determined by establishing binding curves with specific cross-linked antisera. A constant amount of ^{125}I-labeled Ig preparation is reacted with increasing concentrations of cross-linked antiserum, until a maximum of binding is reached. This "plateau" of binding provides an estimate of the proportion of the given allotype.

For iodination, the Chloramine-T method is routinely used (Greenwood et al., 1963). However, in specific cases, the ICl method (McFarlane, 1958) and, more recently, the lactoperoxidase method (Thorell and Johansson, 1971) are also employed.

For each assay, 75 μl of labeled Ig (generally 2000–4000 c.p.m.) is measured into small plastic tubes (Catalog No. 299/4, Ditta Kartell, Binasco, Milano). The ^{125}I-labeled Ig preparation contains 5% BSA (Armour, Cohn fraction V powder) in order to prevent the adherence of labeled antigen to the walls of

---

*   PBS = phosphate-buffered saline = saline containing 0.014 M sodium phosphate, pH 7.9.
†   borate-buffered saline = saline containing 0.035 M sodium borate buffer, pH 7.9.

the tube. Then, 75 μl of antiserum suspension diluted in PBS is added with thorough mixing. Control tubes to which no antiserum suspension is added are included in each experiment. The tubes are incubated at room temperature for 16 hours, with constant mixing provided by placing the racks of tubes on a revolving wheel. The tubes are then centrifuged in a Beckman 152 Microfuge for 4 minutes. Then 75 μl (half the total reaction volume) of supernatant is transferred to another tube of the same kind and both tubes are counted in a well-type gamma scintillation counter. The tube containing only supernatant is called the top tube; the tube which also contains the sediment is called the bottom tube. The percentage of labeled antigen bound to the insoluble antibody is calculated as follows:

$$\text{Percent binding} = \frac{\text{c.p.m. (bottom)} - \text{c.p.m. (top)}}{\text{total c.p.m.}} \times 100$$

In antibody–inhibition assays, i.e., to test the inhibitory ability of a soluble antiserum vs. the binding reaction by a cross-linked antiserum, the reactants are mixed in the following order: (1) cross-linked antiserum, in an amount giving slightly less than maximum binding, (2) soluble antiserum in variable amounts, and, after careful mixing, (3) a fixed amount of labeled antigen. Control tubes to which no cross-linked antiserum is added are also included. In both assays, inhibition is expressed as:

$$\text{Percent inhibition} = 100 - \frac{\text{percent binding with inhibitor}}{\text{percent binding without inhibitor}} \times 100$$

C. Determination of Antigen-Binding Capacity (ABC) of cross-linked Antisera

A quantitative estimate of the activity of a cross-linked antiserum can be given by the procedure and mathematical treatment developed for another "primary binding reaction," namely, the Farr technique. In particular, we adopted the method of Celada (1966) for determining ABC, which is based on a plot of the binding data utilizing the Von Krogh equation. Accordingly, the procedure for the binding reaction was modified for this purpose. (1) The antigen solution contained IgG with the relevant allotype in a concentration of 1 μg/ml, in borate buffer* supplemented with 1% normal chicken serum. A trace amount of the same IgG labeled with ^{125}I was added to provide about 10,000 c.p.m./ml. (2) The antiserum was diluted in borate buffer containing 10% normal chicken serum. (3) The reaction, comprised of 250 μl of antigen solution and 250 μl of antibody suspension, was performed in larger plastic tubes (Catalog No. 1090, NUNC, Roskilde, Denmark). After incubation for 16

---

* Boric acid, 6.184 g; Sodium tetraborate, 9.536 g; and sodium chloride, 4.384 g; per liter; pH 8.2.

hours on a revolving wheel and centrifugation at 2000 X g for 30 minutes, 250 μl of the supernatant was transferred to an identical tube. The counting and calculation of binding were done as described above. The data, plotted as log μl/ml of antiserum $vs.$ log (percent binding/100 - percent binding), show a linear relationship over a broad range of binding proportions. Using the value of the intercept a, i.e., the value of log μl/ml corresponding to 50% binding [and therefore corresponding to log (percent binding/100 - percent binding) = 0], ABC can be calculated since log ABC = $2.70 - a$.

By the same procedure, but varying the antigen concentration, useful parameters of avidity can also be derived (Celada et $al.,$ 1969; Tosi and Celada, 1973).

III. ACTIVITY AND SPECIFICITY OF
CROSS-LINKED ANTISERA

It is desirable to have some quantitative estimate of the activity of a given antiserum after ethyl chloroformate treatment, particularly in terms of specificity and avidity. In quantitative terms, a direct comparison between soluble $vs.$ insoluble antiserum can only be made if the same primary binding reactions are possible with the antiserum in both forms. This is the case of anti-bovine-albumin antisera (anti-BSA) for which a well-established primary reaction (the Farr technique) exists. This reaction was therefore adopted as model system.

A rabbit anti-BSA antiserum obtained after 70 days from a single intramuscular injection of 1 mg BSA in complete Freund's adjuvant was used. An aliquot was precipitated by half-saturated ammonium sulfate, dialyzed against PBS, and labeled with ^{125}I by the Chloramine-T method. A trace amount of this labeled material was added to the antiserum before cross-linking. Being very small, it did not interfere with the ^{125}I-BSA assay and allowed a quantitative estimate of the recovery of antibody in the final antiserum suspension. The untreated anti-BSA antiserum and the cross-linked preparation were then assayed in parallel for their activity against the same BSA solution. The only differences were that no ammonium sulfate was added to the insoluble system and that the incubation time was 16 hours rather than 30 minutes.

By plotting the data according to the Von Krogh equation, a linear relationship is obtained in both cases, as shown in Fig. 1. The slopes are very similar and close to the value of 0.75 found in the mouse anti-BSA system (Celada, 1966). The intercept a is much higher for the insolubilized antiserum, i.e., much more antiserum is required to bind 50% of the antigen. In terms of antigen-binding capacity, the cross-linked antiserum possesses only 5.8% of the activity of the untreated antiserum.

It can be asked whether this antibody activity which is preserved in the cross-linked form can be considered equivalent to the untreated antibody as far

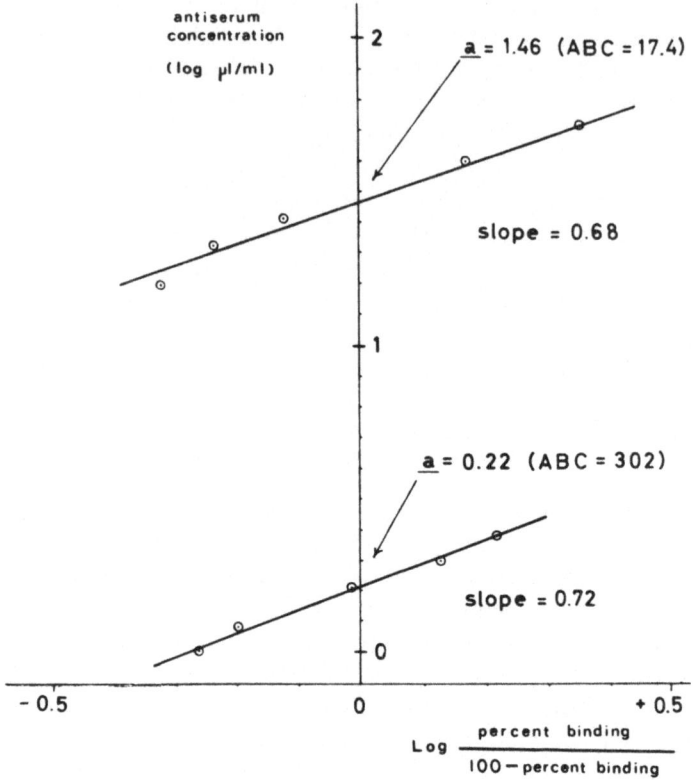

Figure 1. Activity of a rabbit anti-BSA antiserum, untreated (*lower curve*) and cross-linked by ethyl chloroformate treatment (*upper curve*). BSA concentrations = 1 μg/ml, including 10,000 c.p.m./ml of ^{125}I-labeled BSA. Data are plotted according to Celada (1966). Data on the abscissa are calculated for the cross-linked antiserum on the basis of antibody recovery. To determine antibody recovery, an aliquot of antiserum was precipitated with half-saturated ammonium sulfate dialyzed against PBS, and labeled with ^{125}I. 16,000 c.p.m. were added per ml of antiserum before treatment. The final antibody suspension (after ethyl chloroformate treatment, washing, and dilution) contained 720 c.p.m./ml. Therefore 1 ml of final suspension corresponds to 720/16,000 = 0.045 ml of untreated antiserum, in terms of *amount* of antibody recovered in the cross-linked form.

as avidity is concerned. This can be tested by performing binding experiments similar to those shown in Fig. 1, but at varying BSA concentrations. If the values of intercept *a* obtained in each curve are then plotted on a logarithmic scale against the antigen concentration, a relationship is obtained which is characteristic for each antiserum and depends primarily upon its avidity. The general pattern of this relationship includes a rectilinear portion with slopes varying from about 0.3 to 1.0 for different antisera. This linear portion continues up to relatively high antigen concentrations. At very low antigen concentrations, a slope $\simeq 0$ is gradually reached, i.e., the value of intercept a does not decrease below a minimal value. Two avidity indices can be derived from such plots. The first is the slope of the rectilinear portion of the curve. In high-avidity antisera, this slope is very close to 1.0, while in low-avidity antisera, obtained during early stages after immunization, it is only 0.3–0.4. The second is the intercept b, obtained by extrapolation of the rectilinear portion down to the minimal value reached by a. In high-avidity antisera, the value of a keeps decreasing until very low antigen concentrations are reached. In low avidity antisera, a reaches a constant value much earlier. Consequently, the more avid the antiserum, the lower the corresponding value of intercept b. As shown in Fig. 2, both these

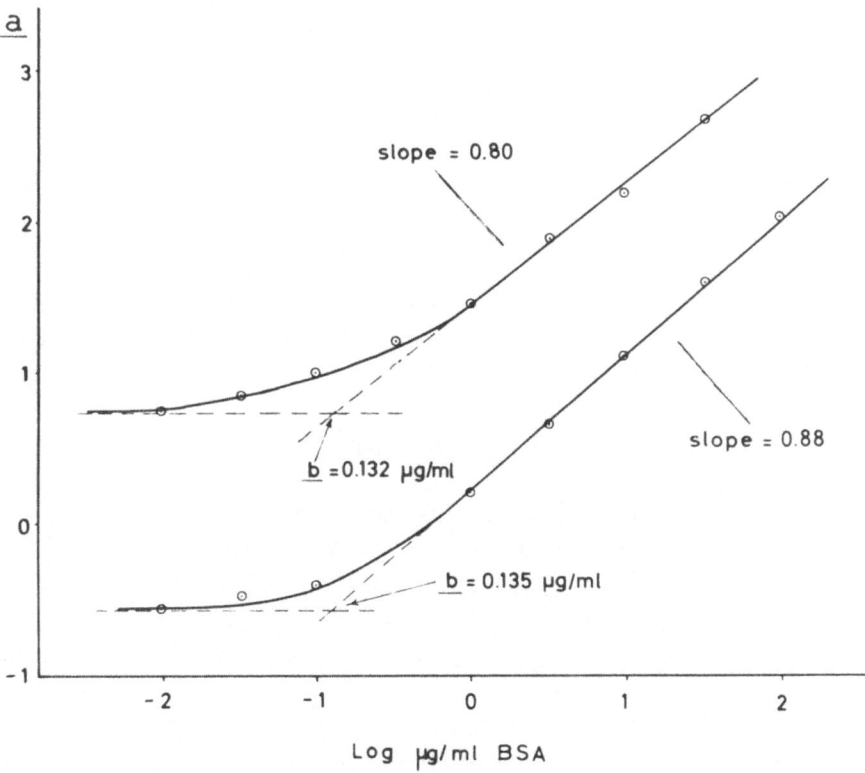

Figure 2. Avidity curve of a rabbit anti-BSA antiserum (same as in Fig. 1), untreated (*lower curve*) and cross-linked (*upper curve*). Data on the abscissa correspond to intercept values determined by experiments similar to those shown in Fig 1. All data are equalized as far as *amount* of antibody is concerned (the *activity* of the cross-linked antibody is of course reduced).

Table I. Specificity of Cross-Linked Antisera*

Allotype of IgG		Maximum percentage of ^{125}I-labeled IgG bound					
		anti-1	anti-2	anti-14	anti-15	anti-human leukocytes	no antiserum added
1/1	14/14	92.0	2.8	80.0	0.2	2.8	1.1
2/2	15/15	1.1	91.9	2.2	92.9	0.4	-0.7

*From Landucci-Tosi et al. (1970)

avidity indices show a close correspondence in the soluble and in the cross-linked systems.

If these results have a general validity, it can be concluded that *the activity of a cross-linked antiserum is quantitatively decreased but qualitatively similar to the activity of the corresponding untreated antiserum.*

A direct comparison between soluble and insoluble forms cannot be made for the anti-allotype sera, to which the above conclusions can be applied only by analogy. However it can be generally stated that anti-allotype antisera retain their specific activity as shown in Table I.

The stability of the cross-linked antibody upon storage at $4°C$ is apparently good. The antibody concentration of the anti-BSA antiserum considered above was described by 15% after 6 months storage. We have several cross-linked anti-allotype antisera that are still very active and specific even four years after their preparation.

IV. APPLICATIONS

A. Typing of the *e*-Group Specificities
by Radioimmunoassay

The *e*-group allotypes 14 and 15 are allelic specificities located on the Fc portion of γ chains (Dubiski, 1969). They are associated with a single amino acid interchange at position 309, where alanine is represented in molecules carrying allotype 15 and threonine in molecules carrying allotype 14 (Appella *et al.*, 1971). These allotypes provide very useful markers, especially in conjunction with the *a*-group allotypes, which are located in the V_H region.

The *e*-group allotypes were originally discovered through antisera agglutinating sheep red blood cells coated with rabbit Ig. Sera of unknown phenotype were typed by inhibition of the agglutination reaction (Dubiski, 1969). Using cross-linked antisera and ^{125}I-labeled IgG, this procedure was tested to see whether it could be simplified by the use of a radioimmunoassay. In fact, anti-14

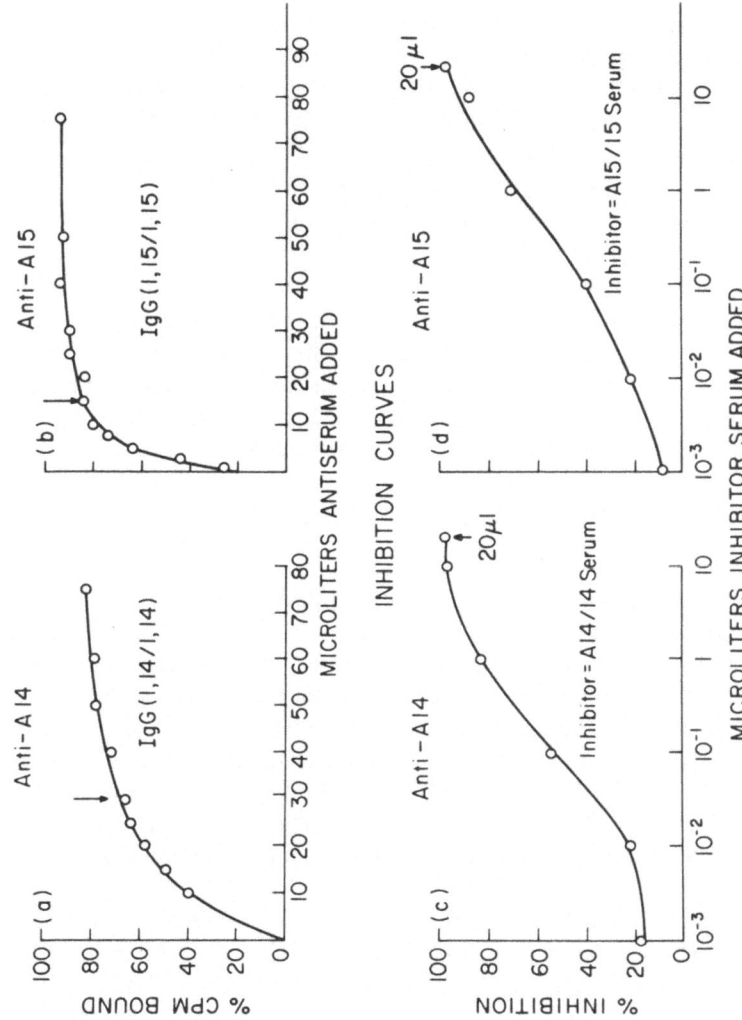

Figure 3. Binding curves (a and b). Increasing volumes of cross-linked antisera were added to a fixed amount of 125I-IgG (about 7000 c.p.m.). Nonspecific binding of 1,15/1,15 IgG by anti-14 antiserum and of 1,14/1,14 IgG by an anti-15 antiserum was less than 5%. Arrows indicate antiserum volume selected for the performance of inhibition curves. Inhibition curves showing inhibition of binding of 125I-IgG by unlabeled antigen (c and d). Increasing volumes of normal rabbit serum (inhibitor) were added to a fixed amount of 125I-IgG. After mixing, the selected antiserum volume (30 μl for anti-14, 15 μl for anti-15) was added. Arrows indicate volume of inhibitor serum chosen for the performance of routine typing. (From Landucci-Tosi and Mage, 1970.)

and anti-15 antisera were found to be active and specific after insolubilization (Fig. 3, a and b) and can be used in sensitive inhibition assays (Fig. 3, c and d). The typing results obtained by the radioimmunoassay were in complete accord with those obtained by hemagglutination-inhibition. The radioimmunoassay has the advantage of being less laborious both in the preparation of the reagents and in the performance of the test (Landucci-Tosi and Mage, 1970).

The same system can be applied to test *antisera* directly for the presence of anti-14 or anti-15 activity, without going through the cross-linking procedure each time. The untreated nonprecipitating antiserum competes with the cross-linked antiserum for the available antigenic sites. A complete inhibition is expected if the antigenic sites recognized by the soluble and cross-linked antibody are the same, or at least spacially close. Since the difference between 14 and 15 is due to a single amino acid interchange, it is likely that there is either one or very few sites recognized by all the antisera with the same specificities. Actually, as shown in Fig. 4, the inhibition by different anti-14 antisera was essentially complete in all antiserum combinations tested. However, if the insolubilized antiserum recognizes one or more determinants in addition to those recognized by the untreated (inhibitor) antiserum, the inhibition should be only partial. Therefore this sytem could be generally useful for evaluating the degree of heterogeneity of antisera directed against the same complex antigen.

B. The Molecular Association of Fc and Fd
Markers of γ Chains

The e-group allotypes 14 and 15 exhibit linked inheritance with the a-group allotypes 1, 2, and 3. One e-group allotype and the corresponding a-group allotype in *cis* position constitute a phenogroup whose inheritance can be traced for many generations with only rare instances of genetic recombination (Mage *et al.,* 1971). It can be asked whether the two allotypes belonging to the same phenogroup contribute exclusively to the same heavy chain. Alternatively, there may exist "recombinant" molecules in which Fc and Fd markers transmitted in repulsion are present. The answer to this question might provide information concerning possible mechanisms by which V-region genes can interact with C-region genes.

The problem was approached by testing ^{125}I-labeled IgG preparations from (a) a doubly heterozygous rabbit (1/2, 14/15) with phenogroups 1-15 and 2-15, (b) a double heterozygous rabbit (1/2, 14/15) with phenogroups1-15 and 2-14, and (c) a rabbit with the same genetic constitution as (a) but allotype-suppressed by neonatal injection of anti-1 antiserum. The preparations were tested for the proportion of molecules carrying each of the four markers by establishing the amount of radioactive counts that could be maximally bound by each specific cross-linked antiserum.

Finding a discrepancy between the quantitative levels of the allotypes

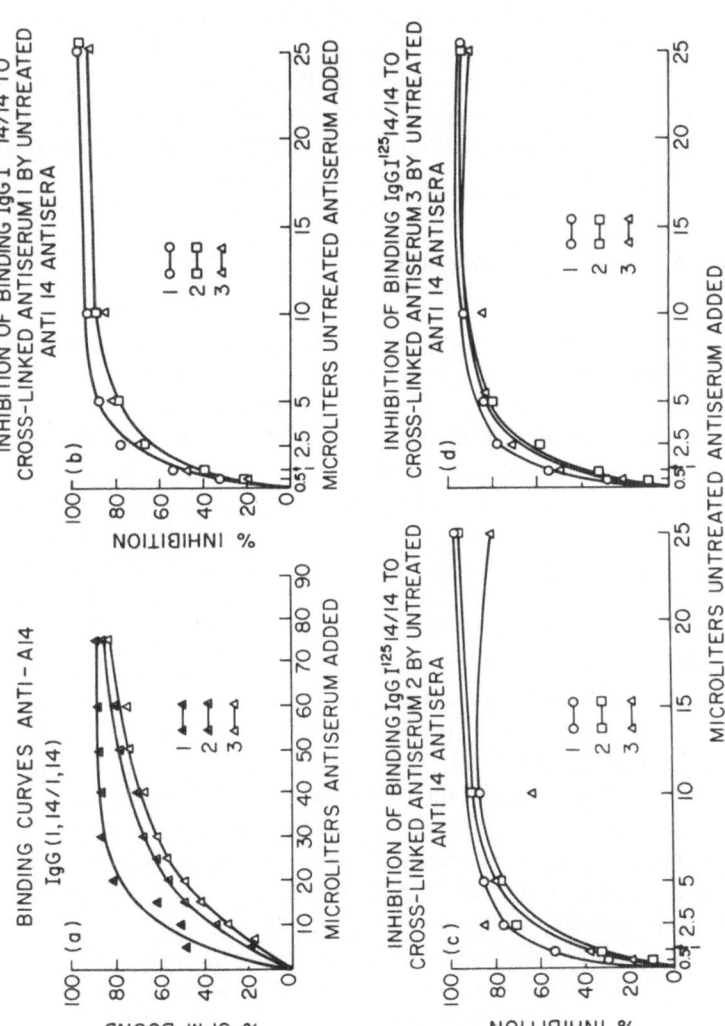

Figure 4. (a) Binding curves obtained with three different anti-14 antisera (listed as No. 1, No. 2, and No. 3). (b), (c), and (d) Inhibition of binding of cross-linked antisera by non-cross-linked antisera. Increasing volumes of untreated antisera were added to a fixed amount (20 μl for antiserum No. 1, 40 μl for No. 2, 50 μl for No. 3) of cross-linked antisera. After mixing, ^{125}I-labeled 1,14/1,14 IgG was added. (From Landucci-Tosi and Mage, 1970.)

belonging to the same phenogroup would be strong evidence in favor of the contribution to the same molecules of markers transmitted in repulsion. Such a discrepancy was not actually found (Landucci-Tosi *et al.,* 1970). The markers transmitted in coupling were shown to have similar quantitative expressions, not only in the two normal rabbits with opposite genetic phase, but also in the allotype-suppressed animal. Therefore, although the existence of a low proportion of "recombinant" molecules cannot be excluded, it appears that the molecular association between the two groups of allotypes reflects very closely their genetic phase. Similar conclusions were reached by other authors, using the other sets of γ-Fc markers: 11 and 12 (Prahl *et al.,* 1970) and 8 and 10 (Hamers and Hamers-Casterman, 1967).

C. Expression of *a*-Group Allotypes on IgG and IgM Isolated From the Same Rabbit

The presence of the *a*-group allotypes 1, 2, and 3 on all major classes of rabbit Ig was first observed by Todd (1963) and has been confirmed by several authors (Feinstein, 1963; Lichter, 1967; Sell, 1967; Pernis *et al.,* 1968; Kindt and Todd, 1969). A satisfactory explanation of this finding is that these markers are associated with a common pool of V genes shared by all heavy chains.

On the other hand, it is known that in heterozygous rabbits the allelic *a*-group markers do not possess the same phenotypic expression. For instance, in 1/2 rabbits, Ig carrying allotype 1 is on the average four times more concentrated than Ig carrying allotype 2 (Mage, 1967). Although the mechanism of this unbalance is not known, it is not unreasonable to think that it may be due to a different susceptibility to selection by antigen conferred by some structure associated with the allotypic determinants. It may be relevant to note that the Fc markers 14 and 15 do not seem to confer an appreciably different phenotypic expression (Landucci-Tosi *et al.,* 1970).

The unbalance between allelic products in rabbits heterozygous for *a*-group markers allows a *functional* test for the presence of the same V genes on IgG and IgM. In other words, it is possible to test not only whether the same allotypic determinants can be demonstrated on the different Ig classes, but also whether they possess the same phenotypic expressions on both IgG and IgM.

To facilitate the purification procedure, IgG and IgM were isolated from the same 1/2 heterozygous rabbits in the form of anti-BSA antibodies by absorption and subsequent elution from an insoluble immunoabsorbent. Also, IgG from the same rabbits, but devoid of anti-BSA activity, was purified by ammonium sulfate precipitation and DEAE-cellulose chromatography. In addition to two normal animals, a rabbit allotype-suppressed for allotype 1 was also examined. Each preparation, after labeling with ^{125}I, was tested for the proportion of molecules carrying either the 1 or the 2 allotype by determining the maximum amount of radioactive counts that could be bound to specific cross-linked antisera.

The results depicted in Fig. 5 show that in each IgG and IgM fraction from a normal rabbit, there were 3–4 times as many molecules with 1 as with 2. The proportion of these markers is reversed in each fraction from the rabbit in which the expression of the 1 allotype was suppressed.

A general conclusion that can be drawn is that not only are the 1 and 2 specificities present on both IgG and IgM, but they also appear to exhibit similar relative phenotypic expressions. The exposure to an anti-allotype serum during fetal and neonatal life appears to cause a suppression of the allotype to about the same extent in IgG and IgM. Thus, our data support the concept that IgG and IgM share the same set of V-region genes, which appear to exhibit similar expression whether they become associated with genes for γ or μ constant regions. It is possible that some or all the cells which produced IgG anti-BSA were derived from cells which produced IgM anti-BSA (Kinkade *et al.*, 1970; Harrod and Warner, 1972). It is therefore conceivable that the expression of *a*-group allotypes on IgG does not have a genetic meaning *per se*, but is only a consequence of the sequence of differentiation events which take place at the

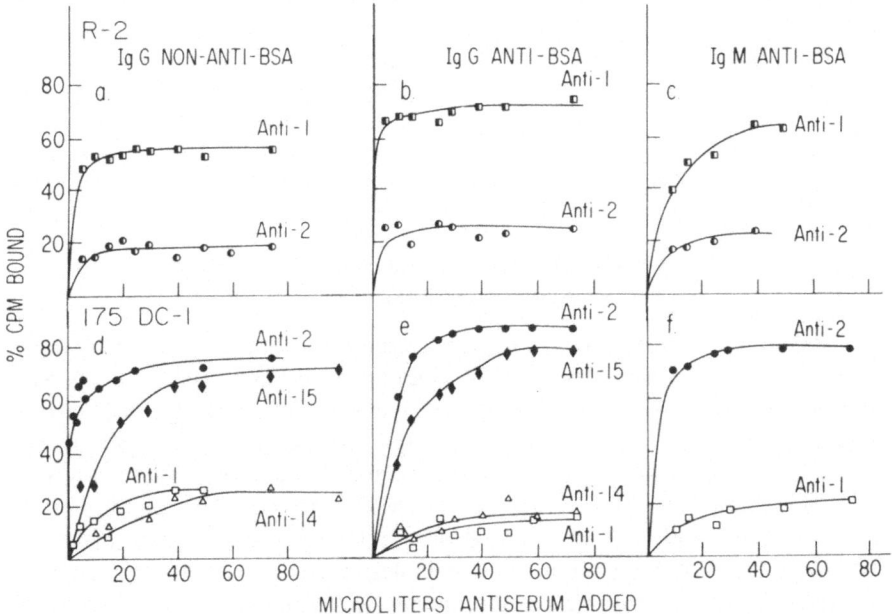

Figure 5. Binding curves obtained with insolubilized antisera and ^{125}I-IgG non-anti-BSA (a and d), IgG anti-BSA (b and e), and IgM anti-BSA (c and f) from two heterozygous 1/2 rabbits. Rabbit R-2 (*top*) was a normal rabbit, whereas rabbit 175 CD-1 (*bottom*) was allotype-suppressed for 1. Both IgG fractions from this animal exhibited suppressed expressions of 1 and also of the Fc marker 14 which is associated with 1. The IgM also exhibited suppressed expression of 1 and did not bind significantly to anti-14 and anti-15. (From Landucci Tosi *et al.*, 1972*b*.)

cellular level. The selection between the two alleles could actually be made when the cell is producing IgM, and would remain "fixed" even when the cell "switches" to IgG synthesis.

D. IgG Molecules Lacking a-Group Allotypes

In normal rabbits, a minor portion of serum IgG, the so-called a-negative molecules, does not carry detectable a-group allotypes. Instead, these molecules carry a different allotypic specificity, A 31, located on the Fab portion (Knight et al., 1970). It may be asked if the same e-group markers which are demonstrable on the Fc region of a-positive molecules are also present on the Fc region of a-negative molecules.

Large amounts of a-negative IgG in almost pure form can be obtained from allotype-suppressed homozygous animals (David and Todd, 1969; Vice et al., 1970). We studied the IgG of a 2/2 homozygous, suppressed animal (rabbit V 303) whose parents were homozygous 15/15. The results (Fig. 6) demonstrate that 90–95% of the IgG molecules of this animal are a-negative, and that most, if not all, of them carry the e-group determinant 15. Moreover, the Fc portion of a-negative IgG was also found to be indistinguishable by peptide mapping from the Fc portion of a-positive IgG (Knight et al., 1971). All this evidence points toward the existence of at least two genetically distinct V-region genes, a-negative (i.e. A 31) and a-positive, each of which can be associated with the same C-region gene. This parallels the conclusions, based on sequence analysis in human, that the same C region can be associated with different V_H subgroups.

E. Reactions of Isoantisera Directed Against Rabbit Allotypes with Hare IgG

Rabbit and hare are not considered by zoologists as closely related species. They belong in the same family (Leporidae) but to different genera (Lepus and Oryctolagus) (Leone, 1968). Nevertheless, heterologous sera directed against rabbit IgG strongly cross-react with hare IgG. We examined a goat anti-rabbit IgG and a sheep anti-rabbit IgG-Fc antiserum for their ability to bind the IgG of the two species. For both antisera, the ABC with hare IgG was found to correspond to about 45% of the ABC with rabbit IgG. This suggests that these two species are not distant from the immunological standpoint. Another piece of evidence in favor of this view is the finding (Kelus and Gell, 1967) that some anti-allotype isoantisera give precipitation lines in Ouchterlony with hare sera.

We decided to reinvestigate this point since it might have some interesting implications concerning the evolution of rabbit allotypes. Both a- and b-group rabbit allotypes are known to be associated with multiple amino acid interchanges (Appella et al., 1969). How multiple differences can accumulate be-

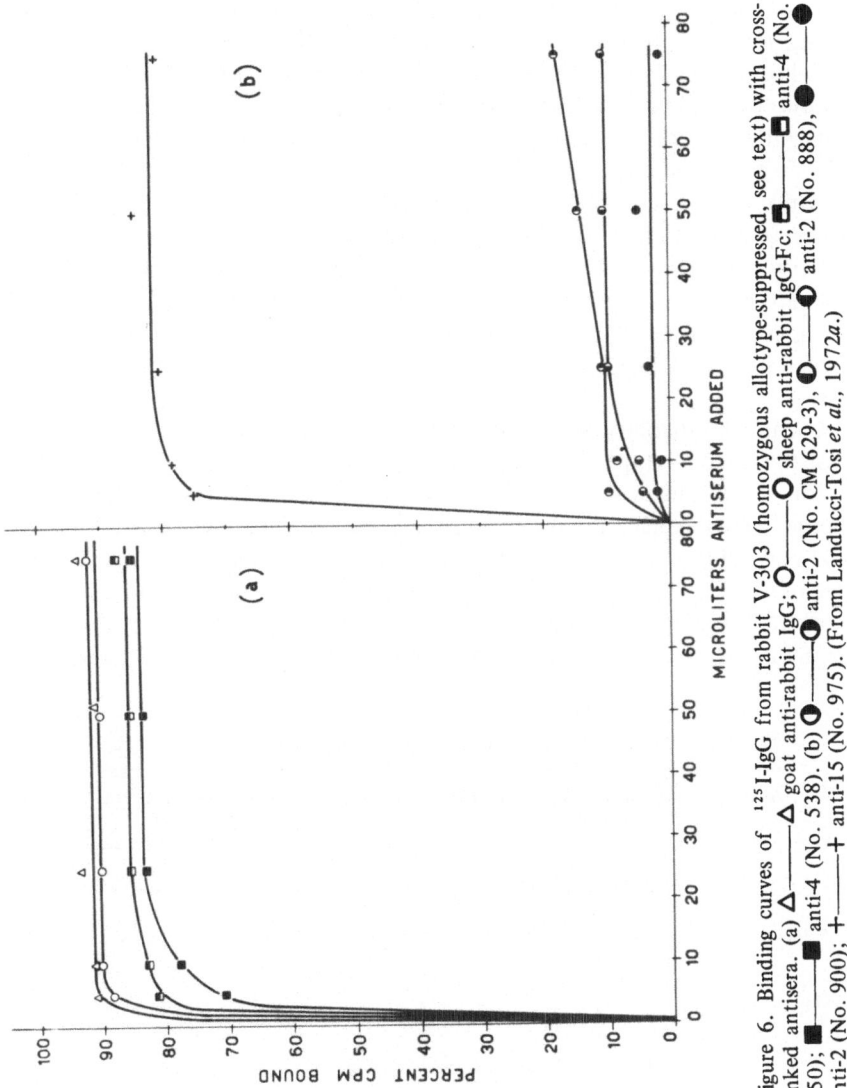

Figure 6. Binding curves of ^{125}I-IgG from rabbit V-303 (homozygous allotype-suppressed, see text) with cross-linked antisera. (a) △———△ goat anti-rabbit IgG; ○———○ sheep anti-rabbit IgG-Fc; ◨———◨ anti-4 (No. 550); ■———■ anti-4 (No. 538). (b) ◑———◑ anti-2 (No. CM 629-3), ◐———◐ anti-2 (No. 888), ●———● anti-4 (No. anti-2 (No. 900); +———+ anti-15 (No. 975). (From Landucci-Tosi et al., 1972a.)

tween alleles during evolution is not clear. It cannot even be excluded that the structural genes for the polypeptide chains characteristic of each allotype are not truly allelic, but coexist on the same chromosome. Allelism would be present at a different (regulatory) locus, which would allow the expression of only one of the structural genes (Bell and Dray, 1971). By examining the situation in the hare, one may hope to gain some insight in the evolutionary process which led to rabbit allotypes, and perhaps to antibody diversification in general.

Four purified hare IgG preparations were labeled with ^{125}I and reacted against different anti-allotype cross-linked isoantisera. A general outline of the results is presented in Table II. The results obtained with the different IgG preparations were similar. Reactions were obtained only with anti-b-group-allotype sera (with the exception of anti-9) and with antisera against the 15 specificity belonging to the e-group. No sizable reaction was observed with any of the anti-a-group-allotype sera, even though they were not weaker (in terms of ABC values) than anti-b-group-allotype sera. The absence of reactions against allotypes 9 and 14 may not be significant since they have low frequencies in rabbit.

A marked variability was observed between the different antisera directed against the same allotype. This was especially true for anti-4 sera, but it was also true for anti-5 and anti-6 sera as far as the maximum percent of binding is concerned. Two explanations of this can be considered. (1) The antisera may be *qualitatively* different, namely they may recognize different determinants included in the same rabbit allotypic specificity. Some of these determinants could be present in the hare and some others not. (2) They may differ only *quantitatively* in terms of activity and avidity. We strongly favor the latter hypothesis

Table II. Reactions of Anti-Allotype Isoantisera with Hare IgG

Allotype group	Allotype specificity	Number of antisera tested	Number of antisera reacting*
a	1	3	0
	2	3	0
	3	3	0
b	4	6	4
	5	3	3
	6	3	3
	9	3	0
e	14	6	0
	15	2	2

*Antisera were considered as nonreacting when they failed to bind at least 10% of the ^{125}I-labeled IgG.

since on quantitative tests it was found that the antisera which are weaker (in terms of ABC) against the rabbit, also react to a lesser extent with the hare, and in some cases are completely negative. In addition, the low binding given by weak antisera can be considerably increased by applying sequential binding reactions.

Figure 7 represents the binding curves obtained by three strongly reacting antisera. It should be noted that the anti-5 antiserum was produced by a rabbit possessing the allotype 6 and *vice versa,* i.e., the anti-6 antiserum was produced by a rabbit possessing allotype 5. Therefore, the well-known cross-reaction between allotypes 5 and 6 does not come into play here.

Inhibition experiments were performed with the same antisera, using as antigen ^{125}I-labeled hare IgG and as inhibitors normal *rabbit* sera of various allotype constitutions. As shown in Table III, the inhibition patterns appear to be totally specific.

Experiments were also performed with the same system, but using as inhibitors normal *hare* sera. These sera were obtained from hares caught in

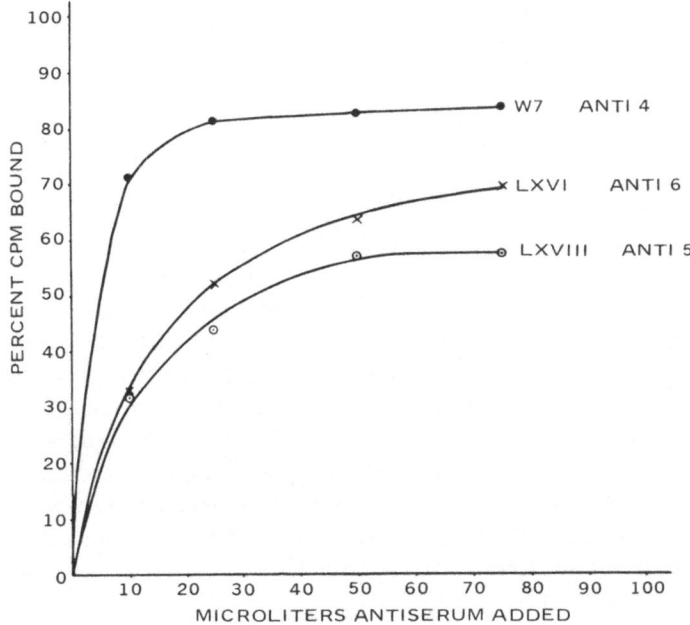

Figure 7. Binding curves of ^{125}I-labeled IgG from hare H 34 by three anti-rabbit allotype isoantisera in cross-linked form. Antiserum W7 (anti-4) was produced by a 5/5 rabbit; LXVIII (anti-5) by a 4/6 rabbit; LXVI (anti-6) by a 5/5 rabbit. These reactions were used for the inhibition experiments shown in Table IV. (From Landucci-Tosi *et al.,* 1973.)

Table III. Specificity of the Reactions of Anti-Rabbit-Allotype Sera with Hare IgG

Inhibitor serum*				Percent inhibition of binding of ^{125}I-hare IgG		
Rabbit	Phenotype			anti-4 (W7)	anti-5 (LXVIII)	anti-6 (LXVI)
S65	1/2	4	12	15	73.9	0	11.2
S66	1	4	12	15	75.0	0	3.8
S67	1/2	4	12	15	100	0	8.7
S8	2/3	5	11/12	15	1.4	74.9	0.2
2260	3	5	12	15	0	74.8	1.1
1708	3	5	11	15	0	100	2.8
680	1	6	12	15	0	5.3	97.1
2053	3	6	11	15	0	4.0	100
1718	3	6	11	15	4.1	4.6	100
2062	3	9	11	15	0	0	0
1653	2	9	12	15	0	6.7	0
2916	3	9	11	15	0	0	0

*A fixed amount (5 μl) of inhibitor serum was used in all the reactions.

different countries. A total of 24 hares were tested, and all were found to inhibit anti-4, anti-5, and anti-6 reactions.

These data strongly suggest that on hare IgG there exist structures which show enough similarity with rabbit group *b* allotypes to give a relatively strong immunological reaction with rabbit isoantisera. Although these structures in the rabbit are controlled by seemingly allelic genes at a single locus, in the hare they appear to be isotypes since they are possessed by all individuals tested as yet. Moreover, from the data shown in Fig. 7, it is apparent that these structures must reside *on the same IgG molecules.* The general significance of these findings is not easily interpretable. When structural similarities are found between different species they can usually be explained by convergent evolution or by common origin. At present, these data are not easily explained by either of the two theories. Nevertheless, we feel that this information may become valuable when more details of rabbit allotype structures are known and when other related species are examined.

V. CONCLUDING REMARKS

It must be clearly pointed out that, although the use of cross-linked antisera appears to present relevant advantages for allotype analysis, this method nevertheless has the limitations which are inherent in the anti-allotype antisera themselves. Thus these antisera are by no means to be considered perfect analytical reagents. They can conceivably cause either an overestimate or an underestimate of the proportion of molecules carrying a given allotypic specificity. Sera with low avidity can give a reduced plateau of binding. We have observed some instances of antisera derived from early bleedings giving much lower plateaus than antisera from the same rabbit after longer immunization periods. A low plateau of binding might conceivably also be due to a lack of antibodies against some of the determinants constituting the complex "family" of allotypic structures. On the other hand, an antiserum nominally recognizing a single allotype may also contain antibodies against an unrelated specificity. It is also possible that such antibodies are not recognized by precipitation reactions but show up in a primary binding reaction. Although the cross-linked antisera generally proved to be highly specific, we sometimes observed a further increase in binding of some antigen preparations after having reached a plateau level. This may be attributable to the presence of a minor antibody against an undetermined specificity. To minimize these variables, several antisera should be tested against the same allotypic specificity.

Bearing these limitations in mind, the general validity of allotype analysis performed by cross-linked antisera seems well established. This approach may be helpful in the future in solving some of the puzzling problems related to allotype structure and genetics.

ACKNOWLEDGMENTS

Much of the work presented here was part of a collaborative program with Dr. Rose Mage, to which the authors wish to express their deep gratitude. The authors also thank Dr. Piero Dassat for his constant encouragement and advice, Dr. Angelo Carbonara and Dr. Alma Luzzati for many helpful discussions, and Dr. Franco Celada for critically revising the manuscript. We also thank Dr. Leonard Herzenberg for having introduced us to the use of cross-linked antisera and having performed the preliminary experiments. Some of the reagents used in this work were kindly provided by Dr. S. Dubiski, Dr. G. Mancini, and Dr. C. Todd.

REFERENCES

Appella, E., Rejnek, J., and Reisfeld, R. A. (1969). *J. Mol. Biol.* **41**: 473.
Appella, E., Chersi, A., Mage, R., and Dubiski, S. (1971). *Proc. Natl. Acad. Sci. U.S.* **68**: 1341.
Avrameas, S., and Ternynck, T. (1967). *J. Biol. Chem.* **242**: 1641.
Baglioni, C. (1970). *Proc. Roy. Soc. B* **176**: 329.
Bell, C., and Dray, S. (1971). *Science* **171**: 199.
Celada, F. (1966). *J. Exp. Med.* **124**: 1.

Celada, F., Schmidt, D., and Strom, R. (1969). *Immunology* **17**: 189.
Centeno, E. R., and Sehon, A. H. (1971). *Immunochemistry* **8**: 887.
Chersi, A., Mage, R., Rejnek, J., and Reisfeld, R. A. (1970). *J. Immunol.* **104**: 1205.
David, G., and Todd, C. W. (1969). *Proc. Natl. Acad. Sci. U.S.* **62**: 860.
Dray, S., and Nisonoff, A. (1963). *Proc. Soc. Exp. Biol. Med.* **113**: 20.
Dray, S., Young, G. O., and Nisonoff, A. (1963). *Nature* **199**: 52.
Dubiski, S. (1969). *J. Immunol.* **103**: 120.
Dubiski, S. (1972). *Med. Clin. N. Am.* **56**: 557.
Feinstein, A. (1963). *Nature* **199**: 1197.
Greenwood, F. C., Hunter, W. M., and Glover, J. S. (1963). *Biochem. J.* **89**: 114.
Hamers, R., and Hamers-Casterman, C. (1967). *Cold Spring Harbor Symp. Quant. Biol.* **32**: 129.
Herrod, H. G., and Warner, N. L. (1972). *J. Immunol.* **108**: 1712.
Hopper, J. E., MacDonald, A. B., and Nisonoff, A. (1970). *J. Exp. Med.* **131**: 41.
Kelus, A. S., and Gell, P. G. H. (1967). *Progr. Allergy* **11**: 141.
Kindt, T. J., and Todd, C. W. (1969). *J. Exp. Med.* **130**: 859.
Kinkade, P. W., Lawton, A. R., Bockman, D. E., and Cooper, M. D. (1970). *Proc. Natl. Acad. Sci. U.S.* **67**: 1918.
Knight, K. L., Gilman-Sachs, A., Hunt, W. L., and Dray, S. (1970). *J. Immunol.* **104**: 550.
Landucci-Tosi, S., and Mage, R. G. (1970). *J. Immunol.* **105**: 1046.
Landucci-Tosi, S., Mage, R. G., and Dubiski, S. (1970). *J. Immunol.* **104**: 641.
Landucci-Tosi, S., Mage, R. G., Gilman-Sachs, A., Dray, S., and Knight, K. L. (1972*a*). *J. Immunol.* **108**: 264.
Landucci-Tosi, S., Mage, R. G., and Lawton, A. R. (1972*b*). *Immunochemistry* **9**: 317.
Landucci-Tosi, S., Tosi, R., and Perramon, A. (1973). *J. Immunol.* **110**: 286.
Leone, C. A. (1968). *The Serological Museum* **39**: 17.
Lichter, E. A. (1967). *J. Immunol.* **98**: 139.
McFarlane, A. S. (1958). *Nature* **182**: 53.
Mage, R. G. (1967). *Cold Spring Harbor Symp. Quant. Biol.* **32**: 203.
Mage, R. G. (1971). In Amos, B. D. (ed.), *Progress in Immunology*, Academic Press, New York, p. 47.
Mage, R. G., Young-Cooper, G. O., and Alexander, C. (1971). *Nature New Biology* **230**: 63.
Pernis, B., Torrigiani, G., Amante, L., Kelus, A. S., and Cebra, J. J. (1968). *Immunology* **14**: 445.
Prahl, J. W., Mandy, W. J., David, G. S., Steward, M. W., and Todd, C. W. (1970). *Protides Biol. Fluids, Proc. Colloq.* **17**: 125.
Sell, S. (1967), *Immunochemistry* **4**: 49.
Smith, G. P., Hood, L., and Fitch, W. M. (1971), *Ann. Rev. Biochem.* **40**: 969.
Thorell, J. E., and Johansson, B. G. (1971). *Biochim. Biophys. Acta* **251**: 363.
Todd, C. W. (1963). *Biochem. Biophys. Res. Commun.* **11**: 170.
Tosi, R., and Celada, F. (1973). Submitted for publication.
Vice, J. L., Gilman-Sachs, A., Hunt, W. L., and Dray, S. (1970). *J. Immunol.* **104**: 550.

Chapter 5

Idiotypic Specificity as a Probe for Investigating Persistence and Changes in Clones of Cells Producing Immunoglobulins

Susan Spring-Stewart* and Alfred Nisonoff

Department of Biological Chemistry
University of Illinois College of Medicine
Chicago, Illinois

I. BACKGROUND

In this article we will review recent work, from other laboratories as well as our own, on the persistence during extended immunization of antibody molecules of a given idiotypic specificity. We will first discuss some of the basic concepts underlying these experiments.

It was first shown by Slater *et al.* (1955) that myeloma proteins possess individually-specific antigenic determinants. For example, if one immunizes a rabbit with a purified human IgG myeloma protein and then absorbs the antiserum with nonspecific IgG and perhaps with another myeloma protein of the same class and subclass, the absorbed antiserum in general reacts only with the immunogen and not with any other human myeloma tested. One can also obtain such specific antisera by immunization with a purified human or rabbit antibody population. The recipient animal can be of the same or a different species than the donor. If a different species, or an animal of the same species but of different allotype, is employed, the antiserum must be appropriately absorbed to render it specific for the immunizing antigen, i.e., for the injected

---

* Recipient of an Arthritis Foundation Postdoctoral Fellowship.

purified antibody population. Oudin (1966) proposed the term "idiotypic specificity" to designate those antigenic specificities in a population of molecules which are not present in other serum proteins of the same animal or in antibody directed to the same antigen but derived from another animal. A further restriction in Oudin's definition is that the antiserum must be prepared in a recipient animal of the same species as the donor; the phrase "individually-specific antigenic determinant" has generally been used in connection with heterologous antisera (Kunkel, 1970). In some recent publications, however, the term, idiotypic specificity, has also been applied to determinants recognized by antisera prepared in a nonhomologous species (Kuettner et al., 1972). This appears to be largely a matter of convenience, since the term "idiotypic determinant" is less cumbersome.

One can raise the question whether homologous and heterologous antisera recognize the same idiotypic determinants. Although a general answer cannot be given to this question, there are instances in which the two types of antiidiotypic antibodies appear to react with the same region of the antibody used as immunogen. For example, the BALB/c myeloma protein, MOPC 315, which has antibody activity against the dinitrophenyl group, was used to elicit antiidiotypic antibodies in rabbits (Brient et al., 1971) or in BALB/c mice (Sirisinha and Eisen, 1971). In both instances the reaction with antiidiotypic antibody was markedly inhibited by haptens containing the dinitrophenyl group, indicating that the hapten-binding region of protein 315 is an important idiotypic determinant recognized by heterologous or isologous antiidiotypic antibody.* Similarly, antiidiotypic antibodies were prepared against the antibenzoate antibody from the same individual rabbit in 2 rabbits and in 2 guinea pigs (Spring-Stewart and Nisonoff, unpublished data). Marked inhibition of the idiotypic reactions by benzoate derivatives was seen in each case, again implicating the active site as an important idiotypic determinant recognized by a homologous or heterologous species.

Antiidiotypic antibodies have been prepared against a variety of myeloma and Bence-Jones proteins (Slater et al., 1955; Korngold and Lipari, 1956; Korngold and Van Leeuwen, 1957a,b; Stein et al., 1963) and against macroglobulins from Waldenstrom's disease (Boerma and Mandema, 1957), as well as against antibodies specific for a variety of antigens, including bacteria (Oudin and Michel, 1963, 1969a,b; Gell and Kelus, 1964; Braun and Krause, 1968; Haber, 1970), blood-group substances (Kunkel et al., 1963; Harboe and Deverill, 1964; Williams et al., 1968), proteins (Oudin and Cazenave, 1971; Schade and Nisonoff, 1972), and haptens (Daugharty et al., 1969; Kuettner et al., 1972).

* It is possible that the hapten causes a conformational change, altering idiotypic determinants outside the active site. If so, such changes must be greatly restricted in scope since they do not affect reactions with anti-Fab or antiallotypic antisera (Brient and Nisonoff, 1970).

II. CROSS-REACTIVITY BETWEEN IDIOTYPIC DETERMINANTS FROM ANTIBODIES OF THE SAME SPECIFICITY FROM DIFFERENT INDIVIDUALS

The original definition of individually-specific or idiotypic determinants did not allow for cross-reactions among related proteins from different individual animals. If one considers human myeloma proteins or antibodies from humans or outbred rabbits, cross-reactions are infrequent and, when they do occur, are generally weak (Braun and Krause, 1968; Hopper *et al.*, 1970; Oudin and Bordenave, 1971). It is now becoming clear, however, that particularly in inbred families or strains, such cross-reactions are a major factor to be considered. For example, Eichmann and Kindt (1971) demonstrated a number of idiotypic cross-reactions among antistreptococcal antibodies produced by rabbits of a family group. The family consisted of a brother—sister mating pair, both able to produce antistreptococcal antibodies of high titer and limited heterogeneity, and their F1 and F2 descendants. In inbred mice, idiotypic cross-reactions are much more frequent although, at present, quite unpredictable. For example, strong idiotypic cross-reactions are observed among the anti-*p*-azophenylarsonate anti-bodies of nearly all hyperimmunized A/J mice. In contrast, there are very weak intrastrain idiotypic cross-reactions among the antiphenylarsonate antibodies of C57/BL or BALB/c mice. There are marked intrastrain cross-reactions, however, among the anti-*p*-azobenzoate antibodies of BALB/c as well as A/J mice (Kuettner *et al.*, 1972).

*Inter*strain idiotypic cross-reactions are similarly unpredictable at the present time. One observes interstrain idiotypic cross-reactions among the anti-*p*-azobenzoate antibodies of A/J and BALB/c mice. The same antiidiotypic antisera do not, however, cross-react strongly with antibenzoate antibodies of DBA or C57/BL mice. In contrast to antibenzoate antibodies, there is very little interstrain idiotypic cross-reaction among the antiphenylarsonate antibodies of A/J and BALB/c mice (Kuettner *et al.*, 1972). Indeed, the only strains showing idiotypic cross-reactions with the antiphenylarsonate antibodies of A/J mice are very closely related to A/J in their genetic background (Pawlak and Nisonoff, unpublished).

A very significant type of cross-reaction is that observed between certain mouse myeloma proteins with antibody activity directed to the same antigen. Thus, Potter and Lieberman (1970) studied 8 BALB/c myeloma proteins which bind phosphorylcholine and found that 5 of the 8 shared common idiotypic determinants.* Of great interest was the observation of Cohn, Notani, and Rice (1969) that some normally induced BALB/c antibodies to pneumococcal C carbohydrate share idiotype with these 5 myeloma proteins. The antipneumococcal antibodies react with phosphorylcholine, which closely resembles a hapten

---

* The light chains of two of these proteins were found to have identical sequences up to residue 23 (Hood *et al.*, 1970).

group that constitutes part of the polysaccharide antigenic structure (Leon and Young, 1971).

III. LOCALIZATION OF IDIOTYPIC DETERMINANTS

As would be predicted, idiotypic determinants are localized in the Fab fragments of immunoglobulins (Grey et al., 1965; Seligmann et al., 1966; Daugharty et al., 1969; Hopper et al., 1970; Wang et al., 1970), and have been found in the variable segment of a human light chain isolated from urine (Tan and Epstein, 1967; Solomon and McLaughlin, 1969) or after enzymatic digestion of a Bence-Jones protein (Solomon and McLaughlin, 1969). The interference of haptens with the reactions of antihapten antibodies with their antiidiotypic antibodies (Brient and Nisonoff, 1970; Brient et al., 1971; Sirisinha and Eisen, 1971) indicates that the antigen-binding site of an antihapten antibody is frequently, if not always, an important idiotypic determinant.[*]

IV. PERSISTENCE OF CLONES OF CELLS PRODUCING IMMUNOGLOBULIN OF A GIVEN STRUCTURE

A. Persistence of Idiotypic Specificities During Prolonged Immunization

The fact that molecules of identical structure persist during prolonged immunization was indicated by the investigations of MacDonald et al. (1969). It has previously been shown by Roholt et al. (1965) that the restoration of hapten-binding activity of an antihapten antibody can be accomplished by the recombination of heavy and light chains, mediated through noncovalent interactions, however, for appreciable restoration of activity, both chains must be derived from the same rabbit, as well as from antibody of the same specificity. This approach was applied to study antibenzoate antibody isolated from the serum of an individual rabbit at six-month intervals. Recombinants of antibody heavy chains from the earlier bleedings with antibody light chains from the latter bleedings, or vice versa, resulted in the restoration of a large fraction of the original antibody activity (MacDonald et al., 1969). It thus appeared that molecules of similar or identical structure were present in the two sets of bleedings. Since the half-life of a rabbit antibody (Taliaferro and Talmage, 1956; Weigle, 1958) is only a few days, and since most antibody-forming cells are similarly short-lived (Schooley, 1961; Makinodan and Albright, 1967), it was proposed that clones of cells, perpetuated by memory cells, persist for long

---

[*] A myeloma protein with antiphosphorylcholine activity was found to be inhibitable by phosphorylcholine only when a deficiency of antiidiotypic antibody was used (Sher et al., 1971; Sher and Cohn, 1972). Also see footnote on p. 100.

periods of time and synthesize molecules of similar or identical structure (MacDonald *et al.*, 1969).

Because of the large amounts of material and effort required, recombination of heavy and light chains is a cumbersome method for studies of the persistence of molecules with a given structure. As an alternative, investigations were initiated of idiotypic specificities of antihapten antibody taken from individual rabbits at varying intervals. For immunization, recipient rabbits were matched to donors with respect to 9 major allotypic specificities. The immunogen was specifically purified anti-*p*-azobenzoate antibody that had been partially poly-merized with glutaraldehyde and incorporated in complete Freund's adjuvant. About 90% of recipient rabbits responded to repeated inoculation with the production of antiidiotypic antibodies. For assays, an indirect precipitation method is used which comprises 0.1–0.5 μg of ^{125}I-labeled F(ab')$_2$ fragments of the purified donor antibody, 10–20 μg of unlabeled rabbit IgG, a slight excess of antiidiotypic antiserum (frequently 5–10 μl), and excess goat anti-rabbit fragment Fc. The presence of cross-reacting idiotype in an unknown sample is determined by measuring its capacity to inhibit the binding of the labeled ligand. Typically, after hyperimmunization, 30–70% of the labeled donor antibody population is bound to antiidiotypic antibodies. When different recipient rabbits are immunized with the same donor (anti-*p*-azobenzoate) prepa-ration, their sera frequently react with approximately the same subfraction of the antihapten antibody population. When one recipient reacts with a larger subfraction than another, the larger population invariably includes the smaller (Hopper *et al.*, 1970). It was tentatively concluded that the immunogenic portion of the donor population comprises a discrete number of homogeneous subpopulations; the nonimmunogenic fraction may be so heterogeneous that it fails to elicit anti-antibodies in any recipient.

By use of the method of inhibition of indirect precipitation, the following major points emerged. Upon repeated challenge with antigen (BGG*-*p*-azobenzo-ate), a set of idiotypic specificities identified during the first few weeks is gradually, or sometimes rapidly, replaced by new idiotypic specificities on the antibenzoate antibody molecules. This effect is illustrated by the data in Figs. 1 and 2. The results in Fig. 1 were obtained with antiidiotypic antisera prepared against antibenzoate antibodies isolated either approximately 2 months (2M) or 8 months (8M) after the onset of immunization with BGG-*p*-azobenzoate. Antibodies isolated after month 5 failed to react with the anti-2M antibodies. On the other hand, molecules with the 8M idiotype persisted from month 5 through 17 (Fig. 1). On a weight basis, optimal inhibition was obtained with the autologous antibodies, i.e., with the population used for immunization (see Figs. 1 and 2 in MacDonald and Nisonoff, 1970).

Similar results were observed in studying the idiotypes of antibenzoate

* BGG = bovine gamma globulin.

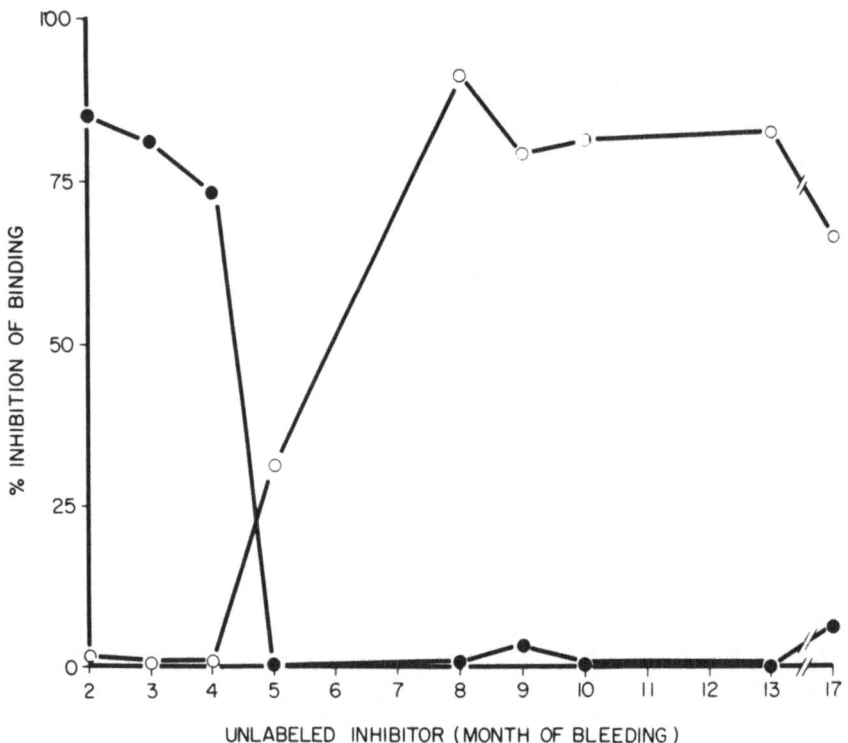

Figure 1. Summary of data obtained with a 60-fold excess by weight of unlabeled competitor (30 μg). *Solid circles:* labeled donor antibodies from month-2 bleedings of rabbit AZ1 reacting with anti-2M (i.e., with antiidiotypic antibody directed against the purified antibody antibenzoate isolated 2 months after the start of immunization). *Open circles:* labeled donor antibodies from month-8 antibodies reacting with anti-8M. Inhibitors are unlabeled, specifically purified, anti-*p*-azobenzoate antibodies from sera of rabbit AZ1 taken at the time specified on the abscissa. Note that the data are plotted as percent inhibition rather than percent of control. (Reprinted, by permission, from MacDonald and Nisonoff, 1970.)

antibodies of several other rabbits (MacDonald and Nisonoff, 1970; Spring *et al.,* 1971). It should be noted that the rabbits were immunized repeatedly at either weekly, biweekly, or monthly intervals, In 2 rabbits studied, the change in idiotype ocurring after the first few weeks was accompanied by an increase in combining affinity for the hapten.

Thus, despite repeated challenge, clones of cells synthesizing antibody of a given idiotype can persist for over a year, although the gradual quantitative change in inhibitory capacity indicates that unrelated clones are slowly but continually initiated.

All of the above discussion refers to IgG antibodies; many of the data were obtained with antibodies specifically purified by a procedure which includes passage through DEAE-cellulose at low ionic strength so that only IgG was eluted. In other experiments, in which whole antibenzoate antiserum was tested as the inhibitor of antiidiotypic antiserum, immunoelectrophoretic experiments failed to reveal the presence of IgM antibenzoate antibodies.

B. Effect of Rest Periods on the Expression of Idiotypic Specificities

Several rabbits that had been subjected to hyperimmunization with BGG-*p*-azobenzoate for 42 to 48 weeks were allowed to rest for slightly less than

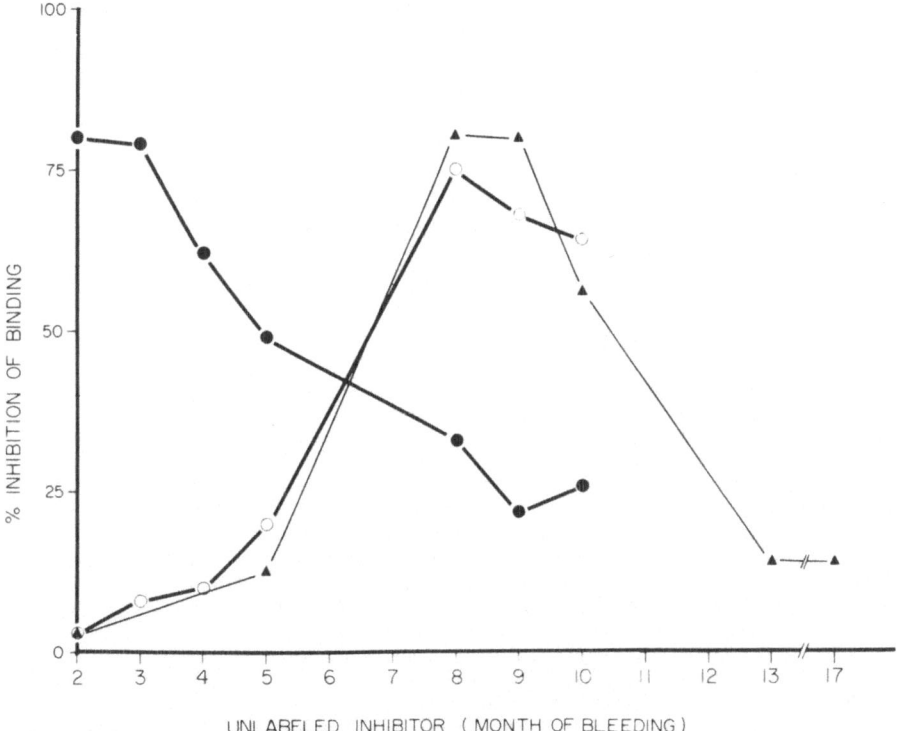

UNLABELED INHIBITOR (MONTH OF BLEEDING)

Figure 2. Summary of data obtained with the highest concentration of inhibitor tested [30 μg, or a 60-fold excess by weight over the ^{125}I-F(ab')$_2$ fragments from the donor antibody (from rabbit AZ5)]. *Solid circles:* donor ^{125}I-F(ab')$_2$ fragments from month-2 bleedings reacging with homologous antiserum, anti-2M (i.e., with antiidiotypic antibody directed against the purified antibody antibenzoate isolated 2 months after the start of immunization): *open circles:* ^{125}I-F(ab')$_2$ fragments from month-8 bleedings reacting with homologous antiserum, anti-8M; *solid triangles:* ^{125}I-F(ab')$_2$ fragments from 10M bleedings reacting with anti-8M. Inhibitors are unlabeled, specifically-purified, anti-*p*-azobenzoate antibodies from bleedings of rabbit AZ5 taken during the month after start of immunization specified on the abscissa. Note that data are plotted as the percent inhibition rather than as percent of control. (Reprinted, by permission, from MacDonald and Nisonoff, 1970.)

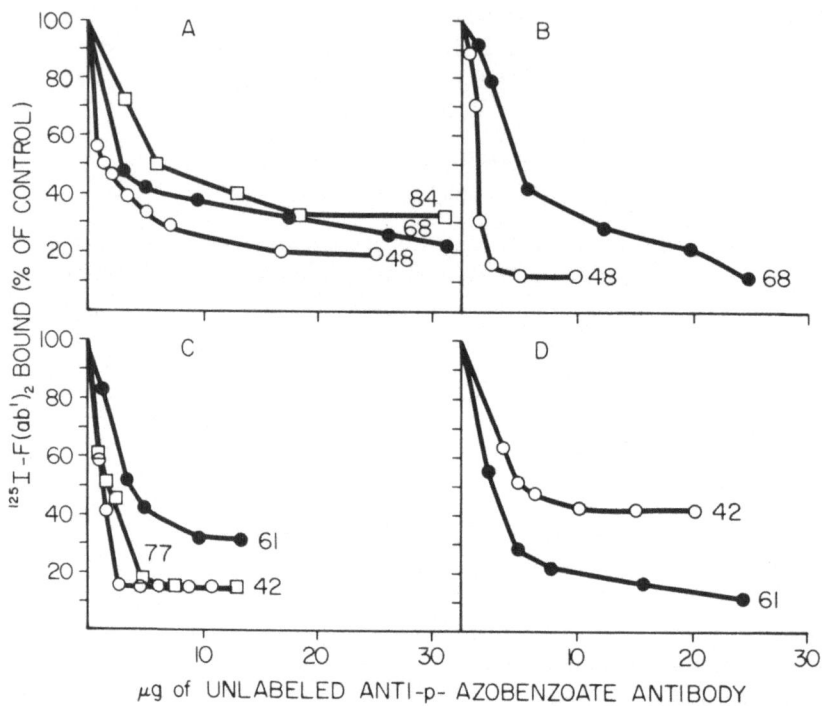

Figure 3. Inhibition of binding of ^{125}I-labeled F(ab')$_2$ fragments (0.5 µg) of anti-p-azobenzoate antibodies to homologous antiidiotypic antisera by anti-p-azobenzoate antibodies present before and after a 5-month rest period. Rabbits 14R (Fig. 3A) and 14S (Fig. 3B) were inoculated every 2 weeks between weeks 1 and 45 with 1 mg of BGG-p-azobenzoate. They were allowed to rest between weeks 45 and 65; during week 66 they were bled and given a booster inoculation. Serum was again collected between weeks 67 and 69. Antiidiotypic antisera were prepared against the antibodies present 48 weeks after the start of immunization. Also, rabbit 14R was allowed a second rest period between weeks 67 and 79. The rabbit was given a booster inoculation during week 79 and antiserum was collected at week 84. Rabbits 16B (Fig. 3C) and 16A (Fig. 3D) were inoculated every 2 weeks between weeks 1 and 37, with 3 mg of BGG-p-azobenzoate. They were allowed to rest between weeks 38 and 58, then were bled and given a booster injection. Antiserum was again collected between weeks 60 and 62. Rabbit 16B was allowed a second rest period between weeks 60 and 72; it was inoculated again at week 73 and bled at week 77. Antiidiotypic antisera were prepared against the antibodies present at week 41 in rabbit 16B and at week 61 in rabbit 16A. The following concentrations of precipitable antibenzoate antibody were present in antisera: Rabbit 14S: week 48, 0.5 mg/ml; week 68, 2.6 mg/ml. Rabbit 14R: week 48, 0.3 mg/ml; week 68, 1.8 mg/ml; week 84, 0.6 mg/ml. Rabbit 16B: week 41, 0.5 mg/ml; week 61, 0.4 mg/ml; week 77, 0.2 mg/ml. Rabbit 16A: week 41, 1.0 mg/ml; week 61, 1.6 mg/ml. The numerals on the curves represent the week of the bleeding used for the inhibition tests. (Reprinted, by permission, from Spring *et al.*, 1971.)

5 months, then challenged again with the antigen (Spring *et al.*, 1971). Prior to this challenge, their sera did not contain precipitating antibody, but the titers were restored after inoculation to levels comparable to those at the start of the

rest period. Figure 3 shows the results of such experiments carried out with 4 rabbits (Spring et al., 1971). Figs. 3A, 3B, and 3C will be discussed first. Here, the antiidiotypic antibodies were prepared against antibenzoate antibodies isolated from sera taken before the rest period. In each case almost complete inhibition of binding was observed with the antibodies present after the booster inoculation which followed the rest period, as well as with the "pre-rest" antibodies. However, the "post-rest" antibodies were somewhat less effective inhibitors on a weight basis. These results indicate that all of the clones contributing to the idiotype detected before the rest period were still present afterwards, but that new clones had also been stimulated; this would account for the lower inhibitory capacity per unit weight of the "post-rest" antibody population.

The results in Fig. 3D are in accord with this view. In this case, the antiidiotypic antibodies were prepared against antibenzoate antibodies isolated after, rather than before, the rest period. About one-third of the antiidiotypic antibody population was not inhibitable by the "pre-rest" population. This finding indicates that new idiotypic specificities had been induced after the rest period; this is not necessarily inconsistent with the conclusion drawn above that all clones present before the rest period were still active.

Experiments relating to persistence of idiotypic specificities have been reported from other laboratories. Oudin and Michel (1969a), using rabbit antisera, studied the idiotypic specificities of anti-Salmonella antibodies in 4 rabbits. Reactions were measured by double diffusion in agar gel. In one rabbit, molecules with cross-reacting or identical idiotype persisted over a period of 29 months, which included a 17-month rest period. In two other rabbits, persistence was shown in a period between 2 and 5 weeks after the start of immunization. In the fourth rabbit, some, but not all, idiotypic specificities initially observed were lost during the first few weeks of immunization.

Persistence of antibody populations during rest periods has also been demonstrated by Eichmann et al. (1970) and by Jaton et al. (1971) for antistreptococcal and antipneumococcal antibodies, respectively. Each of these groups was studying antibody populations of limited heterogeneity. Eichmann et al. (1970) separated a slow and a fast component of antistreptococcal (GroupA) antibody from an individual rabbit on the basis of their distinctive electrophoretic mobilities. Goat antisera were then prepared against each antibody component. Antiidiotypic activity was present in each of the goat antisera, as indicated in Ouchterlony tests with the goat antiserum placed in the center well and the immunogen and nonspecific rabbit IgG placed in adjacent outer wells; in each case, the line formed with the immunogen spurred over that formed with the IgG. Such tests also demonstrated that the fast and slow components had unrelated idiotypic determinants. The persistence of the clone of cells synthesizing the slow component of the antistreptococcal antibody was then studied. The

Table I. Rabbit Antibody

					Residue positions from				
	1	2	3	4	5	6	7	8	9
I	ASP	VAL	VAL	MET	THR	GLX	THR	PRO	ALA
	ALA	PHE	leu	LEU				THR	thr
			met	val					
II	ASP	VAL	VAL	MET	THR	GLX	THR	PRO	ALA
III	ASP	VAL	VAL	MET	THR	GLX	THR	PRO	ALA
	ALA	PHE	pro	leu	val	THR	val	val	pro
				val	leu	val		thr	thr
						leu			val
Nonantibody[†]	ALA	VAL	VAL	THR	THR	THR	GLX	PRO	GLY
	asp	asp	pro	MET	met	glx	PRO	val	pro
		ile		VAL	glx		VAL	gly	ala
								glx	val
								leu	leu

* Underlined residues are those present in the unique sequence of C II. *Capital letters:* concentration < 10% are not listed.
† From Jaton *et al.* (1970).
(Reprinted, by permission, from Jaton *et al.*, 1971.)

rabbit received multiple inoculations over a 3–4 week interval and was then allowed a 7-month rest period followed by one inoculation of antigen. It was then allowed to rest again for a 9-month interval. The idiotypic specificity associated with the slow-migrating component was still present after the booster series of immunizations given at the end of the rest period. No antistreptococcal antibody molecules were detected during the intervals between courses of immunization. A similar set of experiments was carried out with antistreptococcal antibody of another rabbit. These again demonstrated persistence of idiotypic specificities after a 7-month rest period.

Jaton *et al.* (1971) demonstrated the persistence of molecules of related or identical structure in a rabbit inoculated with Type VIII pneumococcal vaccine. This rabbit received three 1-month courses of immunization with a rest period of 1 month after each series of inoculations. Antibodies were isolated after each course and designated C_I, C_{II}, and C_{III}. Three criteria were used to examine each population for the presence of molecules with the same structural character-istics: (1) Antiidiotypic antisera to the C_{II} population were prepared in guinea pigs and used to detect the presence of C_{II} determinants in C_I and C_{III}; (2) peptide maps were prepared from the L chains of each of the 3 antibody populations and compared with those from normal molecules of the same

L-Chain Sequences

the amino terminus*

10	11	12	13	14	15	16	17	18	19	20	21
SER	VAL	SER	GLX	PRO	VAL	GLY	GLY				
thr	ser	glx	ALA	ALA	ala	val	thr				
	thr	thr	thr			ala	ala				
		val									
SER	VAL	SER	GLX	PRO	VAL	GLY	GLY	THR	VAL	THR	ILE
SER	VAL										
thr	thr										
val	leu										
VAL	VAL										
ala	leu										
pro	pro										
leu	ala										
glx	asp										

≥ 25% of residues recovered; *Lower case:* 10–24% of residues recovered; Residues present at

allotype, b4; (3) the amino-terminal sequences of L chains of the 3 antibody populations were compared.

Amino acid sequence obviously is the most definitive criterion for establishing the persistence of antibody molecules with identical structure. The N-terminal sequences of 3 antipneumoccocal antibody populations are presented in Table I. Quantitative data indicated that more than 90% of the molecules of the C_{II} antibody population had the unique sequence listed. In contrast, L chains from the C_I and C_{III} antibody populations were more heterogeneous since they had alternative residues at several positions in the chain. However, the major sequence in both C_I and C_{III} was that of C_{II}. The L-chain sequences from all three antibodies were much more homogeneous and quite different from the first 11 residues of non-antibody L chains of allotype b4.

Quantitative radioimmunodiffusion using guinea pig antiidiotypic antibodies to the C_{II} population indicated that 45% of the molecules in the C_I and C_{III} populations shared idiotype with the C_{II} molecules; a similar value was also determined by quantitative studies of the radio labeled peptide maps of the C_I, C_{II}; and C_{III} antibodies. Both of these values agreed closely with that predictable from the sequence data. It is evident that the persistence of clones of cells producing molecules of a particular idiotypic specificity and structure can be followed by a variety of methods. Moreover, it is apparent from these investigations that while some clones of cells may persist for long periods of time, gradual changes in antibody populations do occur as a result of the stimulation of new and unrelated clones of cells, as indicated above.

C. Factors Effecting the Persistence of Clones of Cells

Two factors which might influence the persistence of clones of cells during the course of immunization would be the dosage of antigen and the frequency of challenge. Experiments designed to investigate these parameters were carried out by Spring *et al.* (1971).

In the first series (Fig. 4), rabbits were inoculated biweekly with 1, 3, or 10

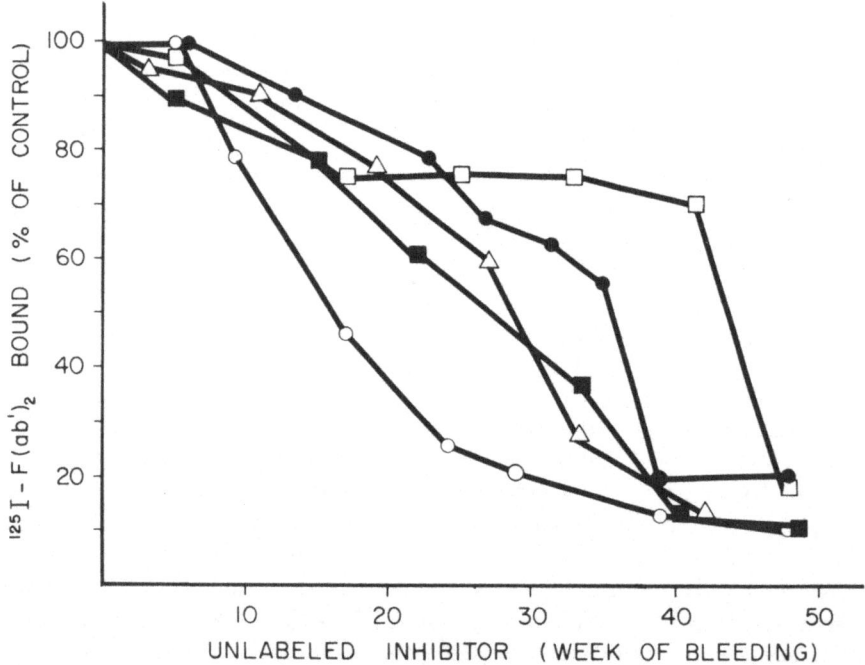

Figure 4. Inhibition of binding of ^{125}I-labeled F(ab')$_2$ fragments (0.5 μg) of anti-*p*-azobenzoate antibodies to the homologous antiidiotypic antiserum by 30 μg amounts of anti-*p*-azobenzoate antibodies present in the serum of the donor rabbit at varying times after the start of immunization. The number of weeks is indicated on the abscissa of the graph. Rabbits 13X (○) and 14U (●) received 10 mg of antigen every 2 weeks; antiidiotypic antisera were prepared against the antibodies present 48 weeks after the start of immunization. Rabbits 14R (□) and 14S (■) received 1 mg of antigen every 2 weeks; antiidiotypic antisera were prepared against the antibodies present at week 48. Rabbit 16B (△) received 3 mg of antigen every 2 weeks; antiidiotypic antiserum was prepared against antibodies present at week 42. (Reprinted, by permission, from Spring *et al.*, 1971.)

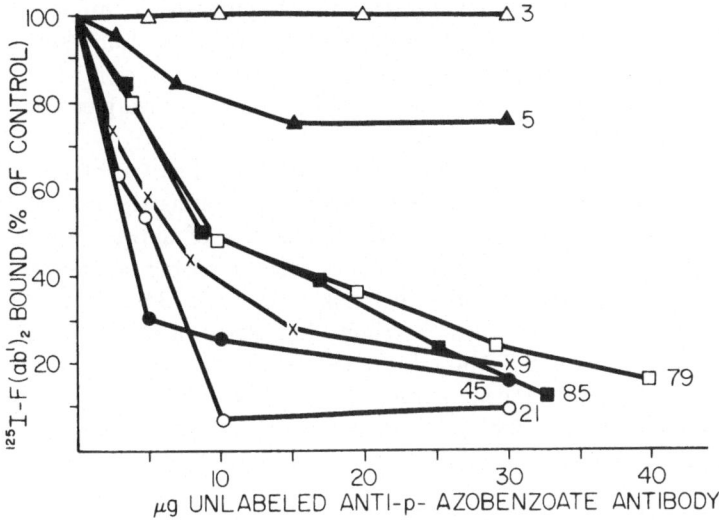

Figure 5. Inhibition of binding of ^{125}I-labeled F(ab')$_2$ fragments (0.5 µg) of anti-p-azobenzoate antibodies from rabbit Z4 to an approximately equivalent amount of antiidiotypic antibodies. The immunogen was anti-p-azobenzoate antibody isolated from the serum of rabbit Z4, 21 weeks after the start of immunization. Rabbit Z4 received 3 mg of BGG-p-azobenzoate every 4 weeks. Competitor molecules are unlabeled specifically purified anti-p-azobenzoate antibodies isolated from bleedings of rabbit Z4 at various times; the number of weeks after the start of immunization is indicated by the numeral on each curve. The following concentrations of precipitable antibenzoate antibody were present in the antisera: week 3, 0.5 mg/ml; week 5, 2.0 mg/ml; week 9, 2.6 mg/ml; week 21, 1.0 mg/ml; week 45, 0.5 mg/ml; week 79, 0.4 mg/ml; week 85, 0.3 mg/ml. (Reprinted, by permission, from Spring *et al.*, 1971.)

mg doses of antigen (a BGG-p-azobenzoate conjugate). Serum was collected prior to each inoculation and an antiidiotypic antiserum was prepared against the anti-p-azobenzoate antibodies present 42 or 48 weeks after the start of immunization. These will be designated week-42 or week-48 antibodies. Antisera from other bleedings were tested for the presence of molecules having the same idiotypic specificity as the week-42 or week-48 antibodies. The indirect precipitation technique (MacDonald and Nisonoff, 1970) summarized in Section IV A. was used. Hyperimmune antisera or known antibody content were tested for their inhibitory capacity in this system.

As indicated by the data in Fig. 4, there appears to be little effect of dosage of antigen administered biweekly on the appearance and persistence of clones of cells synthesizing antibenzoate antibody molecules. The fact that even relatively large doses of antigen administered frequently caused only gradual change in idiotype was attributed to either more effective capture of antigen by memory cells, as compared to unrelated precursor cells, or to the induction of tolerance in those cells which were initially capable of synthesizing anti-*p*-azobenzoate antibodies, but which had not been previously induced to proliferate. The more effective capture of antigen by memory cells could be attributed to a higher affinity of their receptors or, more probably, simply to their greater concentration as compared to precursor cells.

A second series of experiments was performed in essentially the same manner. In this case, however, the effect of increasing the interval between injections to one month was studied; the dosage of antigen was 3 mg per inoculation. The antiidiotypic antibodies were prepared against the anti-*p*-azobenzoate molecules present in the week-21 or week-23 bleedings. The results obtained with antibodies from 3 rabbits inoculated at monthly intervals are shown in Figs. 5, 6, and 7; those for rabbits inoculated at biweekly intervals are in Figs. 8 and 9. It is apparent from these data that the idiotypic populations change more slowly in rabbits inoculated on a monthly schedule than in rabbits inoculated on a biweekly schedule. In two cases (Figs 5 and 6), molecules

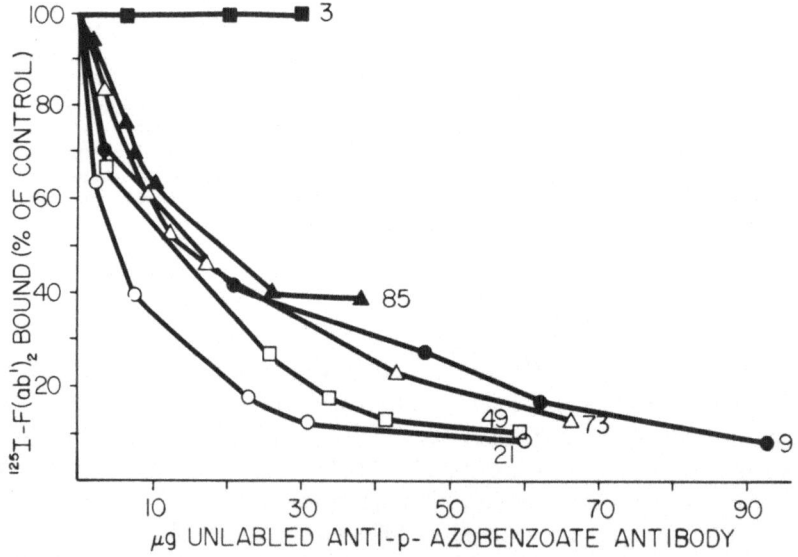

Figure 6. Inhibition of binding of ^{125}I-labeled F(ab')$_2$ fragments (0.5 μg) of anti-*p*-azobenzoate antibodies from rabbit Z6 to an approximately equivalent amount of antiidiotypic antibodies. The immunogen was anti-*p*-azobenzoate antibody isolated from the serum of rabbit Z6, 21 weeks after the start of immunization. Rabbit Z6 received 3 mg of BGG-*p*-azobenzoate every 4 weeks. Competitor molecules are unlabeled specifically-purified anti-*p*-azobenzoate antibodies isolated from bleedings of rabbit Z6 at various times; the number of weeks after the start of immunization is indicated by the numeral on each curve. The following concentrations of precipitable antibenzoate antibody were present in the antisera: week 3, 0.7 mg/ml; week 9, 1.6 mg/ml; week 21, 0.8 mg/ml; week 49, 0.3 mg/ml; week 73, 0.3 mg/ml; week 85, 0.3 mg/ml. (Reprinted, by permission, from Spring *et al.*, 1971.)

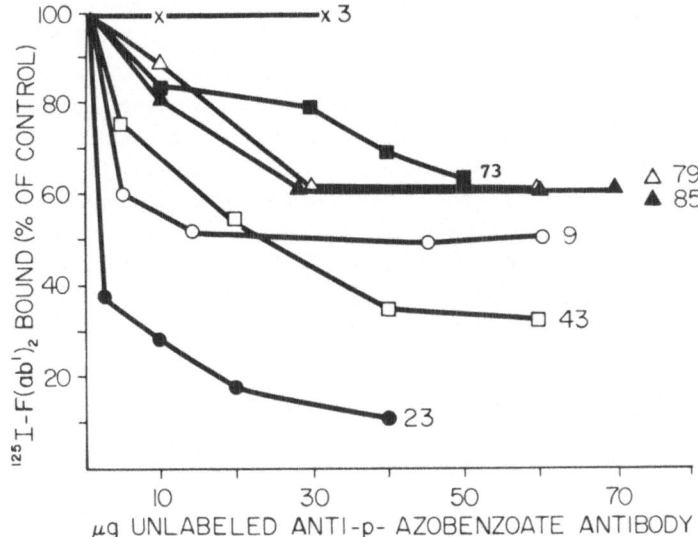

Figure 7. Inhibition of binding of ^{125}I-labeled F(ab')$_2$ fragments (0.5 μg) of anti p-azobenzoate antibodies from rabbit Z9 to an approximately equivalent amount of antiidiotypic antibodies. The immunogen was anti-p-azobenzoate antibody isolated from the serum of rabbit Z9, 23 weeks after the start of immunization. Rabbit Z9 received 3 mg of BGG-p-azo-benzoate every 4 weeks. Competitor molecules are unlabeled specifically-purified anti p-azobenzoate antibodies isolated from bleedings of rabbit Z9 at various times; the number of weeks after the start of immunization is indicated by the numeral on each curve. The following concentrations of precipitable antibenzoate antibody were present in each antiserum: week 3, 0.9 mg/ml; week 9, 2.2 mg/ml; week 23, 0.4 mg/ml; week 43, 0.8 mg/ml; week 73, 0.7 mg/ ml; week 79, 0.7 mg/ml; week 85, 0.3 mg/ml. (Reprinted, by permission, from Spring *et al.*, 1971.)

bearing the same idiotypic specificities were present from 9 to 73–79 weeks after the start of immunization, although concentrations of molecules bearing the idiotype of the immunogen slowly changed. The more gradual change in idiotype seen in rabbits inoculated once a month is in accord with the relatively small quantitative changes in idiotype associated with prolonged rest periods (discussed above).

V. SUMMARY

Persistence of clones of cells, each producing antibody molecules of a unique structure, was suggested by studies of complementation of heavy and light chains of antibodies taken from an individual rabbit at various times during the course of immunization. The concept of idiotypic specificity as a marker for a clone of antibody-producing cells leads to a more convenient method for pursuing investigations of this type. The studies summarized here indicate that clones of cells, undoubtedly mediated by memory cells, may persist for long periods of time and are only gradually replaced by new clones, despite repeated challenge by large amounts of antigen. Mechanisms to account for this finding are suggested. The rate of replacement of clones appears to be influenced somewhat more by the frequency of challenge with antigen than by the amount administered, and is minimized by a prolonged rest period, although some new clones are then stimulated by a single injection of antigen. The study of idiotypic specificities appears to be a useful technique for following certain events occurring in immunologically competent lymphoid cell populations.

ACKNOWLEDGMENT

This work was supported by grants from the National Institutes of Health (AI 06281 and AI 10220).

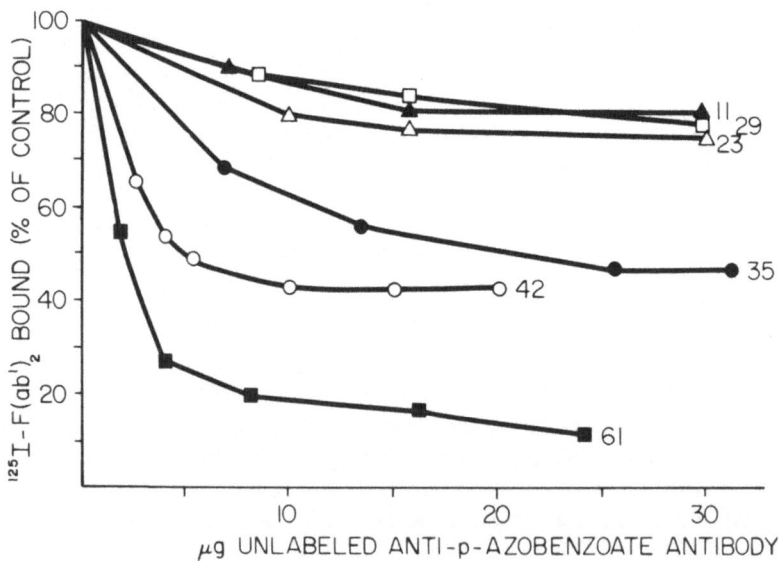

Figure 8. Inhibition of binding of ^{125}I-labeled F(ab')$_2$ fragments (0.5 μg) of anti-*p*-azobenzoate antibodies from rabbit 16A to an approximately equivalent amount of antiidiotypic antibodies. The immunogen was anti-*p*-azobenzoate antibody isolated from the serum of rabbit 16A, 61 weeks after the start of immunization. Rabbit 16A received 3 mg of BGG-*p*-azobenzoate every 2 weeks. Competitors are unlabeled antisera taken from bleedings of rabbit 16A at various times; the number of weeks after the start of immunization is indicated by the numeral on each curve. The following concentrations of precipitable antibody were present: week 11, 2.4 mg/ml; week 23, 1.5 mg/ml; week 29, 1.6 mg/ml; week 35, 1.3 mg/ml; week 42, 1.0 mg/ml; week 61, 1.6 mg/ml; (Reprinted, by permission, from Spring *et al.*, 1971.)

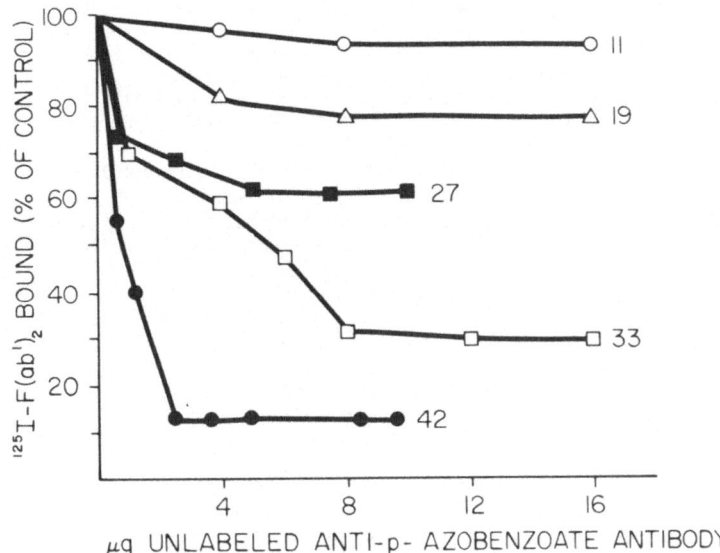

Figure 9. Inhibition of binding of ^{125}I-labeled F(ab')$_2$ fragments (0.5 μg) of anti-g-azobenzoate antibodies from rabbit 16B to an approximately equivalent amount of antiidiotypic antibodies. The immunogen was anti-p-azobenzoate antibody isolated from the serum of rabbit 16B, 42 weeks after the start of immunization. Rabbit 16B received 3 mg of BGG-p-azobenzoate every 2 weeks. Competitors are unlabeled antisera taken from bleedings of rabbit 16B at various times; the number of weeks after the start of immunization is indicated by the numeral on each curve. The following concentrations of precipitable antibenzoate antibody were present: week 11, 1.6 mg/ml; 19, 0.8 mg/ml, week 27, 0.5 mg/ml; week 33, 0.8 mg/ml; week 42, 0.5 mg/ml. (Reprinted, by permission, from Spring *et al.*, 1971.)

REFERENCES

Boerma, F. W., and Mandema, E. (1957). *J. Lab. Clin. Med.* **49**: 358.
Bordenave, G., and Oudin, J. (1971). *Ann. Inst. Pasteur* **120**: 265.
Braun, D. G., and Kruase, R. M. (1968). *J. Exp. Med.* **128**: 969.
Brient, B. W., and Nisonoff, A. (1970). *J. Exp. Med.* **132**: 951.
Brient, B. W., Haimovich, J., and Nisonoff, A. (1971). *Proc. Natl. Acad. Sci. U.S.* **68**: 3136.
Cohn, M. G., Notani, G., and Rice, S. (1969). *Immunochemistry* **6**: 111.
Daugharty, H., Hopper, J. E., MacDonald, A. B., and Nisonoff, A. (1969). *J. Exp. Med.* **130**: 1047.
Eichmann, K., and Kindt, T. J. (1971). *J. Exp. Med.* **134**: 532.
Eichmann, K., Braun, D. G., Feizi, T., and Krause, R. M. (1970). *J. Exp. Med.* **131**: 1169.
Gell, P. G. H., and Kelus, A. S. (1964). *Nature* **201**: 687.
Grey, H. M., Mannik, K. M., and Kunkel, H. G. (1965). *J. Exp. Med.* **121**: 561.
Haber, E. (1970). *Federation Proc.* **29**: 66.
Harboe, M., and Deverill, J. (1964). *Scand. J. Haematol.* **1**: 223.
Hood, L. E., Potter, M., and McKeon, D. J. (1970). *Science* **170**: 1207.
Hopper, J. E., MacDonald, A. B., and Nisonoff, A. (1970). *J. Exp. Med.* **131**: 41.
Jaton, J. C., Waterfield, M. D., Margolies, M. N., and Haber, E. (1970). *Proc. Natl. Acad. Sci. U.S.* **66**: 959.

Jaton, J. C., Waterfield, M. D., Margolies, M. N., Bloch, K. J., and Haber, E. (1971). *Biochemistry* 10: 1583.
Korngold, L., and Lipari, L. (1956). *Cancer* 9: 183.
Korngold, L., and Van Leeuwen, G. (1957a). *J. Exp. Med.* 106: 467.
Korngold, L., and Van Leeuwen, G. (1957b). *J. Exp. Med.* 106: 477.
Kuettner, M. G., Wang, A. C., and Nisonoff, A. (1972). *J. Exp. Med.* 135: 579.
Kunkel, H. G. (1970). *Federation Proc.* 29: 55.
Kunkel, H. G., Mannik, K. M., and Williams, R. C., Jr. (1963). *Science* 140: 1218.
Leon, M., and Young, M. N. (1971). *Biochemistry* 10: 1424.
MacDonald, A. B., and Nisonoff, A. (1970). *J. Exp. Med.* 131: 583.
MacDonald, A. B., Alescio, L., and Nisonoff, A. (1969). *Biochemistry* 8: 3109.
Makinodan, T., and Albright, J. F. (1967). *Prog. Allergy* 10: 1.
Nisonoff, A., MacDonald, A. B., Hopper, J. E., and Daugharty, H. (1970). In "Sump. Exp. Approaches to Homogeneous Antibody Populations," *Federation Proc.* 29: 72.
Oudin, J. (1966). *Proc. Roy. Soc. (London), Ser. B.* 166: 207.
Oudin, J., and Bordenave, G. (1971). *Nature* 231: 86.
Oudin, J., and Cazenave, P. A. (1971). *Proc. Natl. Acad. Sci. U.S.* 68: 2616.
Oudin, J., and Michel, M. (1963). *C. R. Acad. Sci.* 257: 86.
Oudin, J., and Michel, M. (1969a). *J. Exp. Med.* 130: 595.
Oudin, J., and Michel M. (1969b). *J. Exp. Med.* 130: 619.
Potter, M., and Lieberman, R. (1970). *J. Exp. Med.* 132: 737.
Roholt, O. A., Radzimski, G., and Pressman, D. (1965). *Science* 147: 613.
Schade, S. Z., and Nisonoff, A. (1972). *J. Immunol.* 108: 1295.
Schooley, J. C. (1961). *J. Immunol.* 86: 331.
Seligmann, M., Meshaka, G., Hurez, D., and Mihaesco, C. (1966). *Immunopathol. Intern. Symp. 4th 1965*, p. 229.
Sher, A., and Cohn, M. (1972). *J. Immunol.* 109: 176.
Sher, A., Lord, E., and Cohn, M. G. (1971). *J. Immunol.* 107: 1226.
Sirisinha, S., and Eisen, H. N. (1971). *Proc. Natl. Acad. Sci. U.S.* 68: 3130.
Slater, R. J., Ward, S. M., and Kunkel, H. G. (1955). *J. Exp. Med.* 101: 185.
Solomon, A., and McLaughlin, C. L. (1969). *J. Biol. Chem.* 244: 3393.
Spring, S. B., Schroeder, K. W., and Nisonoff, A. (1971). *J. Exp. Med.* 134: 765.
Stein, S., Nachman, R. L., and Engle, R. L., Jr. (1963). *Nature* 200: 140.
Taliaferro, W. H., and Talmage, D. W. (1956). *J. Infect. Diseases* 99: 21.
Tan, M., and Epstein, W. (1967). *J. Immunol.* 98: 568.
Wang, A. C., Wilson, S. K., Hopper, J. E., Fudenberg, H. H., and Nisonoff, A. (1970). *Proc. Natl. Acad. Sci. U.S.* 66: 337.
Weigle, W. O. (1958). *J. Immunol.* 81: 204.
Williams, R. C., Jr., Kunkel, H. G., and Capra, J. D. (1968). *Science* 161: 379.

Chapter 6

Immunoglobulins and Antibodies in Pigs

Jaroslav Rejnek and Ludmila Prokesová

Department of Immunology
Institute of Microbiology
Czechoslovak Academy of Science
Prague, Czechoslovakia

I. INTRODUCTION

Studies on the ontogenetic development of the antibody response have played an important role in the rapid advances made in immunology during the past fifteen years. Such investigations have permitted a better understanding of the results obtained using adults. This is so because antigenic stimulation in adults results in a response whose level is dependent on the intensity of previous uncontrolled antigenic contacts. In the newborn, on the other hand, the prior antigenic knowledge of an experimental animal can be kept to a minimum or eliminated, thereby allowing a clearer picture of the response.

When choosing an experimental model suitable for developmental studies of immune reactions, many factors, i.e., maturity of animals at the time of birth, passive transfer of maternal antibodies, and metabolism of immunoglobulins and other serum proteins which may influence the results, must be taken into consideration. The animal which would best suit such studies should be without antibodies acquired either passively or as a result of uncontrolled immunization (Sterzl and Silverstein, 1967), should be fairly mature at birth, and should be convenient for experimentation at a young age. These requirements can be fulfilled using the pig as the experimental animal. No passive transfer of immunity occurs in pig embryos during their intrauterine life (Brambell *et al.*, 1951). All serum proteins, including immunoglobulins, are synthetized in the fetus, which means that the immune reactions develop without the presence and influence of maternal antibodies. Furthermore, piglets can be delivered by hysterectomy or Caesarean section under sterile conditions, then kept in sterile isolators and fed a diet of nonantigenic character (Trávnícek *et al.*, 1966). Thus, germfree piglets represent a very suitable approach to the study of immuno-globulins of nonantibody character and the dynamics of antibody formation. It is the aim of this short review to discuss the data obtained when using pigs as the experimental animal model in the study of immunoglobulins and antibody response.

II. THE PROTEINS OF PIG SERUM

Pig serum contains approximately 7% proteins. Sokol *et al.* (1954) found the value of 7.2–7.42%; Lecce and Matrone (1960), 6%; and Porter (1969*b*), 6.84 ± 0.33%. Immunoelectrophoretic characterization of pig serum proteins was described by Brummersted-Hansen (1961), Brummersted-Hansen and Hirschfeld (1961), Wellmann and Engel (1963), Rejnek *et al.* (1966), and Karlsson (1966*a*). The porcine blood serum spectrum shows the same main distribution of precipitation lines as those of man and other mammalian species. Precipitation arcs were obtained in the prealbumin, albumin, alpha 1-, alpha 2-, beta 1-, beta 2-, and gamma-globulin regions. A number of precipitation lines were found in alpha- and beta-globulin regions while the main components present in highest concentrations were albumin and immunoglobulins. Compari-son of human and pig serum showed that the concentration of immunoglobulins in pig serum was significantly higher.

Baumstark (1968) compared the behavior of pig and human serum proteins in chromatography on DEAE cellulose and in gel filtration, and measured molecular weights and electrophoretic mobilities of some serum proteins. The chromatogram obtained after separation on DEAE cellulose was similar in shape to the chromatogram obtained for human serum. One of the main differences between human and pig serum appeared to be a higher concentration of proteins in the transferrin region of the DEAE-cellulose chromatogram of pig serum. Some of the proteins of pig serum possessed electrophoretic mobilities almost identical to their human counterparts, while the general trend appeared to favor a somewhat lower mobility. The slightly lower mobilities exhibited by the pig serum proteins explain their earlier appearance in the DEAE-cellulose column effluent. Gel filtration of pig serum on a Sephadex G-200 column resulted in three main fractions similar to those of human serum, but some quantitative differences have been found. Pig serum contains a higher concentration of proteins with molecular weights of the order of 150,000–800,000 than does human serum.

Even paper or agar gel electrophoresis of pig serum demonstrates a wide zone in the gamma-globulin region, indicating the presence of a large amount of immunoglobulins. A myelomalike disease producing large amounts of homogene-ous immunoglobulins has never been found in pigs. All data concerning pig immunoglobulins were obtained by studying the heterogeneous immunoglobulins of normal or artificially-immunized pigs. Three main immunoglobulin classes (IgG, IgM and IgA) have been described in pig serum so far, and all three are clearly visible upon immunoelectrophoretic analysis of pig serum. These three classes are analogous to corresponding immunoglobulins known in man and other mammals. This comparison has been made on the basis of their molecular weight, electrophoretical mobility, composition of the molecules of heavy and light chains, and antigenic cross-reactivity with immunoglobulins of other animal species.

Isolation and identification of pig IgG, IgM, and IgA led to their quantitative estimation in serum and other body fluids. Porter (1969b) employed single radial immunodiffusion for this purpose, using specific antisera to single immunoglobulin classes. According to his results, the concentration of immunoglobulins in pig serum was as follows: IgG, 2.15 ± 0.24%; IgA, 0.18 ± 0.05%; and IgM, 0.11 ± 0.03%. Curtis and Bourne (1971) used the same technique for estimating immunoglobulins in pig serum and found the following values: IgG, 18.31 ± 0.67 mg/ml (IgG2, 12.41 ± 0.48 mg/ml); IgA, 1.44 ± 0.12 mg/ml; IgM, 3.15 ± 0.19 mg/ml. The same authors found slightly different values in the serum of pregnant sows: IgG, 24.33 ± 0.94 mg/ml (IgG2, 14.08 ± 0.49 mg/ml); IgA, 2.37 ± 0.20 mg/ml; IgM, 2.92 ± 0.18 mg/ml. According to these results, immunoglobulins represent approximately one-third of all pig serum proteins.

A. Immunoglobulin G

IgG forms 85–90% of all immunoglobulins present in pig serum. The comparison of human and pig IgG using sedimentation analysis showed that both immunoglobulins have molecules of corresponding sizes. The molecular weight of pig IgG can be lowered by splitting disulfide bonds, thus demonstrating its multichain structure (Franek 1961). N-terminal amino acids of pig IgG have been determined by several authors (Table I).

The number of disulfide bonds in IgG molecules was determined by amperometric titration in the presence of sodium sulfite. Franek and Lankas (1963) showed that oxidative sulfitolysis in the absence of disaggregating agents splits 8

Table I. N-Terminal Amino Acid Residues in Pig IgG

N-terminal amino acid (mole/mole)						Reference
Glu	Ala	Ser	Thr	Val	Leu	
1.99	1.04					Eriksson and Sjöquist, 1960
1.57	0.65					Putnam et al., 1962
1.32	0.70	0.17	0.05	0.10	0.10	Colacicco, 1963

disulfide bonds in the pig IgG molecule. All disulfide bonds were split in 5.5 M guanidinehydrochloride (20.2 S–S bonds), while in 10 M urea only 18.2 disulfide bonds were detectable. The total amount of cysteic acid estimated in pig IgG after hydrolysis was 39.4 ± 2.0 mole/mole.

Isolation of heavy (H) and light (L) polypeptide chains of pig IgG can be achieved by oxidative sulfitolysis followed by gel filtration on Sephadex G-100 in 0.05 M formic acid and 6 M urea. This procedure leads to good separation of polypeptide chains in high yields, and the products are quite soluble. If this procedure is carried out in normal buffers without the presence of disaggregating agents, 8 disulfide bridges per IgG molecule are split. Under these conditions, approximately 7% of IgG molecules remain incompletely split and are eluted during gel filtration as the first peak followed by γ- and L-chain peaks (Franek and Keil, 1964; Franek and Zikán, 1964, Franek, 1965). Pig IgG is composed of 67% γ chains and 33% light chains [extinction coefficient for γ chains is 16% higher than for light chains (Franek and Zikán, 1964)]. According to Franek (1966), the molecular weight of pig γ chains is 50,000; that of light chains, 24,000. The γ and L chains differ in amino acid compositions, peptide maps, and N-terminal amino acid residues. Franek (1965) estimated the N-terminal amino acids in the chains of pig IgG and found glutamic acid for the γ chains. The amino terminal of the L chains was either blocked or contained alanine.

The amount of incompletely split molecules of pig IgG originating during oxidative sulfitolysis depends on the pH of the reaction mixture, on the duration of the reaction, and on the concentration of sodium sulfite (Franek and Zikán, 1964; Franek, 1965). These incompletely split molecules are composed of two molecular types. One is formed of one heavy chain and one light chain (half a molecule of the original IgG) having a molecular weight of 70,000. The other one contains two heavy chains and one light chain and its molecular weight is 122,000. These two subunits can be separated by repeated gel filtration (Franek, 1965, 1966).

It can be assumed that pig IgG contains molecules with interchain disulfide bonds of varying stability, and that the higher stability of some IgG molecules results in higher molecular weight subunits formed after oxidative sulfitolysis. Pig IgG preparations can be separated into two fractions using zinc acetate precipitation. The fraction which is soluble in 0.02 M zinc acetate solution can be split completely into γ and L chains without any detectable presence of any of the higher subunits. On the other hand, the fraction which precipitates at 0.02 M concentration of Zn ions, after sulfitolysis, gives rise to a relatively large proportion of high molecular weight subunits (Rejnek et al., 1967).

Heavy and light chains of pig IgG correspond in their physiocochemical characteristics to those derived from the IgG of other animal species. However, after oxidative sulfitolysis, and even after reduction and alkylation (using 2-mercaptoethanol or dithiothreitol), another structural subunit was found which has not yet been fully characterized. This subunit, containing γ-chain antigenic determinants, was found in L-chain fractions obtained after splitting interchain disulfide bonds and gel filtration of serum or colostrum IgG. The subunit could not be separated even after repeated rechromatography of the L-chain preparation. Sedimentation analysis of the fraction of L chain in which the above-mentioned component was enriched showed that this component had a molecular weight corresponding approximately to that of L chains. Other evidence showing the difference between γ chains and the component present in light-chain preparations came from electrophoretic analyses, where the component migrated faster than γ chains. Absorption experiments showed that the L-chain-like component contained antigenic determinants specific for both Fc and Fd fragments. When the component was digested by papain, only Fc determinants were demonstrated. This led to the suggestion that the Fd part of the component was too small for a precipitation reaction with corresponding antiserum. These results suggest that the L-chain-like component represents part of the γ chain, but its origin remains obscure (Rejnek et al., 1967). The presence of a component related to heavy chains in pig light-chain preparations was also described by Yamashita et al. (1968). They called the component ρ chain and claimed that it represented a separate light-chain type rather than a heavy-chain fragment.

The heterogeneity of pig IgG is similar to that found in other animal species. It can be separated according to charge heterogeneity into two fractions, fast-migrating IgG and slow-migrating IgG, using DEAE-cellulose chromatography (Metzger and Fougereau, 1967; Zikán et al., 1970). Both fractions have the same molecular weight, sedimentation constant, and carbohydrate content (2%); but differ in electrophoretic mobility and antigenic properties. Differences in antigenic structure are localized on the Fc fragment (Metzger and Fougereau, 1967). Similar results were obtained by Zikán et al. (1970) who used chromatography on DEAE-Sephadex to separate pig IgG into two fractions which differed in their negative charge. The slow-migrating fraction IgG I and fast-migrating fraction IgG II also differed in amino acid composition, mainly in the content of glutamic acid and tyrosine. Using a fingerprint technique, the authors identified 3 peptides specific for IgG I and 5 peptides specific for IgG II. The differences were mainly localized in the γ-chains. Further comparison of pig IgG I and IgG II also showed differences in the resistance to enzymatic splitting. IgG I is less resistant to papain digestion in the presence of a reducing agent than IgG II. The two fractions, IgG I and IgG II, also differed in their biological activities, as was shown by studying antibodies to sheep red blood cells. These differences will be discussed later. The differences between IgG I and IgG II are probably localized on the Fc fragment, but not in its terminal octadecapeptide which is identical in both IgG I and IgG II (Zikán et al., 1970).

Primary structure studies, i.e., the studies of the amino acid sequence of pig IgG, encounter many difficulties, as no myelomalike disease (connected with the production of homogenous immunoglobulins known in men and mice) has been found in pigs; all the studies therefore have been performed on normal hetero-genous IgG. Only the C-terminal part of pig γ chains has been studied in some details thus far. Zikán *et al.* (1970) described the amino acid sequence of the C-terminal octadecapeptide and compared it to the sequence of γ-chain octa-decapeptides of other animal species. Only slight differences were found (e.g., a 4 amino acid residue difference between pig and human γ-chain octadecapep-tides), suggesting that only a few variations occurred in this part of the γ chain during phylogenetic evolution.

More data have been accumulated on the structure of light chains. Pig IgG contains two basic types of light chains which correspond to κ and λ chains found in other animal species (Franek, 1966; Franek and Zorina, 1967; Hood *et al.*, 1967; Novotný and Franek, 1968). Pig κ and λ chains can be separated by SE-Sephadex chromatography. The light chains having a lower positive charge correspond to the λ type and can be more easily split off the original IgG molecule. This indicates that the disulfide bridge connecting λ and γ chains is more labile than that of κ chains (Franek, 1966). According to Franek and Zorina (1967), pig serum IgG contains 60—70% λ chains and 30—40% κ chains. Similarly, Hood *et al.* (1967), who studied light chain types of various animal species, estimated the ratio of κ chains to λ chains in pigs to be one·to one.

No detectable amino-terminal residue has been found in pig λ chains. It was suggested that the N-terminal was blocked in a similar fashion as in rabbit, human, or murine λ chains (Franek and Zorina, 1967; Hood *et al.*, 1967; Mage *et al.*, 1970). Pig λ chains contain two intrachain disulphide bridges. The amino acid sequence around these bridges has been studied in greater detail. It was found that this sequence was very homologous to the sequence of corresponding areas described in human Bence-Jones proteins of the λ type (Franek *et al.*, 1968). The similarity between pig and human λ chains was further confirmed while studying the sequence of the variable part of pig λ chains. Franek *et al.* (1969) established the sequence of 22 amino acids between positions 73 and 94, comparing it to the sequence of a corresponding area of Bence-Jones proteins. Out of 22 positions, 8 were invariable and identical in both pig and human λ chains. In most of the variable positions, at least one common amino acid residue existed in both species compared. Only positions 92 and 94 differed completely (Franek *et al.*, 1969).

The C-terminal amino acid sequence has also been studied in pig λ chains. Hood *et al.* (1967) described the sequence of C-terminal octapeptides as being: Thr—Val—Thr—Pro—Ser—Glu—Cys—Ala. The presence of a cysteine residue next to the C-terminal residue is a characteristic feature of λ chains.

Studying the primary structure of pig κ chains revealed a high degree of homology with κ chains of other animal species (Novotný *et al.*, 1970). As has been mentioned above, the N-terminal amino acid in pig κ chains is alanine. The sequence of the first 24 amino acids, beginning with the amino terminal, was determined, and a marked homology with human Bence-Jones proteins of the κ type was found. The analyzed peptide exhibited approximately the same degree of homology with the peptides of all three known subgroups of human κ chains (Novotný et al., 1970). As far as the constant portion of pig κ chains is concerned, the sequence of residues 155–206 was studied. 62% of these residues were identical when compared with human Bence-Jones κ proteins, as opposed to 60% when compared with murine Bence-Jones κ proteins. The similarity between pig and human κ chains was even higher than between human and murine κ chains, where 50% homology was found (Novotný and Franek, 1970).

The C-terminal sequence of pig κ chains reported by Hood et al. (1967) and Novotný et al. (1969) was Asp—Glu—Cys—Glu—Ala, while κ chains of all other animal species studied so far had C-terminal cysteine. The C-terminal dipeptide Glu—Ala has not been found in any other light chain type investigated thus far, but the rest of the C-terminal sequence up to the cysteinyl residue corresponds to the κ chain C-terminal peptides of mice, men, and rabbits. It has been suggested that the pig κ chain represents a peculiar developmental stage, and that in other animal species deletion of the Glu—Ala dipeptide took place (Novotný et al., 1969).

There is very little known about the carbohydrate component of pig IgG other than that published by Niedermeier et al. (1971). These authors reported that pig IgG contains about 2% carbohydrates, which are bound mainly to γ chains, but a small portion of carbohydrates was present even in L-chain preparations. Of course, the L-chain preparation might have been contaminated with a small amount of γ chains. An indication of the heterogeneity of the carbohydrate component is the fact that, in certain cases, less than one molecule of a given carbohydrate per molecule of IgG was determined. The carbohydrate composition of pig immunoglobulin G is demonstrated in Table II (according to Niedermeier, 1971).

The mannose—galactose ratio (5.3) is relatively high when compared with that for human IgG (2.1).

Table II. The Carbohydrate Composition of Pig IgG*

Carbohydrate	Protein (mole/mole)		
	γ chain	L chain	IgG
Fucose	0.5	—	1.1
Mannose	2.3	0.3	5.3
Galactose	0.4	0.2	1.0
Glucosamine	4.5	0.2	9.0
Sialic acid	0.2	0	0.4

*According to Neidermeier, 1971.

B. Immunoglobulin M

Pig antibodies of macroglobulin character were first described by Kabat (1939) in his study of antipneumococcal antibodies, the molecular weight of which was estimated to be 910,000–930,000. Vaerman (1970) recently showed the existence of cross-reactivity between pig and human IgM. However, only limited data concerning structural and chemical properties of pig IgM are available. The primary cause of this limitation is that no macroglobulinemia-like disease which would produce homogenous IgM in large amounts has been discovered in pigs. Still, the restricted results obtained in the studies of pig IgM showed no significant structural differences when compared with human IgM which has been far more intensively studied.

The fact that techniques used to isolate the IgM of other animal species can be applied in a like manner to isolate IgM from pig serum (Franek, 1962; Prokesová, 1969; Porter, 1969b) confirms the physiochemical similarity of pig and other mammalian IgM. Franek (1962) reported the basic molecular characteristics of pig IgM. The sedimentation coefficient was 19.2S (extrapolated to zero concentration), intrinsic viscosity 0.11 dl/g, and molecular weight 870,000. Besides 19S IgM, faster-sedimenting IgM molecules were also found in pig serum (Franek, 1962; Prokesová, 1969). During our study of pig IgM polypeptide chains, we came to the conclusion that the methods which are successful for the preparation of IgG polypeptide chains are less effective in the case of IgM. When disulfide bonds of IgM were split using either 0.1 M β-mercaptoethanol or oxidative sulfitolysis in normal buffers, a certain amount of incompletely split molecules or aggregates arose which were not separated from μ chains on Sephadex G-100 columns equlibrated in 6 M urea containing 0.05 M formic acid. Better separation was achieved when G-200, instead of G-100, Sephadex was used. Gel filtration of reduced and alkylated IgM on G-200 Sephadex resulted in the separation of three fractions. In the first peak, incompletely split molecules composed of both μ and L chains were eluted. This fraction contained several components of different molecular size. The second peak contained μ chains slightly contaminated with molecules formed by both μ and L chains. In the third peak, L chains were eluted. Better results were attained when oxidative sulfitolysis was employed. In this instance, a lesser amount of higher molecular weight subunits was formed so that the μ-chain preparation included only traces of L-chain-containing subunits. Furthermore, the yield of L chains was about twice as high as in the case of reduction and alkylation, and both μ- and L-chain preparations were quite soluble (Prokesová, 1969).

As in other mammalian species, pig μ chains migrate more slowly in electrophoresis on acid starch gel containing 6 M urea than do γ chains, and their molecular weight, estimated by the sedimentation equilibrium technique, is 78,000 (Prokesová, 1969).

Another interesting result was obtained by immunochemical investigation of

L-chain preparations derived from pig IgM. These preparations contained polypeptide chains similar to L chains from pig IgG except that they did not carry antigenic determinants characteristic of light chains but reacted with antisera to heavy, i.e., μ, chains. The fact that this component did not represent contamination with μ chains was proved in experiments which showed that the component's electrophoretical mobility differed from that of μ chains and could not be removed by rechromatography. The origin of this component is not yet clear. The existence of this light-chain component carrying μ-chain antigenic determinants was not observed in other animal species studied and its origin remains obscure (Prokesová, 1969).

When the splitting of disulfide bonds is accomplished in either 6 M urea or another disaggregating solution, oxidative sulfitolysis gives less satisfactory results. The polypeptide chains are less soluble and their antigenic and electrophoretic properties are altered. Better results, i.e., more soluble and less altered chains, can be obtained if 0.3 M β-mercaptoethanol is employed in the disaggregating solution. But even in this case, changes in the antigenic structure of single polypeptide chains were found. This means that conformational changes occurred during the splitting of disulfide bonds in disaggregating solutions. Polypeptide chains with all their disulfide bonds broken are convenient for primary structure studies, but not for the study of immunological and physicochemical properties.

C. Immunoglobulin A

The existence of IgA in pig body fluids was definitely confirmed only recently, although it has long been assumed. A number of authors called attention to the precipitation line in the immunoelectrophoretic picture of pig serum and colostrum or milk, which was reminiscent of human IgA (Kim *et al.*, 1966; Karlsson, 1966*a,b,c*; Tormo *et al.*, 1967; Brummerstedt-Hansen, 1967; Surján, 1969) and which bound radioactively-labeled antigen in serum and colostrum from immunized animals (Rejnek *et al.*, 1966). On the basis of immunoelectrophoretic analyses of fractions obtained after separation of pig serum on DEAE cellulose, Baumstark (1968) designated one of the fractions as IgA.

A more detailed study of IgA in pigs was performed by Bourne (1969*a,b*) who isolated a protein from pig serum and milk possibly corresponding to IgA. Further characterization showed that it had several properties in common with IgA of other animal species. It migrated to the beta 2 region in electrophoresis, was present not only in serum but also in external secretions, and exhibited molecular polymorphism, having sedimentation constants of 7*S*, 11*S*, and 18*S*. In immunochemical analysis, this protein gave a reaction of partial identity with IgG and IgM which meant that it had specific determinants as well as determinants in common with immunoglobulins G and M. Further proof confirming the homology of the studied protein with IgA was given by showing antigenic differences between the protein isolated from colostrum and that isolated from serum. Double diffusion tests in agar gels showed that the precipitation line of the colostral protein formed a spur over the line of the serum protein, suggesting the presence of a secretory component characteristic of secretory IgA (Bourne, 1969*b*).

Porter (1969*b*) described the presence of a protein homologous to human IgA in pig colostrum. He isolated the protein using gel filtration and DEAE-cellulose chromatography, and showed that it was composed of molecules with sedimentation constants of 6.2*S*, 8.6*S*, and 10.8*S*. The molecules with the higher sedimentation constants (8.6 and 10.8) were the most prevalent. A similar protein was found in serum, milk, saliva, intestinal secretion, and urine, and most of the antibody activity to *E. coli* present in colostrum was carried by this fraction (Porter, 1969*a*).

Final proof of the existence of an immunoglobulin in pigs corresponding to human IgA was given by Vaerman *et al.* (1969) on the basis of cross reactivity between human and pig IgA. He tested the ability of 43 rabbit and goat antisera specific to human IgA to cross-react with serum and milk of other animal species. Pig serum and milk reacted with three of the antisera tested, and the precipitate obtained from the reaction was used for the preparation of antiserum to pig IgA.

Vaerman (1970) summarized the current understanding of pig IgA in an excellent review on IgA immunoglobulins in man and animals. He reported that the charge properties of pig IgA correspond roughly to that of human IgA. Upon DEAE-cellulose chromatography of pig serum, IgA is eluted after the main part of IgG, but before IgM. In gel filtration on Sephadex G-200, IgA is eluted between the peaks of IgM and IgG. It appears in two peaks, the first of which is significantly higher than the second and corresponds to polymeric forms, possibly dimers (9−10*S*). The second, smaller, peak corresponds to monomers. In human serum, in contrast to pig serum, most of the IgA exists in monomeric form. The double-peak distribution in gel filtration of pig serum IgA has also been described by Cerná and Rejnek (1971).

The results obtained from gel filtration experiments are in accord with those obtained from gradient ultracentrifugation where pig serum IgA was separated again into two peaks. The heavier component was present in larger amounts and sedimented faster than IgG, but more slowly than human milk 11*S* IgA. This component probably represents an IgA dimer, which differs from human 11*S* IgA by the absence of secretory component. The slowly-sedimenting component apparently had the same sedimentation velocity as IgG.

Pig serum IgA has an electrophoretic mobility of the same order as IgM, in contrast to human IgA which migrates faster than IgM. On the other hand, pig

IgA behaves like human IgA when fractionated with zinc ions. When pig serum is precipitated with zinc sulfate to a final concentration of 0.025 M, the majority of IgA remains in the supernatant fluid (Vaerman and Heremans, 1970).

The character and properties of pig IgA polypeptide chains were studied only in colostral IgA because of difficulties connected with obtaining serum IgA in suitable amounts.

III. THE IMMUNOGLOBULINS OF PIG COLOSTRUM AND MILK

Colostrum and milk are the only sources of maternal immunity for newborn piglets since no transfer of maternal antibodies occurs during intrauterine life. These sources are essential for the survival of piglets in a conventional environment where they contact infectious microorganisms against which they have no specific defense mechanisms of their own. Colostral antibodies are transferred directly to the blood circulation of the newborn during the first 24–36 hours after birth. After closure of the intestinal barrier, both colostral and milk antibodies act locally as coproantibodies in the intestinal tract, where they protect the newborn piglet against gastrointestinal infections.

Colostrum represents a very concentrated protein solution, 16.5% (Karlsson, 1966c), and, besides serum proteins, is composed of proteins specific for colostrum and milk which are locally synthetized in the mammary gland. The proteins corresponding to serum proteins originate partly from blood serum and partly from indigenous synthesis in the mammary gland itself. The protein composition of colostrum and milk varies considerably during the course of lactation. The high protein concentration present in colostrum at the time of birth decreases during three to four weeks after birth and then starts to increase again, so that the protein concentration at the end of lactation is higher than in the middle. The concentration of carbohydrates varies in a similar manner (Karlsson, 1966c).

Colostrum and milk contain especially large amounts of immunoglobulins and albumin. Immunoglobulins are present in higher concentration than found in blood serum, while albumin in any stage of lactation does not exceed the level of blood serum albumin. Colostrum and milk also contain a number of proteins in the alpha- and beta-globulin region. Immunoelectrophoretic analyses showed the presence of at least 8 protein fractions in colostrum and milk which were not detectable in blood serum. The main colostrum and milk specific proteins are beta lactoglobulin, which migrates in the prealbumin region (serum prealbumin was not detected), alpha lactalbumin, and casein. These proteins were present (like other proteins) in higher amounts in colostrum than in mature milk, but their relative concentration increases in the mature milk (Karlsson, 1966c).

Immunoglobulins represent more than one-third of all colostral proteins, but their concentration decreases more rapidly during the first 24 hours than does the concentration of other proteins. The conversion of colostrum into milk develops gradually, depending on the gradual variations in mammary gland protein secretions. It occurs sooner in pigs than, for example, in humans. According to Neuhaus (1961), colostrum converts into milk between the fourth and seventh day after birth, while Karlsson (1966c) described it as occurring between the second and third day.

Pig colostrum contains all three immunoglobulin classes (IgG, IgM, and IgA) which have been described in pigs. In contrast to many other mammalian species, the main immunoglobulin component of pig colostrum is IgG; but when compared with the IgG population present in blood serum, colostrum contains primarily fast-migrating molecules (Rejnek et al., 1966). The concentration of colostral IgG decreases after birth more rapidly than the concentration of IgM and IgA. This decrease of immunoglobulin concentration also occurs in the colostrum of other mammalian species but is not as rapid as in pigs and cows, where IgG represents the main immunoglobulin component.

A comparison of the immunoglobulin spectra of mother's and newborn's sera and colostral whey implies that colostral immunoglobulins purposefully complete the immunoglobulins in the newborn's serum. In animals which receive IgG during intrauterine development from the mother's circulation, e.g., in humans, the level of IgG in the cord serum corresponds roughly to that of maternal serum. In this case, colostrum does not represent the source of immunoglobulins for the newborn's circulation, but has a local protective effect in the intestinal tract of the newborn. Therefore, the main component of human colostrum is not IgG but IgA and IgM, which are not transferred in detectable amounts during intrauterine life.

On the other hand, in pigs, in which no immunoglobulin transfer occurs before birth and in which immunoglobulin synthesis in the fetus itself is negligible, the transfer of immunoglobulin via colostrum is quite essential. This might be the reason why pig colostrum contains predominantly IgG at the time of birth, and why the IgG concentration decreases after the intestinal barrier is closed for absorption of immunoglobulins. The decrease of IgG is followed by a relative increase of IgA and IgM, which are exactly the immunoglobulins acting in the immunologic defense of the intestinal tract (Rejnek et al., 1966).

Porter (1969b) performed a quantitative estimation of colostral immuno-globulins at the time of birth, using the single radial immunodiffusion technique, and compared the results with the amount of immunoglobulins found in pig serum. According to his results, immunoglobulins represent 49.2–75.9% of pig colostral proteins and IgG represents 65.3–89.6% of colostral immunoglobulins. The concentration of all immunoglobulin classes is higher in colostrum than in serum, but their mutual ratios are different. IgA accounts for a much higher proportion of the immunoglobulin in the colostrum than in the serum (Porter, 1969b).

The concentration of immunoglobulins present in pig milk decreases during the first week of lactation to one-fifth of its original concentration. The decrease is caused mainly by the decrease of IgG and IgM, the level of which decreases approximately 10 times, while the level of IgA decreases only 2–3 times. Thus, IgA becomes the main immunoglobulin component of pig milk after 72 hours of lactation and represents 70% of the milk immunoglobulins and 30% of the milk whey proteins (Porter and Noakes, 1969; Porter *et al.*, 1970*b*).

It has been shown that all immunoglobulin classes present in pig colostrum carry antibody activity. Rejnek *et al.* (1966) demonstrated antibodies to tetanus toxoid in colostral IgG and IgM; Porter *et al.* (1970*b*) found anti-*E. coli* antibodies in colostral IgA and IgM and incomplete antibodies in IgG. The dynamics of colostral antibodies did not correspond to that of immunoglobulins. Antibodies of IgA and IgM class decreased after the first day of lactation, while the titer of incomplete antibodies increased during the course of lactation.

In order to understand the relation between serum immunoglobulins and their colostral counterparts, attempts have been made to compare their structural and immunochemical properties. Rejnek *et al.* (1965) studied the polypeptide chains of pig serum and colostrum IgG obtained after oxidative sulfitolysis and gel filtration on Sephadex G-100 in 6 M urea containing 0.05 M formic acid. He found that the light chains of colostral IgG can be separated into two fractions. The first one (L_1), which represented the bulk of light chains, corresponded to light chains of pig serum IgG. But the second (L_2), which was eluted at a higher elution volume, was not detected in serum IgG preparation. L_2 chains had higher mobility in starch gel electrophoresis than L_1 chains, but both reacted with antisera to light chains of pig serum IgG.

Sedimentation analyses showed that the main part of pig colostral IgA behaves like human milk IgA. However, its sedimentation velocity is higher than that of pig serum IgA (Vaerman, 1970). Its sedimentation constant is $11S$ ($11S$, Bourne, 1969*a*; $11.25S$, Richardson and Kelleher, 1970; $10.6S$, Cerná and Rejnek, 1971); the molecular weight determined by sedimentation equilibrium corresponds to $420,000 \pm 15,000$ (Cerná and Rejnek, 1971). Besides the $11S$ component, other IgA molecular forms were also described in pig colostrum and milk. Bourne (1969*a*) described the presence of $18S$ and $7S$ components, and Vaerman (1970) described the presence of an $8.9S$ component.

The existence of a secretory component in pig IgA is not yet clear. Bourne (1969*b*) showed that pig colostral IgA carries determinants not present in serum IgA. The evidence of specific determinants in colostral IgA strongly supports the possibility of the existence of a secretory component in pig IgA. This opinion is further supported by the fact that pig milk IgA sediments at the same velocity as human milk IgA in which the secretory component has been found.

A differing opinion was reported by Richardson and Kelleher (1970) who deny the existence of a secretory component in pig colostral IgA. They showed that pig colostral IgA can be split into $6.5S$ subunits by reduction with 0.2 M β-mercaptoethanol, and that its resistance to reduction is much lower than that of human or rabbit colostral IgA, in which the existence of a secretory component was proven (Tomasi et al., 1965; Cebra and Robbins, 1966). These authors found no component among the subunits obtained after splitting which could possibly correspond to the secretory piece. They further claim that there are no antigenic differences between colostral IgA and serum IgA, and that the differences described by Bourne (1969b) were probably caused by the polymeric structure of colostral IgA. However, this objection is hardly acceptable as most pig serum IgA exists in dimeric form. According to them, no secretory component exists in the colostral IgA of those animals whose offspring absorb immunoglobulins through the intestinal wall after birth since the absence of the secretory component might improve the dissociation of IgA molecules and enable the transfer across the intestinal wall. This idea was supported by the finding of Porter (1969a) that only low-molecular-weight IgA was detected in the serum of suckling piglets. However, this hypothesis is contradictory to the fact that a secretory component was found in the colostral IgA of cows (Mach and Pahud, 1971; Porter, 1971), sheep, and goats (Pahud and Mach, 1970), i.e., in animals whose newborns receive maternal immunoglobulins exclusively after birth by absorption through the intestinal tract. Polypeptide chains of pig colostral IgA were studied by Cerná and Rejnek (1971). After splitting the IgA with dithiothreitol in 5 M guanidine hydrochloride, the chains were separated by gel filtration on Sephadex G-100 in 6 M urea containing 0.05 M formic acid. The molecular weight estimated by sedimentation equilibrium in 5 M guanidine hydrochloride, was 61,000 for a chains and 25,000 for light chains. The light chain preparation reacted with specific antisera to pig IgG light chains, but contained a fast-migrating component, demonstrable in starch gel electrophoresis or disc electrophoresis, which resembled the J chain described in human colostral IgA (Halpern and Koshland, 1970). Vaerman (1970) assumes that pig milk also contains an IgA subclass which corresponds to the IgA2 present in human milk, where light chains are not covalently bound to a chains. This IgA subclass has been described in men, rabbits, sheep, mice, horses, and dogs.

IV. THE TRANSFER OF IMMUNITY FROM MOTHER TO NEWBORN

A. Impermeability of Pig Placenta

During the initial period of life, all newborns derive their immunity to disease from the mother through the passive transfer of antibodies. In some mammals, the transfer takes place before birth via the placenta or yolk sac (Bangham et al., 1958; Brambell, 1966). But in other mammals, some immunity is transmitted before birth while the rest of it is transmitted after birth throughout the greater part of lactation (Halliday, 1955; Brambell, 1966). In those mammalian species whose placentae are impermeable for macromolecules, the antibodies are transferred exclusively after birth via the colostrum. The transfer from mother to fetus depends upon the type of placenta, as summarized by Hemmings and Brambell (1961), Amoroso (1961), and Sterzl and Silverstein (1967). In primates with hemochorial placentae, antibodies can pass from the maternal to the fetal circulation across the placental membranes, even though the antibodies transferred are predominantly of IgG class (Gitlin *et al.*, 1963; Du Pan *et al.*, 1959). IgM and IgA are considered incapable of transplacental passage. The very low level of IgM detectable in cord serum is of fetal origin (Schultze and Heremans, 1966). Similarly, IgA is synthetized by the fetus in such limited amounts that it can be detected in cord serum only when using highly sensitive techniques (Vyas *et al.*, 1970). Hemoendothelial and endotheliochorial pacentae (rabbit, guinea pig, rat, mouse, cat, dog) also permit the transfer of antibodies *in utero* (Sterzl and Silverstein, 1967). In rabbits, immunity is transmitted from the maternal to the fetal circulation entirely before birth, perhaps by way of the fetal yolk sac rather than the placenta (Brambell, 1966). Rabbit IgM is transmitted almost as readily as IgG, but only a small part of the protein absorbed by the fetal cells is transmitted to the fetal circulation as intact immunoglobulin; the rest is degradated in cells. Thus, the selectivity of the transport does not depend on discriminative uptake by cells, but rather on the proportion of absorbed protein which is transmitted to the circulation intact.

In both rat and mouse, some immunity is transferred before birth, but most of it is transmitted after birth throughout most of lactation (Halliday, 1955). The transfer occurring in the rat before birth is mainly by way of the yolk sac, as in the rabbit.

Five layers of syndesmochorial placenta, which separate the mother and fetus of sheep, goat, and cow, prevent the transfer of significant amounts of antibodies before birth. The protein composition of lamb serum before and after suckling of colostrum was described by Charlwood and Thomson (1948). Johnson and Pierce (1959) noted the presence of a small amount of immunoglobulin in precolostral calf serum which they considered to be synthetized by the newborn organism.

The pig and horse have six-layer epitheliochorial placentae which also do not allow any transfer of immunoglobulin molecules. The newborns can acquire maternal immunity only after birth by ingestion of maternal colostrum, and even this transmission of immunity is of very short duration.

Newborn piglets do not receive any traces of antibodies from the mother's circulation, as was shown by Sterzl *et al.* (1960*a,b*; 1966). The observation of Meyers and Segre (1963) that antibody activity could be found in concentrated sera of piglets whose mother was actively immunized was not confirmed, although the same antigens and concentration procedures were used (Sterzl *et al.*, 1966). In the sera of newborn piglets, small amounts of immunoglobulin were found (Sterzl *et al.*, 1960*a,b*; Franek *et al.*, 1961; Karlsson, 1966*c*; Sokol and Durkovic, 1967; Prokesová *et al.*, 1969; Porter, 1969*b*), but it was demonstrated that these were actively synthetized by the newborn organism (Prokesová *et al.*, 1970*a,b*; Prokesová and Rejnek, 1971).

B. Intestinal Absorption of Antibodies

The above-mentioned relationships between immunoglobulins in colostrum and serum suggest that colostrum usually contains prevalently those classes of immunoglobulins which do not cross the placenta and are not transferred to offspring during their intrauterine life. At the time of birth, piglets are almost entirely devoid of all immunoglobulins (except for very small amounts of IgG and IgA, which will be discussed later); pig colostrum, which is the only source of natural antibodies, contains all three main classes of immunoglobulins as the serum, even through the absolute amounts of single immunoglobulins are higher in colostrum (Porter, 1969*b*). This is also true of horses, cattle, and sheep, where no diaplacental transfer of maternal proteins to the fetus occurs (Rouse and Ingram, 1970; Vaerman, 1970; Vaerman, 1971). On the other hand, in animals with placentae which are permeable to macromolecules, e.g., the human, the main components of colostrum are IgA and IgM, IgA being the major immuno-globulin (Gugler and von Muralt, 1959; Rejnek *et al.*, 1960; Hanson and Johansson, 1962); these two immunoglobulins do not cross the placenta. IgG, which enters the fetal circulation via the placenta, is present in colostrum only in relatively small amounts.

Colostrum thus appears to be a source from which the newborn organism obtains all those immunoglobulin classes not received during intrauterine life. However, this assumption contradicts the fact that intestinal transfer of antibodies has never been demonstrated in man (Kuttner and Ratner, 1923; Boorman *et al.*, 1958). Similarly, Porter (1969*a*) has shown that some antibody classes are not transferred across the intestinal wall in piglets. These findings indicate the possibility that antibodies present in colostrum and milk might protect the newborn organism not only after being transferred into the circulation but also while in the intestinal tract, which is the first place of microbial invasion. This possibility is supported by experiments in which precolostral newborn piglets reared under germfree conditions were employed (Rejnek *et al.*, 1968*a,b*). This model was chosen because pigs receive no antibodies via the placenta (Sterzl *et al.*, 1966) and die if reared under conventional conditions on an antibodyfree diet (Trnka *et al.*, 1959) or if inoculated with a pathogenic strain of bacteria under germfree conditions. Another advantage of these animals is that their intestinal barrier is permeable to macromolecules only during a limited time after birth. According to Brambell (1958), Lecce and Matrone (1960), and Payne and Marsh (1962), piglets fed milk or any other heterologous proteins lose their ability to absorb antibodies from the intestinal tract during the first 48 hours after birth. Thus, it is possible to study the effect of antibodies on gastrointestinal infection in an animal with no antibodies of its own and whose capacity for antibody transfer across the intestinal tract can be artificially stopped. The control group of piglets delivered by hysterectomy and kept under germfree conditions was fed modified cow's milk for 72 hours, then infected perorally with a living *E. coli* 055 suspension in amounts of 10^9 bacterial cells. All these animals died within 24 hours after infection. Experimental animals were contaminated with the same dose as the controls, and two hours later were orally given either normal or hyperimmune colostrum or serum in various amounts. The results shown in Table III demonstrate that oral administration of 50 ml of normal pig serum or colostrum led to 50% survival of the experimental animals. Lesser amounts of the same material caused only a slight delay in the lethal effect. This was in conformity with the low titer of "natural" antibodies to *E. coli* 055 present in normal serum and colostrum. On the other hand, 100% survival was achieved when hyperimmune serum or colostrum was employed, even though a lesser amount was administered. The question of whether the experimental animals were protected by the direct action of antibodies in the intestinal tract or whether some of the antibodies passed into the circulation, even though the intestinal barrier was closed by feeding the animals modified cow's milk for 72 hours after birth, was solved by checking the antibody titer in experimental animal sera collected before and two hours after administration of serum and colostrum. The results obtained by passive hemagglutination assay show (Table III) that no antibody activity was detected in the blood stream even in piglets which received hyperimmune serum or colostrum containing high titers of antibodies.

These results indicate that the peroral administration of antibodies can protect against gastrointestinal infection even when no transfer of antibodies into the circulation can be proved. The comparison of normal and hyperimmune colostrum and serum indicates that specific antibodies are responsible for the protective effect since the effect is proportional to the antibody titer. Because no antibodies were found by passive hemagglutination in the serum of piglets which received hyperimmune serum or colostrum orally after the intestinal barrier was closed, attempts have been made to detect such antibodies using more sensitive methods. Tlaskalová *et al.* (1970c) tested a group of 72-hour-old germfree piglets which were orally administered 12.5 ml of either serum or colostrum obtained from sows immunized by formalized suspension of *E. coli* 055. Six hours later, the animals were infected intravenously with *E. coli* 055, using a dose of 5×10^8 living cells. The antibody titer was estimated before injecting the bacteria using a very sensitive bactericidal method (Sterzl *et al.,* 1964). The clearance of living bacteria from the blood stream was estimated by plating blood samples on Endo's medium (Miler *et al.,* 1968). The serum of

Table III. Effect of Orally Administered Colostrum and Serum on Survival of Germfree Piglets Contaminated Per-orally with *E. coli* 055

Groups of animals	Animal No.	Dose in ml	Protein administered	Titer of antibodies in protein administered	Titer of antibodies in piglet serum		Time of death in hours (S = survived)
					before protein administration	after protein administration	
I	1	50	Normal colostrum	1 : 32	0	0	S
	2	50	"	1 : 32	0	0	48
	3	50	"	1 : 32	0	0	S
	4	50	"	1 : 32	0	0	48
	5	50	"	1 : 32	0	0	72
	6	50	"	1 : 32	0	0	S
	7	50	"	1 : 32	0	0	S
	8	50	"	1 : 32	0	0	S
II	1	25	"	1 : 32	0	0	24
	2	25	"	1 : 32	0	0	72
	3	25	"	1 : 32	0	0	24
	4	25	"	1 : 32	0	0	24
III	1	50	Normal serum	1 : 128	0	0	S
	2	50	"	1 : 128	0	0	72
	3	50	"	1 : 64	0	0	48
	4	50	"	1 : 64	0	0	S

IV	1	25	Normal serum	1 : 64	0	0	0	72
	2	25	"	1 : 64	0	0	0	24
V	1	50	Immune colostrum	1 : 25,600	0	0	0	S
	2	25	"	1 : 25,600	0	0	0	S
	3	25	"	1 : 25,600	0	0	0	S
	4	12.5	"	1 : 25,600	0	0	0	S
	5	12.5	"	1 : 25,600	0	0	0	S
VI	1	50	Immune serum	1 : 51,200	0	0	0	S
	2	25	"	1 : 51,200	0	0	0	S
	3	12.5	"	1 : 51,200	0	0	0	S
	4	12.5	"	1 : 51,200	0	0	0	S
Controls	1	—	—	—	—	—	—	24
	2	—	—	—	—	—	—	24
	3	—	—	—	—	—	—	24
	4	—	—	—	—	—	—	24
	5	—	—	—	—	—	—	24
	6	—	—	—	—	—	—	24
	7	—	—	—	—	—	—	24
	8	—	—	—	—	—	—	24

control animals contaminated with *E. coli* 055 suspension without administration of either serum or colostrum did not contain any antibodies, even though a very sensitive bactericidal method was used for detection (Table IV). The course of clearance in controls confirmed that the *E. coli* 055 used was a typical S strain not phagocytosed in the absence of antibodies (Miler *et al.*, 1968). These animals died with signs of massive bacteriemia shortly after contamination.

Serum from experimental piglets which received specific antibodies perorally (in the form of immune serum or colostrum) contained antibodies detectable by a bactericidal method, although in very low titers. 50% of these animals survived; the survival was dependent upon the titer of antibodies present in their sera. Simiarly, the rate of clearance was well correlated with the antibody titer. In piglets which did not survive, increasing numbers of living bacteria were found in the circulating blood during the last few hours before death. In the survivors, the blood stream was free of microorganisms within 10 hours after contamination. The bactericidal reaction was the only one capable of detecting antibodies in the serum of these piglets, as passive hemagglutination did not show the presence of any antibody activity in the same samples.

It can be concluded from these results that antibodies present in colostrum and milk can pass through the intestinal wall in very small amounts in some piglets even after the closing of the intestinal barrier. However, the fact that the protective effect of orally administered antibodies was much higher in animals infected perorally than in animals infected intravenously confirms that antibodies present in colostrum and milk act directly in the intestinal tract itself.

These experiments show that germfree piglets are a satisfactory model for studying the transfer of antibodies across the intestinal barrier during the immediate postnatal period. At the time of birth, piglets have practically no immunoglobulins in their circulation, except for a very small amount of IgG and IgA (Sterzl *et al.*, 1960a,b; Prokesová *et al.*, 1969, 1970a,b; Prokesová and Rejnek, 1971). After the first ingestion of colostrum, antibodies pass through the intestine wall for only a relatively short period of time. This period differs a little, according to different authors who have studied the problem. According to Brambell (1958), the postnatal period for the passive transfer of immunity is 36 hours. Other authors, such as Barrick, Matrone, and Osborne (1954), Olsson (1959), and Lecce and Matrone (1960), showed that intestinal absorption stops completely within 48 hours. These results were also confirmed by the studies of Asplund, Grummer, and Phillips (1962) and Speer *et al.* (1959). Payne and Marsh (1962) made a detailed study of the permeation of immunoglobulins and the closure of the intestinal barrier, and found that if piglets were fed either colostrum or modified cow's milk, absorption stopped 12 hours after birth, when the epithelial cells of the intestinal mucosa filled with immunoglobulins or other soluble protein. If the animals were left to starve, however, the barrier did not close and absorption of immunoglobulin was still found 106 hours after

Table IV. Effect of Orally Administered Immune Colostrum and Serum on Survival of Germfree Piglets Contaminated Intravenously with *E.coli* 055

Group of animals	Animal No.	Protein administered	Titer of bactericidal antibodies in protein administered	Titer of bactericidal antibodies in piglet serum		Time of death in hours (S = survived)
				before protein administration	after protein administration	
I	1	Immune colostrum	10^{-12}	0	10^{-4}	S
	2	"	10^{-12}	0	1:2	14
	3	"	10^{-12}	0	10^{-1}	S
II	1	Immune serum	10^{-15}	0	0	7
	2	"	10^{-15}	0	10^{-2}	44
	3	"	10^{-15}	0	10^{-3}	S
	4	"	10^{-15}	0	1:2	10
	5	"	10^{-15}	0	10^{-2}	S
Controls	1	–	–	–	–	6
	2	–	–	–	–	8

birth. Similar results were obtained by Lecce and Morgan (1962) who studied the permeability of the intestine in neonatal pigs and lambs for polyvinylpyrrolidone, which is similar to serum proteins in its molecular weight and osmotic properties. They found that piglets fed colostrum lost the ability to absorb polyvinylpyrrolidone 24—36 hours after birth, while starving piglets did absorb polyvinylpyrrolidone even after 86 hours. The same was true for newborn lambs, which absorbed polyvinylpyrrolidone, bovine serum proteins, and ovoproteins even after 48 hours if starved. In lambs fed heterologous colostrum, the absorption stopped after 24 hours. The closure of the intestinal barrier was irreversible, since the ability to absorb proteins was not renewed if animals were left to starve after cessation of absorption.

The results of the experiments by Tlaskolová et al. (1970c), described above, show that germfree piglets intravenously contaminated with the highly virulent strain E. coli O55 died during the first 24 hours after contamination. 50% of these animals could be protected by peroral administration of immune serum or colostrum even after the intestinal barrier was closed for macromolecules. Unlike the works describing the complete cessation of immunoglobulin absorption from colostrum during the first 24—48 hours after birth, these authors have shown the passage of a small amount of antibodies through the intestinal barrier.

Porter (1969a) studied the ability of the newborn piglet intestinal tract to absorb different classes of colostral immunoglobulins and antibodies present after the initial ingestions of colostrum. He found that a considerable portion of antibodies to E. coli O141 and E. coli O8 in porcine colostrum were associated with IgA, but these IgA antibodies were not detected in sow serum, where the antibody activity was mainly connected with IgM. When studying the transfer of immunoglobulins and antibodies across the intestinal wall in newborn piglets, he demonstrated that, although IgA was absorbed from the colostrum, colostral IgA antibodies to E. coli were not transferred into the circulation as part of the passive immunity. The absorbed antibodies were associated with IgM. He suggested that the lack of absorption of colostral IgA antibodies could be due to the presence of a secretory piece in colostral IgA molecules. On the other hand, Bourne et al. (1971b), who studied natural antibodies to E. coli in pigs, found antibody activity in IgM, IgG, and IgA, and claimed that this antibody activity in all classes was transmitted to the serum of suckling piglets.

Thus, these findings merely underline the question of the function of the antibodies contained in colostrum and milk which, although they are the only source of maternal antibodies for the newborn piglet, can be transferred into the blood stream only for a limited time after birth, while some types of antibodies are possibly not transferred at all. Owen et al. (1961) studied the effect of the administration of immunoglobulins on survival and on the serum protein spectrum in colostrumfree piglets reared under conventional conditions. They found that the animals survived much better if antibodies were administered perorally, even at a time when proteins were no longer absorbed from the intestinal tract. They assumed that these antibodies acted as coproantibodies. Similarly, Salajka (1966), who studied the aethiopathogenesis of colienterotoxemia in weaned piglets, showed that the prevalence of hemolytic specific pathogenic serotypes of *E. coli* in young pigs after weaning was associated with the disappearance of immunoglobulins transferred in the maternal milk. He assumed that the growth of specific pathogenic strains in the alimentary tract of suckling pigs was inhibited by antibodies contained in the milk. Similar conclusions can be made from the above mentioned data of Rejnek *et al.* (1968*a,b*) and Tlaskalová *et al.* (1970*c*), which showed that perorally administered antibodies would protect newborn piglets from gastrointestinal infection at a time when antibodies are either not transferred into the blood circulation or are transferred in quantities so minute that they could hardly result in a pronounced protective effect. It must therefore be assumed that antibodies in colostrum and milk can protect against gastrointestinal infection directly within the intestinal tract itself.

Another problem connected with the action of antibodies in the intestinal tract is the question of the effectiveness of antibodies belonging to single immunoglobulin classes. There are not enough experimental data to show to what extent passively-acquired single antibody classes take part in the protection against gastrointestinal infection. Their significance can be discussed only on the basis of the results obtained in the studies of immunoglobulins and antibodies present in the intestinal tract of adult animals, where the antibodies are actively synthetized by the given organism.

Tomasi and Bienenstock (1968) demonstrated that a number of antibacterial and antiviral antibodies were associated with secretory IgA in human colostrum, parotid saliva, and nasal secretions; but much less is known about immunoglobulins in the alimentary tract. Berger *et al.* (1967) described the presence of specific IgA polio antibodies and IgA anti-*E. coli* antibodies in gastrointestinal secretions, often in high titers, and stated that these antibodies were distributed differently among the immunoglobulin classes found in serum. Immunofluorescent studies also have demonstrated the predominance of IgA-containing plasma cells in the lamina propria of the small intestine.

Allen and Porter (1970) studied the localization of immunoglobulin in pig intestinal tissue. They found IgG occurring as an extravascular component in the intestine and demonstrated the presence of both IgA and IgM in cryptepithelium. They proposed that these two immunoglobulins might play a complementary role as antibodies in intestinal secretions. Porter *et al.* (1970*a*), when studying intestinal secretion of immunoglobulins and antibodies in pigs, have shown the presence of all three immunoglobulin classes, although antibodies to *E. coli* were entirely associated with IgA. They also investigated the molecular size of the secreted immunoglobulins using gradient centrifugation and gel filtration, and found that intestinal IgM had characteristics of a 7S immunoglobulin. Bourne *et al.* (1971*a*) described the presence of IgG, IgA, and IgM in the small intestine, IgA being the major component. IgG and IgM were present in lesser amounts. IgA had antigenic determinants characteristic for secretory IgA.

When studying the protective effect of passively transferred antibodies into the intestinal tract of germfree piglets, Rejnek *et al.* (1968*a,b*) found that most of the antibody activity to *E. coli* O55 present in hyperimmune serum and colostrum, as determined by radioimmunoelectrophoresis with ^{51}Cr-labeled lipopolysaccharide, was associated with IgM. This means that, in this case, the protective effect was connected with antibodies of IgM class.

In summary, it seems probable that both IgA and IgM antibodies play an important role in the defense mechanism acting in the intestinal tract.

V. ANTIBODIES IN ARTIFICIALLY IMMUNIZED PIGS

Immunoelectrophoretic analysis showed that considerably more protein can be detected in the immunoglobulin region of pig serum than in the same region of human serum. In order to determine which of the precipitation lines correspond to immunoglobulins, Rejnek *et al.* (1966) immunized adult pigs and sows with tetanus toxoid and examined the binding activity of single serum protein fractions by means of radioimmunoelectrophoresis. The results obtained by this approach showed that antibody activity was present in three immunoelectrophoretically distinguishable IgG fractions, in the IgM fraction, and in another fraction which was thought to be IgA. The presence of IgA in pig serum has since been confirmed by Vaerman (1970). He assumed that in pigs as well as in other mammalian species, antibodies are carried mainly by the three basic immunoglobulin classes, IgG, IgM, and IgA, and that the antibodies of the IgG class are probably composed of several subclasses. Similarly, Matthaeus and Korn (1967) studied the neutralizing antibodies in the serum of pigs immunized with hog cholera virus. They found neutralizing activity in high-molecular-weight antibodies of the IgM class, in 7S antibodies of the IgG class, and in antibodies migrating to the γ1-globulin region. Zikán *et al.* (1970) studied pig IgG antibodies to sheep red blood cells separated into two fractions on a DEAE-Sephadex column according to charge differences. L chains separated from the IgG I and IgG II fractions showed little structural differences, while many differences were localized in the heavy chains. The two fractions had different biological activities. The slow-migrating fraction IgG I participated in hemolysis and complement fixation, while the fast-migrating fraction IgG II was not effective in these biological reactions. However, both fractions reacted similarly in hemagglutination. These results showed that pig antibodies exhibit heterogeneity of biological properties, similar to what has been found in other mammals, e.g., guinea pig, rat, and hamster, where the fast-migrating fraction IgG II fixes to the skin of the homologous species and does not fix complement, while the slow-migrating fraction IgG I of all these species fixes to the skin of heterologous species and is capable of fixing complement (Bloch *et al.*, 1963; Ovary *et al.*, 1963; Benacerraf *et al.*, 1963; Gray, 1969).

Pig antibodies, especially antibodies to haptens, have been used for the study of localization and properties of the antibody binding site. Franek *et al.* (1965) showed that antibodies to the dinitrophenyl group can be obtained in high yields from pigs. After repeated immunization by dinitrophenylated bovine IgG in adjuvant, antibodies were formed at an average concentration of 1 mg/ml. The amount of antibodies to the carrier protein was only rarely higher than 5% of the total amount of antibodies to the immunizing antigen. The yield of purified antibodies was 60–70%. Since it is advantageous to have high amounts of antibodies from a single source in order to perform immunochemical and chemical studies, the pig represents an ideal experimental animal from which 1 g of purified antibodies to the DNP group can be obtained.

The problem of localizing the binding site of an antibody molecule has been investigated by many authors (Edelman *et al.*, 1961; Porter, 1962; Franek and Nezlin, 1963; Karush and Utsumi, 1965; Metzger and Mannick, 1964). There are different opinions on the basic question concerning the functional significance of heavy and light chains of the antibody molecule which form the active site. According to some authors, either L chains or H chains were involved in antibody specificity; however, according to others, both types of chains were needed for the formation of the active site. Franek *et al.* (1965) studied this problem using heavy and light chains from porcine and bovine antibodies to dinitrophenyl groups. They followed the antibody activity in recombined molecules formed after mixing heavy and light polypeptide chains prepared either from specific anti-DNP antibodies or from nonspecific nonantibody IgG molecules. They found that free heavy and light chains obtained without mutual contamination had no significant binding activity demonstrable by equilibrium dialysis. When specific heavy chains were mixed with either specific or nonspecific light chains, the resulting molecules were active, whereas the molecules formed from nonspecific heavy chains and specific light chains were inactive. The authors considered heavy chains to be the "inactive form," which can be activated by either specific or nonspecific light chains.

Zikán and Kotýnek (1968) studied the interaction of pig anti-DNP antibodies. They isolated chains using ε-DNP-lysine and found that, in either sulfitolysed antibodies or recombined molecules (mixture of heavy and light chains), the binding heterogeneity was greatly lowered or entirely removed when compared to that of the original antibodies. At the same time, the amount of active proteins in the sample decreased by approximately one-half. But the association constant of the modified antibodies was of the same order as the average association constants of the original antibodies. They also reported that antibody heavy chains can be nonspecifically reactivated by light chains, and that the amount of hapten bound by the complex of heavy and light chains increases with the increasing excess of light chains. The limiting value of the amount of hapten bound when using antibody light chains was higher than in the case of nonspecific light chains.

Similar results were obtained with pig antibodies to tetanus toxoid and human serum albumin (Rejnek, unpublished results). In this case, the binding activity in isolated chains and recombined molecules (mixture of heavy and light chains) was followed by binding radioactively labeled antigen to the immune precipitate, i.e., using radioimmunoelectrophoresis and radioimmunodiffusion techniques. With this approach, low antibody activity was demonstrated in isolated specific heavy chains, while markedly higher activity was found in recombined molecules formed by mixing specific heavy chains with either specific or nonspecific (nonantibody) light chains. The molecules containing specific heavy chains and specific light chains showed slightly higher binding activity than those containing nonspecific light chains. In isolated light chains and in recombined molecules containing nonspecific heavy chains, no antibody activity was found.

All the above-mentioned results suggest that the demonstration of binding activity in isolated heavy chains depends on the method used to detect the activity. Therefore, Zikán and Sterzl (1967) compared the activity of single polypeptide chains and recombined molecules of single polypeptide chains and recombined molecules of anti-DNP antibodies by the use of polarography (Zikán, 1966) and passive hemagglutination. In polarographic determination, no antibody activity was found in isolated heavy chains, but after mixing these chains with light chains, the activity markedly increased. When passive hemagglutination was used, however, relatively high binding activity was detected in isolated heavy chains, but practically no increase in binding activity was demonstrated when these chains were mixed with light chains. These findings seem to support the hypothesis proposed by Singer *et al.* (1965) that both chains contribute to the antibody binding site; heavy chains determine the specificity of the binding capacity while light chains enhance the binding capacity in a relatively nonspecific manner, i.e., L chains mainly determine the proper conformation of the binding site. This can be seen from the fact that the effect of light chains on binding site formation can be substituted in the passive-hemagglutination system by the reaction of heavy chains with antigen bound to the surface of red blood cells.

A further study of the antibody binding site, utilizing pig antibodies as a model, has been made by Franek (1971) using the affinity-labeling method. Pig antidinitrophenyl antibodies were labeled by *m*-nitrobenzenediazonium fluoroborate. The amount of bound hapten was determined in isolated light and heavy chains. 10% of the light and 21% of the heavy chain molecules were labeled. The localization of labeled tyrosine was studied in isolated λ chains; it was found that the main part of the label was present on tyrosine in position 33 and a lesser part on tyrosine in position 93. The author suggested the possibility that both labeled tyrosine residues participate in the antibody binding site, as they are located in those sections of the chain where hypervariability was observed. However, he was well aware of the fact that other acceptable explanations, like nonspecific labeling of tyrosine 93, can be found.

VI. IMMUNOGLOBULINS AND ANTIBODIES IN NEWBORN PIGLETS

A. Character and Properties of Newborn Piglet Immunoglobulin

As has been shown above, no transfer of immunoglobulins and antibodies occurs in piglets during their intrauterine life. The same is true also for other serum proteins and, therefore, the serum protein spectrum at birth reflects active synthesis of serum proteins during intrauterine ontogenesis. Proteins of newborn piglet serum differ from adult serum proteins in both qualitative and quantitative aspects. The total concentration of proteins in piglet serum is relatively low, 25–30 mg/ml (Lecce and Matrone, 1960; Trávníček and Mandel, 1971), and the proteins do not form any visible precipitate with trichloracetic acid. The low concentration of serum proteins is caused mainly by the low concentration of albumin and immunoglobulins. The newborn piglet serum protein spectrum differs from that found in newborn calves, goats, and lambs. No transfer of serum proteins from the maternal to fetal circulation occurs before birth in these animals either, yet they have six times as much albumin in their sera as is found in piglets. The picture of newborn piglet serum proteins is reminiscent of that found in sheep and goat fetuses at the end of the first third of gestation (Lecce et al., 1961a).

Alpha globulins represent more than 50% of all serum proteins in newborn piglets. This fraction includes a specific fetal protein, fetuin, which has not been found in the serum of adult animals. The fetuin concentration reaches its maximum level on the 62nd day of gestation, then slowly decreases, and finally disappears approximately four weeks after birth. On the other hand, adult pig serum contains proteins which are not detectable in newborn piglet serum (Sokol et al., 1954; Lecce and Matrone, 1960; Lecce et al., 1961a,b; Karlsson, 1966b; Trávníček and Mandel, 1971).

The concentration of immunoglobulins in piglet serum is so low that a number of authors who analyzed unconcentrated piglet sera claimed that newborn precolostral piglet serum did not contain any immunoglobulins (Earle, 1935; Jacobsen and Monstgaard, 1950; Barrick et al., 1954; Rutqvist, 1958; Lecce and Matrone, 1960). However, analyses of concentrated piglet sera employing sensitive immunochemical techniques showed the presence of small amounts of immunoglobulin of the IgG class (Sterzl et al., 1960a,b; Franek et al., 1961; Karlsson, 1966c; Sokol and Durkovic, 1967; Porter, 1969b). In contrast to the above-mentioned authors, Kim *et al.* (1964, 1966) did not find any immunoglobulins, even in concentrated piglet sera. This difference might be caused by the use of different experimental animals, i.e., Minnesota miniature piglets, by these authors. In our laboratory, serum of two different species of newborn miniature piglets were examined, and in both a small amount of IgG was found (Prokesová and Rejnek, unpublished results).

Piglets, therefore, represent a good experimental model since they are free of maternal serum proteins. To avoid even a small contamination which could be caused by ingestion of maternal blood or secretions during delivery, the piglets can be obtained surgically by hysterectomy or Caesarean section performed under sterile conditions 2–3 days before term (112th day of gestation). Piglets thus obtained can be kept in isolators for germfree breeding and fed an artificial sterile diet (Trávníček *et al.*, 1966) in order to prevent microbial contamination which would otherwise cause death in piglets reared without ingestion of maternal colostrum (Trnka *et al.*, 1959).

The presence of IgG in the serum of piglets obtained by hysterectomy on the 112th day of gestation can be shown by single radial immunodiffusion in agar gel containing antibodies to adult pig γ chains. It can also be detected by double diffusion tests following repeated administration of the serum sample into the starting well, and by immunoelectrophoresis after concentration of the globulin fraction of the serum. IgG concentrations in individual piglet sera display significant differences; the average value is approximately 50 μg/ml (Prokesová *et al.*, 1969; 1970*b*; 1972). Intensive concentration of a piglet serum globulin fraction enabled us to prove that serum of newborn piglets contained not only IgG, but also IgA. The analysis was performed in double diffusion tests using specific antisera to adult pig a chains. The concentration of IgA in piglet serum is 25–50 times lower than the concentration of IgG (Prokesová and Rejnek, 1971).

Although every effort has been made, no IgM has been detected in newborn piglet serum. This fact is rather surprising since, according to results obtained in other animal species, the first immunoglobulin formed in ontogeny is IgM (Thorbecke and Van Furth, 1967). It seems improbable that pigs would differ so markedly from other animal species, and the question of the existence of IgM in newborn piglet sera deserves further investigation.

The questions of whether the trace amounts of immunoglobulins present in piglet serum are actively synthetized in the newborn organism or not has been intensively studied. The first successful experiments were performed by Sterzl *et al.* (1960*a,b*) who studied the incorporation of ^{35}S-methionine into piglet serum proteins *in vivo*. Prokesová *et al.* (1970*a,b*) and Prokesová and Rejnek (1971) used a ^{14}C protein hydrolysate for the same purpose. Piglets obtained by hysterectomy were given 2.6 mCi of ^{14}C-labeled protein hydrolysate in three doses during the first three days of extrauterine life. The incorporation of labeled material was followed by radioimmunoelectrophoresis, permitting the detection of radioactivity in single protein fractions. Radioactivity was found in all serum proteins, including IgG and IgA, which means that these two immunoglobulins, like other serum proteins, are actively synthetized in the newborn organism and probably also during its untrauterine life. The questions of immunoglobulin ontogeny in pigs are discussed in more detail elsewhere (Prokešová et al., 1973).

The existence of both IgG and IgA in piglet serum has been demonstrated on the basis of its cross-reactivity with the corresponding immunoglobulins of adult animals. Immunochemical analyses employing specific antisera to single polypeptide chains of pig immunoglobulins showed that piglet IgG carried antigenic determinants of both γ and L chains, and that piglet IgA carried determinants of a and L chains. Some experiments suggest that the antigenic structures of piglet and adult pig immunoglobulins are not completely identical, but the possible differences have not yet been properly characterized.

The study of piglet immunoglobulins comparing them with those of adult animals showed that their heterogeneity was of similar order, even though some differences were found. Radioimmunoelectrophoretic analyses of piglet sera obtained after incorporation of ^{14}C-labeled amino acids, to which nonradioactive adult pig IgG was added, demonstrated that the main part of labeled piglet IgG migrated together with the fast-migrating fraction of adult IgG; only a small part of it was found in the slow-migrating-IgG region (gamma 2). (These sera were not subjected to any concentration or fractionation procedures so that the heterogeneity of the immunoglobulins was not altered.) In concentrated preparations of piglet IgG, however, an anodically-migrating component was found which had the antigenic determinants of γ chains but not of L chains, and which was not present in adult serum or IgG preparations. Differences in charge heterogeneity between piglet and adult IgG are also apparent in DEAE-cellulose chromatography. Only 30% of piglet IgG can be eluted with the low-ionic-strength buffer which elutes the majority of the IgG present in adult serum. The rest can be obtained only if a higher-ionic-strength buffer is used. Summarizing these results, it can be concluded that for the majority of piglet IgG charge is similar to that of fast-migrating adult pig IgG.

Piglet IgA has been studied less intensively than IgG as its concentration in piglet serum is extremely low. However, it was shown by using immunochemical techniques and DEAE-cellulose chromatography that its antigenic and charge properties are characteristic for the IgA class and significantly different from those of IgG.

The most pronounced differences between piglet IgG and adult pig IgG were found in molecular size. Adult pig IgG is rather homogeneous from this point of view, all molecules being about the same molecular weight, 160,000. Franek et al. (1961) studied proteins of newborn piglet sera and described the presence of an immunoglobulin which had a sedimentation constant of 5.1S. In our laboratory, purified piglet IgG (isolated on immunoadsorbent to which antibodies to pig γ chains were bound) was subjected to gel filtration on Sephadex G-100 in tris buffer, pH 8.0, and separated into three fractions. These fractions were analyzed immunochemically and their molecular weights were determined by gel filtration and by sedimentation equilibrium analysis performed in 5 M guanidine HCl. The material in the first fraction, which represented about 40% of the analyzed IgG, migrated cathodically in immunoelectrophoresis and carried antigenic determinants of both γ and L chains. Its antigenic properties and molecular weight correspond to adult pig IgG. The second fraction contained protein which had similar electrophoretic mobility and antigenic structure, but had significantly lower molecular weight, 75,000—90,000. The molecular weight and the presence of both polypeptide-chain types suggested that the protein could represent half-molecules of IgG. The molecular weight of the material present in the third fraction was 40,000—55,000, and this fraction was composed of at least two components. One component gave a characteristic picture of L chains in immunoelectrophoresis and did not contain γ-chain antigenic determinants. The other component migrated anodically and carried only γ-chain determinants. Its migration velocity was similar to Fc fragment of pig IgG, but its exact relation to γ chains remains to be determined.

It can be concluded from the above-mentioned results that the population of piglet IgG molecules is composed of at least 4 different molecular types, but their origin and relationship to each other remain obscure. According to the experiments carried out so far, these differently sized molecules do not originate artificially during the isolation and separation procedures.

The level of immunoglobulins in the sera of precolostral piglets kept under germfree conditions increases so slowly that IgM is not detectable until the 20th day of life (Porter and Kenworthy, 1970; Trávnícek and Mandel, 1971; Porter and Hill, 1970). The long-term study of postnatal ontogeny of piglet immunoglobulins meets many difficulties since precolostral piglets kept under conventional conditions die shortly after birth and the breeding of germfree piglets in sufficient number for a long time is technically very difficult.

The absorption of colostral proteins which takes place immediately after birth in conventionally bred piglets markedly alters their blood serum protein spectrum so that the serum protein level increases rapidly during first 24 hours of life. This increase is caused mainly by absorption of a large amount of immunoglobulins, whose level reaches, in this short time period, that of maternal serum immunoglobulins or even higher (Sokol et al., 1954; Karlsson, 1966b). A similar increase can be observed in the albumin level. Specific colostral proteins, such as alpha lactalbumin, beta lactoglobulin, and casein, are also detectable in piglet sera. After closure of the intestinal barrier, the piglet serum protein level starts to decrease due to catabolism and to dilution by the increasing extracellular fluid volume of the growing organism. After a certain minimum is reached, the level of the serum proteins starts increasing again as a consequence of increased synthesis in the organism itself (Karlsson, 1966*b*).

The serum protein development in piglets after ingestion of colostrum has been studied by several authors. According to Sokol *et al.* (1954), immunoglobulins reach their highest concentration in piglet serum between the first and third day after birth. The concentration starts to decline between the third and the fifth day, and the lowest values are reached around the 30th day of life. Then, the immunoglobulin level increases slowly up to the time of weaning, when it reaches the values of adult animals.

Karlsson (1966*b*) showed the presence of an IgG precipitation line in immunoelectrophoretic analysis of nonconcentrated piglet serum 105 minutes after the first ingestion of colostrum, and IgA and IgM lines 6 hours after ingestion. On the 3rd or 4th day of life, the precipitation line of IgM becomes diffuse and remains in this state for the next two weeks. During the third week, IgM is rarely detectable in piglet sera. During the fourth week the line usually reappears, but even after 19 weeks it is still less intensive than in adult sera. The intensity of the IgG precipitation line decreases during the first five or six weeks of life, then gradually increases; but it does not reach that of adult serum IgG even after 10 weeks. Similarly, the IgA precipitation line weakens during the early period of life. During the fourth week it is scarcely visible, and it becomes more intense again only after 10 weeks.

IgM is the first immunoglobulin whose concentration increases, due to active synthesis in the newborn organism (this fact stresses the importance of macroglobulin antibodies for the developing organism). After this comes the increase in the concentration of IgA followed by that of IgG. The specific colostrum proteins disappear quickly from piglet circulation. Beta lactoglobulin, especially, is rapidly excreted, and is rarely detectable in piglet serum two days after birth. Alpha lactalbumin is usually detectable for the first six days of life, and the presence of casein can also be demonstrated in some piglets for the first six days after birth. The concentration of lipoproteins in precolostral piglet sera is very low, like that in colostrum. This means that the ingestion of colostrum does not influence lipoprotein content in piglet serum and that its level increases later in postnatal life when it is synthetized by the developing organism (Karlsson, 1966*b*).

Curtis and Bourne (1971) also studied serum-protein development in suckling piglets. They found that 24 hours after birth the concentration of IgM in serum of colostrum-fed piglets is 1.06–2.02 mg/ml, while the concentration in the mother's serum is 2.92 ± 0.18 mg/ml. After two days, IgM levels start to decrease, reaching the lowest level between the 8th and 14th day of life. Then a slow increase occurs, and in the 12th week of life, the concentration of IgM is equal to 3/5 of that of adult serum. IgA concentration increases rapidly during the first 24 hours up to the level of 2.12–8.57 mg/ml (the concentrations of IgA in maternal serum are 2.37 ± 0.20 mg/ml), then a rapid decrease takes place so that on the 19th–22nd day the concentration falls to 0.13 mg/ml. Following this, slow increase occurs. In the 12th week of life, IgA concentration is equal to 1/2 that of adult serum; in the 16th week, 3/5 of the adult concentration.

During the first 24 hours, the IgG concentration reaches a level of 18.69–39.06 mg/ml (the concentration in mother's serum, 24.33 ± 0.94 mg/ml). The minimum concentration (6.23 mg/ml) is found between the 36th and 40th day of life. By the 12th week, 1/2 the adult level of serum IgG concentration was demonstrable in piglet sera; by the 16th week, 3/4 of the adult level was demonstrable.

The rate of decrease of maternal immunoglobulins transferred via colostrum to newborn piglets depends on their catabolic half-life. According to Curtis and Bourne (1971), the half-life of pig immunoglobulins is as follows: IgM, 4.5 days; IgA, 3.5 days, and IgG, 14.2 days.

B. Early Antibodies in Newborn Piglets

The fact that newborn precolostral piglet serum contains an IgG which differs from the IgG of adult pigs raises the question of whether this immuno-globulin was synthetized as a consequence of antigenic stimulation, or whether it was synthetized spontaneously only on the basis of genetic information. No antibody activity has been found in newborn piglet immunoglobulins, although a wide spectrum of bacterial, viral, protein, and tissue antigens has been used for detection (Sterzl et al., 1960b; 1965). However, these negative results cannot be considered as proof of the existence of a nonantibody ("nonsense") immuno-globulin in the serum of newborn piglets as it is not possible to test all the antigens which might stimulate the antibody response in piglets during their intrauterine life, even if the pig fetuses are well protected by their placentae, which are impermeable for macromolecules against contacting antigens present in the maternal circulation. Furthermore, newborn piglets are immunologically competent and respond to artificial antigenic stimulation even during their intrauterine life (Sterzl et al., 1960a,b, 1965; Kim et al., 1964, 1966; Sokol, 1968; Sokol et al., 1968; Hájek et al., 1969; Sokol et al., 1970; Tlaskalová et al., 1970a,b; Porter and Kenworthy, 1970; Hájek and Mandel, 1971; Sterzl, unpub-lished results). The results showing the ability of pig fetuses and newborn precolostral piglets to respond to antigenic stimulation were reviewed by Pro-kesová et al. (1973). Likewise, it is not known whether antigens which may possibly stimulate the antibody response in the fetal organism (e.g., autoanti-gens) are immunogenic enough and present in sufficient amounts, since higher doses of antigens are needed in the early stages of ontogeny for stimulation of antibody response than are commonly used for immunization of adult individ-uals.

Attempts have been made to solve the question of the origin of newborn piglet immunoglobulins by comparing their properties with those of early antibodies formed after immunization of newborn precolostral piglets. When studying the antibody response to sheep red blood cells, the first antibodies detectable in the serum of immunized piglets are 19S IgM, even though IgM has never been found in the serum of these animals prior to immunization. Slowly sedimenting antibodies of the IgG class are present two or three days later (Prokesová et al., 1969, 1970b). However, the increase of IgG formation appeared in immunized piglet serum before the antibody activity in this immunoglobulin was detected. This fact again stresses a similar question of whether the initial rise of IgG concentration represents nonantibody immunoglobulins formed under the pressure of antigenic stimulation or whether it represents early antibodies in which the antigen-binding ability is so low that it is not detectable by commonly used techniques. Gradient-ultracentrifugation experiments suggest that the antibody activity to sheep red blood cells is also present in more slowly sedimenting fractions than those corresponding to 7S molecules (Prokesová et al., 1973).

The ontogeny of antibodies to soluble protein antigen was studied in germfree piglets which were immunized with human serum albumin (HSA) in incomplete adjuvant immediately after delivery. The level of immunoglobulins of the three basic classes (IgG, IgM, IgA), as well as the antibody activity, was followed by the radioimmunodiffusion technique (Rejnek, 1971) for 35 days after immunization. The results representing the average of the values obtained in individual animals, showed that the amount of IgG increases rapidly during the first 20 days after immunization, from the basic level of 50 μg/ml on day zero (this amount corresponds to the IgG content commonly found in sera of newborn precolostral piglets) up to the level of 2200 μg/ml found on day 20. Between the 20th and 25th day, a slight decrease occurs, followed by a moderate increase during the last 10 days. Antibody activity carried by immunoglobulins of the IgG class was first detected between the 5th and 11th day and increased during the whole period studied. The level of IgM increased during the first days after immunization, reaching its maximum on the 15th day. Then, the amount of IgM slowly decreased. The antibody activity carried by IgM appeared at approximately the same time as antibody of the IgG class. The antibody activity increased until day 15, then a slight decrease occurred which was followed by a slow increase starting on day 20. The amount of IgA increased during the whole period studied, starting with a very low concentration (1–2 μg/ml) on day zero [thus confirming the finding of Prokesová and Rejnek (1971) that the sera of newborn precolostral piglets contain this immunoglobulin]. The antigen-binding activity of IgA was very low and did not reach a significant level before the end of the period.

The properties of the early anti-HSA antibodies were studied in the sera of immunized animals bled on the 11th day after immunization. The antibodies were isolated by passing the serum through a column of Sephadex immuno-adsorbent with bound HSA. The absorbed antibodies were eluted with glycine-HCl buffers. This preparation contained antibodies of all three immunoglobulin classes, but the amount of IgM and IgA antibodies was so low that only IgG antibodies were followed in further experiments. The antibody preparation was subjected to gel filtration on Sephadex G-200 and separated into four fractions which differed in their sedimentation properties. It was shown that all four fractions contained antibodies belonging, according to their antigenic specificity, to the IgG class, but having different sedimentation constants, varying from 7S to 2.5S. This molecular heterogeneity of piglet IgG antibodies resembled that found in the IgG of nonimmunized newborn precolostral piglets and differed significantly from that found in adult anti-HSA antibodies, where the molecular size heterogeneity was more restricted. This finding supports the idea that the small amount of IgG which is synthetized in the newborn precolostral piglet organism is of antibody origin.

REFERENCES

Allen, W. D., and Porter, P. (1970). *Immunology* 18: 799.
Amoroso, E. C. (1961). *Brit. Med. Bull.* 17: 81.
Asplund, J. M., Grummer, R. H., and Phillips, P. H. (1962). *J. Animal Sci.* 21: 412.
Bangham, D. R., Ingram, P. L., Roy, J. H. B., Shillam, K. W. G., and Terry, R. J. (1958). *Proc. Roy. Soc. (London) Ser. B.* 149: 184.
Barrick, E. R., Matrone, G., and Osborne, J. C. (1954). *Proc. Soc. Exp. Biol. Med.* 87: 92.
Baumstark, J. S. (1968). *Arch. Biochem. Biophys.* 125: 837.
Benacerraf, B., Ovary, Z., Bloch, K. J., and Franklin, E. C. (1963). *J. Exp. Med.* 117: 937.
Berger, R., Ainbender, E., Hodes, H. L., Zepp, H. D., and Hevizy, M. M. (1967). *Nature* 214: 420.
Bloch, K. J., Kourilsky, F. M., Ovary, Z., and Benacerraf, B. (1963). *J. Exp. Med.* 117: 965.
Boorman, K. E., Dodd, B. E., and Gunther, M. (1958). *Arch. Diseases Childhood* 33: 24.
Bourne, F. J. (1969a). *Biochim. Biophys. Acta* 181: 485.
Bourne, F. J. (1969b). *Biochem. Biophys. Res. Commun.* 36: 138.
Bourne, F. J., Pickup, J. and Honour, J. W. (1971a). *Biochim. Biophys. Acta* 229: 18.
Bourne, F. J., Honour, J. W., and Pickup, J. (1971b). *Immunology* 20: 433.
Brambell, F. W. R. (1958). *Biol. Rev. Cambridge Phil. Soc.* 33: 488.
Brambell, F. W. R. (1966). *Lancet* 2: 1087.
Brambell, F. W. R., Hemmings, W. A., and Henderson, M. (1951). *Antibodies and Embryos*, Athlone Press, London.
Brummerstedt-Hansen, E. (1961). *Acta Vet. Scand.* 2: 254.
Brummerstedt-Hansen, E. (1967). In *The Serum Proteins of the Pig. An Immunoelectrophoretic Study*, Munksgaard Publ. Co., Copenhagen, p. 85.
Brummerstedt-Hansen, E., and Hirschfeld, J. (1961). *Acta Vet. Scand.* 7: 317.
Cebra, J. J., and Robbins, J. B. (1966). *J. Immunol.* 97: 12.
Cerná, J., and Rejnek, J. (1971). *Folia Microbiol. (Prague)* 16: 535.
Charlwood, P. A., and Thomson, A. (1948). *Nature* 161: 59.
Colacicco, G. (1963). *Nature* 198: 784.
Curtis, J., and Bourne, F. J. (1971). *Biochim. Biophys. Acta* 236: 319.
Du Pan, R. M., Wenger, P., Koechli, S., Scheidegger, J. J., and Roux, J. (1959). *Clin. Chim. Acta* 4: 110.
Earle, J. P. (1935). *J. Agr. Res.* 51: 479.

Edelman, G. M., Benacerraf, B., Ovary, Z., and Poulik, M. D. (1961). *Proc. Natl. Acad. Sci. U.S.* **47**: 1751.

Eriksson, S., and Sjöquist, J. (1960). *Biochim. Biophys. Acta* **45**: 290.

Franek, F. (1961). *Biochem. Biophys. Res. Commun.* **4**: 28.

Franek, F. (1962). *Collection Czech. Chem. Commun.* **27**: 2808.

Franek, F. (1965). *Collection Czech. Chem. Commun.* **30**: 1947.

Franek, F. (1966). *Collection Czech. Chem. Commun.* **31**: 1142.

Franek, F. (1971). *European J. Biochem.* **19**: 176.

Franek, F., and Keil, B. (1964). *Collection Czech. Chem. Commun.* **29**: 847.

Franek, F., and Lankas, V. (1963). *Collection Czech. Chem. Commun.* **28**: 245.

Franek, F., and Nezlin, R. S. (1963). *Biochimija* **28**: 193.

Franek, F., and Ríha, I., (1964). *Immunochemistry* **1**: 49.

Franek, F., and Zikán, J. (1964). *Collection Czech. Chem. Commun.* **29**: 1401.

Franek, F., and Zorina, O. M. (1967). Collection Czech. Chem. Commun. **32**: 3229.

Franek, F., Ríha, I., and Sterzl, J. (1961). *Nature* **189**: 1020.

Franek, F., Simek, L., and Kotýnek, O. (1965). *Folia Microbiol. (Prague)* **10**: 335.

Franek, F., Keil, B., Novotný, J., and Sorm, F. (1968). *European J. Biochem.* **3**: 422.

Franek, F., Keil, B., and Sorm, F. (1969). *European J. Biochem.* **11**: 170.

Gitlin, D., Kumate, J., Urrusti, J., and Morales, C. (1963). *J. Pediat.* **63**: 871.

Grey, H. M. (1969). *Advan. Immunol.* **10**: 51.

Gugler, E., and Muralt, G. von (1959). *Schweiz. Med. Wochschr.* **89**: 925.

Hájek, P., Kovárů, F., and Kruml, J. (1969). *Folia Microbiol. (Prague)* **14**: 492.

Hájek, P., and Mandel, L. (1971). *Folia Microbiol. (Prague)* **16**: 58.

Halliday, R. (1955). *Proc. Roy. Soc. (London) Ser. B* **143**: 408.

Halpern, M. S., and Koshland, M. E. (1970). *Federation Proc.* **29**: 2228.

Hanson, L. A., and Johansson, B. G. (1962). *Intern. Arch. Allergy Appl. Immunol.* **20**: 65-79.

Hemmings, W. A., and Brambell, F. W. R. (1961). *Brit. Med. Bull.* **17**: 96.

Hood, L., Gray, W. R., Sanders, B. G., and Dreyer, W. J. (1967). *Cold Spring Harbor Sym. Quant. Biol.* **32**: 133.

Jacobsen, P. E., and Monstgaard, J. (1950). *Nord. Veterinarmed.* **2**: 812.

Johnson, P., and Pierce, A. E. (1959). *J. Hyg.* **57**: 309.

Kabat, E. A. (1939). *J. Exp. Med.* **69**: 103.

Karlsson, B. W. (1966*a*). *Acta Pathol. Microbiol. Scand.* **67**: 83.

Karlsson, B. W. (1966*b*). *Acta Pathol. Microbiol. Scand.* **67**: 237.

Karlsson, B. W. (1966*c*). Ph.D. thesis, *Studentlitteratur,* Lund, Sweden.

Karush, F., and Utsumi, S. (1965). In *Molecular and Cellular Basis of Antibody Formation, Proc. of a Symp.,* Publ. House Czech. Acad. Sci., Prague, p. 145.

Kim, Y. B., Bradley, S. G., and Watson, D. W. (1964). *Federation Proc.* **23**: 346.

Kim, Y. B., Bradley, S. G., and Watson, D. W. (1966). *J. Immunol.* **97**: 52.

Kuttner, A., and Ratner, B. (1923). *Am. J. Diseases Children* **25**: 413.

Lecce, J. G., and Matrone, G. (1960). *J. Nutr.* **70**: 13.

Lecce, J. G., and Morgan, D. O. (1962). *J. Nutr.* **78**: *263.*

Lecce, J. G., Matrone, G., and Morgan, D. O. (1961*a*). *Ann. N.Y. Acad. Sci.* **94**: 250.

Lecce, J. G., Matrone, G., and Morgan, D. O. (1961*b*). *J. Nutr.* **73**: 158.

Mach, J. P., and Pahud, J. J. (1971). *J. Immunol.* **106**: 552.

Mage, R. G., Young, G. O., Rejnek, J., Reisfeld, R. A., Dubiski, S., and Apella, E. (1970). *Protides Biol. Fluids, Proc. Colloq. 17 (1969),* p. 215.

Matthaeus, W., Korn, G. (1967). *Zentr. Bakt. Paras. Inf. Hygiene* **204**: 173.

Metzger, H., and Mannik, M. (1964). *J. Exp. Med.* **120**: 765.

Metzger, J. J., and Fougereau, M. (1967). *C. R. Acad. Sci. Paris* **265**: 724.

Miler, I., Tlaskalová, H., Mandel, L., and Trávnícek, J. (1968). *Folia Microbiol. (Prague)* **13**: 472.

Myers, W. L., and Segre, D. (1963). *J. Immunol.* **91**: 697.

Neuhaus, U. (1961). *Tierzucht, Züchtungsbiologie* **75**: 160.

Niedermeier, W., Kirkland, T., Acton, R. T., and Bennett, J. C. (1971). *Biochim. Biophys. Acta* **237**: 442.

Novotný, J., and Franek, F. (1968). *FEBS Letters* 2: 93.
Novotný, J., and Franek, F. (1970). *FEBS Letters* 9: 33.
Novotný, J., Franek, F., Keil, B., and Sorm, F. (1969). *FEBS Symp.* 15: 193.
Novotný, J., Franek, F., and Sorm, F. (1970). *European J. Biochem.* 14: 309.
Olsson, B. (1959). *Nord. Veterinarmed.* 11: 1.
Ovary, Z., Benacerraf, B., and Bloch, K. J. (1963). *J. Exp. Med.* 117: 951.
Owen, B. D., Bell, J. M., Williams, C. M., and Oakes, R. G. (1961). *Can. J. Animal Sci.* 41: 236.
Pahud, J. J., and Mach, J. P. (1970). *Immunochemistry* 7: 676.
Payne, L. C., and Marsh, C. L. (1962). *J. Nutr.* 76: 151.
Porter, P. (1969a). *Immunology* 17: 617.
Porter, P. (1969b). *Biochim. Biophys. Acta* 181: 381.
Porter, P. (1971). *Biochim. Biophys. Acta* 236: 664.
Porter, P., and Hill, I. R. (1970). *Immunology* 18: 565.
Porter, P., and Kenworthy, R. (1970). *J. Comp. Pathol. Therap.* 80: 233.
Porter, P., and Noakes, D. E. (1969). *Biochem. J.* 113: 68.
Porter, P., Noakes, D. E., and Allen, W. D. (1970a). *Immunology* 18: 909.
Porter, P., Noakes, D. E., and Allen, W. D. (1970b). *Immunology* 18: 245.
Porter, R. R. (1962). In Gelborn, A., and Hirshberg E. (eds.), *Symposium on Basic Problems of Neoplastic Disease* Columbia University Press, New York, p. 177.
Prokesová, L. (1969). *Folia Microbiol. (Prague)* 14: 82.
Prokesová, L., and Rejnek, J. (1971). *Folia Microbiol. (Prague)* 16: 476.
Prokesová, L., Rejnek, J., Sterzl, J., and Trávnícek, J. (1969). *Folia Microbiol. (Prague)* 14: 372.
Prokesová, L., Rejnek, J., Kostka, J., and Trávnícek, J. (1970a). *Folia Microbiol. (Prague)* 15: 337.
Prokesová, L., Rejnek, J., Sterzl, J., and Trávnícek, J. (1970b). In Sterzl, J., and Riha, M. (eds.), *Developmental Aspects of Antibody Formation and Structure* Academic Press, New York, p. 757.
Prokesová, L., Rejnek. J., and Sterzl, J. (1973). In *Research in Immunochemistry and Immunobiology,* University Park Press, Baltimore, Maryland (in press).
Putnam, F. W., Easley, C. W., and Lynn, L. T. (1962). *Biochim. Biophys. Acta* 58: 279.
Rejnek, J. (1971). In Ambrosius, H., Malberg, K., and Schäffner, H. (eds.), *Antigen–Antibody Reactions. Contributions to the IVth Symp. on Immunology of the Gesellschaft für Allergie und Immunitätsforschung der DDR* VEB Gustav Fischer Verlag Jena, p. 69.
Rejnek, J., Skvaril, F., and Dolezal, A. (1960). *Cesk. Pediatrie* 15: 97.
Rejnek, J., Kotýnek, O., and Kostka, J. (1965). *Folia Microbiol. (Prague)* 10: 327.
Rejnek, J., Kostka, J., and Trávnícek, J. (1966). *Folia Microbiol. (Prague)* 11: 173.
Rejnek, J., Kotýnek, O., and Kostka J. (1967). *Folia Microbiol. (Prague)* 12: 31.
Rejnek, J., Trávnícek, J., Kostka, J., Sterzl, J., and Lanc, A. (1968a). *Folia Microbiol. (Prague)* 13: 36.
Rejnek, J., Trávnícek, J., Lanc, A., and Tlaskalová, H. (1968b). *Wiss. Z. Friedrich-Schiller-Univ. Jena, Math. Naturwiss. Reihe* 17: 149.
Richardson, A. K., Kelleher, P. C. (1970). *Biochim. Biophys. Acta* 214: 117.
Rouse, B. T., and Ingram, D. G. (1970). *Immunology* 19: 901.
Rutqvist, L. (1958). *Am. J. Vet. Res.* 19: 25.
Salajka, E. (1966). *Vet. Med.* 11: 537.
Schultze, H. E., and Heremans, J. F. (1966). In *Molecular Biology of Human Proteins with Special Reference to Plasma Proteins, Vol. I,* Elsevier Publ. Co., Amsterdam, p. 529.
Singer, S. J., Wofsy, L., and Good, A. H. (1965). In *Molecular and Cellular Basis of Antibody Formation. Proc. of a Symp.,* Publ. House Czech. Acad. Sci., Prague p. 135.
Sokol, A. (1968). *Folia Microbiol. (Prague)* 13: 561.
Sokol, A., Rosocha, J., and Milár, A. (1954). *Vet. Casopis* 4: 139.
Sokol, A., and Durkovic, V. (1967). *Folia Microbiol. (Prague)* 12: 411.
Sokol, A., Koppel, Z., Hrusovský, F., and Eisingerová, M. (1968). *Folia Microbiol. (Prague)* 13: 561.

Sokol, A., Jamrichová, O., and Hrusovský, F. (1970). *Folia Microbiol. (Prague)* 15: 233.
Speer, V. C., Brown, H., Quinn, L., and Catron, D. (1959). *J. Immunol.* 83: 632.
Sterzl, J., and Silverstein, A. M. (1967). *Advan. Immunol.* 6: 337.
Sterzl, J., Kostka, J., Ríha, I., and Mandel, L. (1960*a*). *Folia Microbiol. (Prague)* 5: 29.
Sterzl, J., Kostka, J., Mandel, L., Ríha, I., and Holub, M. (1960*b*). In *Mechanism of Antibody Formation, Proc. of a Symp.*, Publ. House Czech. Acad. Sci., Prague p. 130.
Sterzl J., Pesák, V., Kostka, J., and Jílek, M. (1964). *Folia Microbiol. (Prague)* 9: 284.
Sterzl. J., Mandel, L., Miler. I., and Ríha, I. (1965). In *Molecular and Cellular Basis of Antibody Formation, Proc. of a Symp.*, Publ. House Czech. Acad. Sci., Prague, p. 351.
Sterzl, J., Rejnek, J., and Trávnícek, J. (1966). *Folia Microbiol. (Prague)* 11: 7.
Surján, J. (1969). *Acta Microbiol. Acad. Sci. Hung.* 16: 107.
Thorbecke, G. J., and Van Furth, R. (1967). In *Ontogeny of Immunity*, University of Florida Press, Gainesville, Florida, p. 173.
Tlaskalová, H., Kamarýtová, V., Mandel, L., Prokesová, L., Kruml, J., Lanc, A., and Miler, I. (1970*a*). *Folia Biol. (Prague)* 16: 177.
Tlaskalová, H., Sterzl, J., Hájek, P., Pospísil, M., Ríha, I., Marvanová, H., Kamarýtová, V., Mandel, L., Kruml, J., and Kovárů, F. (1970*b*). In Sterzl, J., and Ríha, M. (eds.), *Developmental Aspects of Antibody Formation and Structure, Vol. II*, Academic Press, New York, p. 767.
Tlaskalová, H., Rejnek, J., Trávnícek, J., and Lanc, A. (1970*c*). *Folia Microbiol. (Prague)* 15: 372.
Tomasi, T. B. Jr., Tan, E. M., Solomon, A., and Prendergast, R. A. (1965). *J. Exp. Med.* 121: 101.
Tomasi, T. B. Jr., and Bienenstock, J. (1968). *Advan. Immunol.* 9: 2.
Tormo, J., Chordi, A., Rodriguez-Burgos, A., and Diaz, R. (1967). *Vet. Rec.* 81: 392.
Trávnícek, J., Mandel, L., Lanc, A., and Růzicka, R. (1966). *Cesk. Fysiologie* 15: 240.
Trávnícek, J., and Mandel L. (1971). *Folia Microbiol. (Prague)* 16: 92.
Trnka, Z., Sterzl, J., Lanc, A. and Mandel, L. (1959). *Giorn. Malatie Infektive Parasitarie, II.* Fasc. p. 330.
Vaerman, J. P. (1970). In *Studies on IgA Immunoglobulins in Man and Animals*, Sintal-Louvain,
Vaerman, J. P. (1971). *Immunology* 21: 443.
Vaerman, J. P., and Heremans, J. F. (1970). *Int. Arch. Allergy Appl. Immunol.* 38: 561.
Vaerman, J. P., Heremans, J. F., and Van Kerckhoven, G. (1969). *J. Immunol.* 103: 1421.
Vyas, G. N., Levin, A. S., Fudenberg, H. H. (1970). *Nature* 225: 275.
Wellmann, G., and Engel, H. (1963). *Zentr. Bakteriol. Parasitenk.* 190: 243.
Yamashita, T., Franek, F., Skvaril, F., and Simek, L. (1968). *European J. Biochem.* 6: 34.
Zikán, J. (1966). *Collection Czech. Chem. Commun.* 31: 4260.
Zikán, J., and Sterzl, J. (1967). *Nature* 214: 1225.
Zikán, J., and Kotýnek, O. (1968). *Biopolymers* 6: 681.
Zikán, J., Blazek, J., and Cerná, J. (1970). In Sterzl, J., and Ríha, M. (eds.), *Developmental Aspects of Antibody Formation and Structure*, Academic Press, New York, p. 411.

Chapter 7

Activation of the Complement System

Neil R. Cooper*

Department of Experimental Pathology
Scripps Clinic and Research Foundation
La Jolla, California

I. INTRODUCTION

The complement system is a mediator of a number of biologically important reactions which range from cytotoxicity of antibody-sensitized cells, bacteria, and viruses to mediation of inflammatory processes. The components of the system are a number of normal serum proteins which are present in the circulation as functionally inactive precursor molecules. Activation is the term applied to the process which enables these proteins to participate in a complement reaction. Activation is not a single event, rather it is a dynamic process, as each component must be activated under appropriate conditions in a certain sequence in order to sustain an ongoing complement reaction.

Most of the biologically significant activities of the complement system occur during activation of the third through ninth components (C3–C9)†. As a result of activation, C3 and C5 are cleaved and a fragment having the ability to mediate histamine release and to induce migration of leukocytes is released from each component; reactive sites which have the ability to trigger other reactions such as phagocytosis are simultaneously generated on the major fragments. Cytolytic potential is a property of the activated fifth through ninth components. Recently it has become clear that there are several mechanisms of

* Recipient of United States Public Health Service Research Career Development Award No. 5-K4-AI-33,630-02.
† Terminology conforms to the recommendations of the World Health Organization Committee on Complement Nomenclature (*Bull. World Health Organ.* 39: 939, 1968). Terminology employed for the proteins of the alternate pathway is as in Müller-Eberhard and Götze, 1972.

activation of the late-reacting complement components (Fig. 1). Two of these mechanisms, termed the classical and alternate pathways, consist of several interacting serum proteins. Individual components, such as C3 and C5, and also the entire late-reacting portion of the sequence may be activated by noncomplement enzymes. It is the purpose of this chapter to discuss the various mechanisms of activation of the complement components and to consider how these processes enable the physiochemically-distinct complement proteins to become members of a functionally meaningful system.

II. MECHANISM OF ACTION OF COMPLEMENT

Before proceeding to a consideration of complement activation, an overview of the reaction mechanism and biological implications of the activation process is in order. There are several pathways which lead to activation of the biologically significant terminal portion of the complement sequence (Fig. 1). The classical activation pathway consists of C1, C4, and C2 (reviewed in Müller-Eberhard, 1969; Cooper et al., 1971), while the alternate pathway of complement initiation includes an unknown number of proteins of which three [C3 proactivator convertase (C3PAse), activated hydrazine sensitive factor (HSFa) and C3 proactivator (C3PA)], have been identified (Götze and Müller-Eberhard, 1971; Müller-Eberhard and Götze, 1972). The individual components of each of these pathways are activated by a series of enzyme—substrate and protein—protein interactions. The later components may also be directly activated by the noncomplement enzymes trypsin and plasmin (Arroyave, 1972).

The classical pathway is initiated on conversion of the first component into an active enzyme, $C\bar{1}$ (Lepow et al., 1956; Becker, 1956). This newly formed enzyme in turn cleaves C4 and C2 and mediates the union of the larger fragment of each molecule into a new complement enzyme, $C\overline{4,2}$, or C3 convertase (Müller-Eberhard et al., 1967). C3 convertase has the ability to activate C3 and participate in the formation of yet another enzyme, $C\overline{4,2,3}$, which has C5 as its substrate (Cochrane and Müller-Eberhard, 1968; Cooper and Müller-Eberhard, 1970; Shin et al., 1971).

Only a minor proportion of the molecules of the components entering into these enzymatic reactions become bound to acceptor molecules or to membranes. The vast majority accumulate as inactive conversion products after being turned over by the various complement enzymes. Since these products of the activation process do not register in hemolytic measurements of the components, activation of the complement system in serum may be detected by showing a quantitative loss of hemolytic activity of the various components. Activation at the C1 step is characterized by reduced levels of hemolytically active C2 and C4, C3, and C5 due to the action of $C\bar{1}$, $C\overline{4,2}$, and $C\overline{4,2,3}$, respectively, as shown in Fig. 2. In this study, activated $C\bar{1}$ was added to a sample of serum and the levels of the individual components remaining after 1 hour at 37°C were determined.

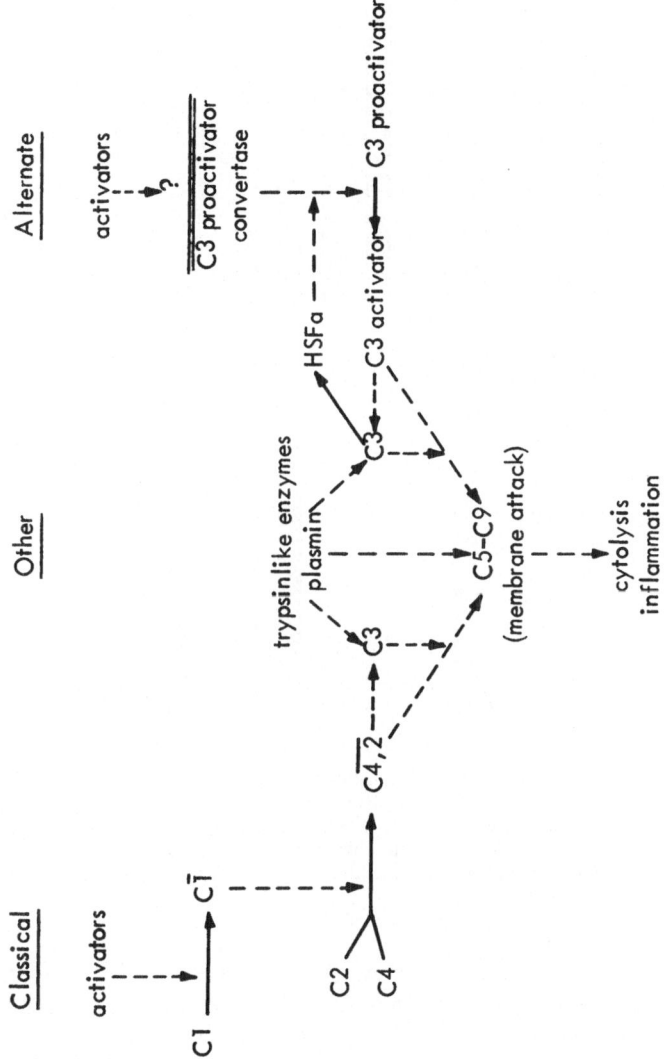

Figure 1. Mechanisms of activation of the complement system.

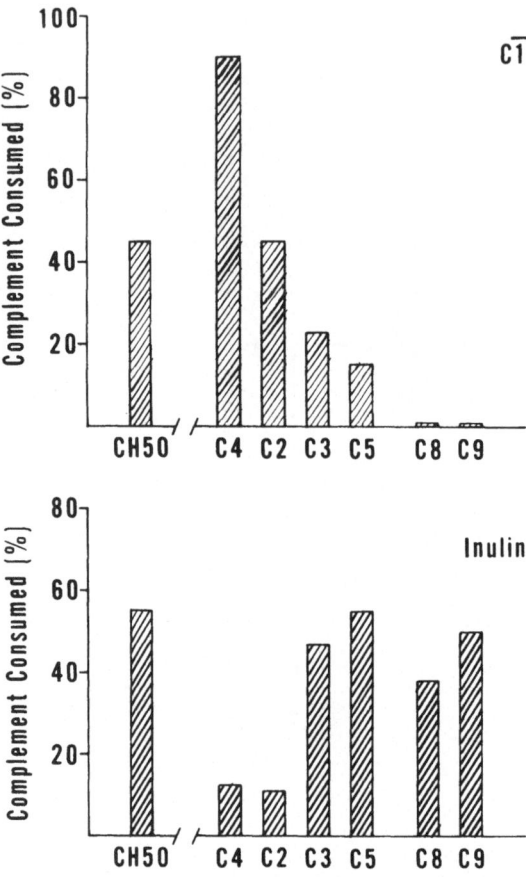

Figure 2. Pattern of loss of complement-component hemolytic activity on addition of C1̄ or inulin to serum. 1×10^{13} effective molecules of C1̄ or 20 mg of inulin were added to 1 ml of serum. After 1 hour at 37°C, the levels of the complement components were determined from the results of quantitative hemolytic titrations.

Activation of the alternate pathway is characterized by formation of a protein, HSFa, which enables the enzyme C3PAse to act on C3PA and mediate its activation (Müller-Eberhard and Götze, 1972). Intermediate steps, which have not yet been defined, are involved in generation of HSFa and perhaps C3PAse. Activated C3 proactivator is an enzyme which cleaves and activates C3, its natural substrate (Götze and Müller-Eberhard, 1971). In this process one must assume that a new enzyme composed of C3PA and C3 is formed, for C5 and later components are activated on triggering of the alternate pathway at the level of C3 proactivator (Gewurz *et al.,* 1968; Sandberg *et al.,* 1970; Frank *et al.,* 1971). Quantitative hemolytic titrations reveal a reduction in hemolytic activity of the components beginning with C3 on activation by inulin of the alternate pathway in serum as shown in Fig. 2. Little C4 and C2 is consumed under these conditions.

The terminal components C5–C9 are described as a functional unit, termed the attack system of complement (Müller-Eberhard, 1969; Kolb *et al.,* 1972), since it is this portion of the complement reaction which effects membrane damage and cytolytic phenomena. Following activation of C5, which is normally produced by enzymatic means, C5 is able to interact with C6 and C7, a process which is undoubtedly characterized by formation of a complex of C5 with C6 and C7 (Nilsson and Müller-Eberhard, 1967; Lachmann and Thompson, 1970; Arroyave, 1972). Next, C8 and, finally, C9 react. Experimental data suggest that C8 reacts with the C5,6,7 complex and C9 reacts with C8 (Kolb *et al.,* 1972; Haxby and Kolb, 1972). Although membrane alterations are apparent following the reaction of C5, these are nonlytic lesions and efficient cytolysis requires the participation of all of the terminal components (Polley *et al.,* 1971). The mechanism by which C5–C9 produce membrane damage is unknown. Among the possibilities is enzymatic attack, however, attempts to demonstrate such processes have been equivocal (Smith and Becker, 1968; Inoue and Kinsky, 1970). It is also considered quite possible that the lytic event is secondary to hydrophobic interactions of the components of the attack mechanism with membranes in analogy to the mode of action of the polyene antibiotics (Kinsky *et al.,* 1967).

The cytolytic potential of the complement system for antibody-coated cells has been known since the early years of this century. Appreciation of the broader biological significance is relatively recent. In particular, knowledge of the inflammation-producing properties of the complement system has come only with the ability to study the isolated complement components. Several types of biological phenomena are mediated by complement. Particularly important are the low-molecular-weight split products of C3 and C5, C3a and C5a, respectively, which induce histamine release and thereby cause smooth muscle contraction and enhanced vascular permeability (Jensen, 1967; Dias da Silva *et al.,* 1967; Cochrane and Müller-Eberhard, 1968). These same factors are chemotactic and thus stimulate the migration of leukocytes into an area of complement activation (Bokisch *et al.,* 1969; Shin *et al.,* 1968; Ward and Newman, 1969). In addition, during complement activation new sites are uncovered or generated on the surface of some of the complement components which facilitate interactions with other effector cells such as phagocytic cells and lymphocytes (Bianco *et al.,* 1970; Cooper, 1972c). It is apparent from this brief summary that activation of the complement system is a prerequisite for biological action.

III. MECHANISMS OF COMPLEMENT COMPONENT ACTIVATION

A. Binding Reactions and Allosteric Interactions

Activation of C1 follows attachment to various substances which include a number of polyanions and certain lymphocyte and viral membranes (Cooper, 1972b) (Table I). There is no evidence that the anionic substances provide specific receptors for C1, rather it is probable that they interact by ionic means with C1q, which is an extremely basic protein. Activation of C1 following binding of the C1q subunit results, in all likelihood, from conformational changes within the C1 molecule induced by the binding reaction.

Certain of the complement proteins exhibit weak attractions for each other which may be demonstrated in sucrose gradient ultracentrifugation analyses of the proteins; thus, monomeric immunoglobulins bind $C\overline{1}$ (Augener et al., 1971), C5 interacts with C6 and C7 (Nilsson and Müller-Eberhard, 1967; Arroyave, 1972), and C8 complexes with C9 (Haxby and Kolb, 1972). These interactions, although readily demonstrable, are quite weak and do not lead to activation of the components unless the activating agent itself has first been activated or

Table I. Mechanisms of Complement Component Activation

Activation by Complex Formation

General formulation:	acceptor + component $\longrightarrow$ activated acceptor–component complex
Nonspecific acceptors:	DNA, polyinosinic acid, certain lymphocyte and viral membranes
Component activated:	C1
Specific acceptors:	Immunoglobulin, C5
Components activated:	C1, C6, C7, C8, C9

Activation by Enzymatic Mechanisms

	enzyme
General formulation:	component $\xrightarrow{\hspace{1cm}}$ activated component
Intrinsic activating enzymes:	$C\overline{1r}$, $C\overline{1s}$, $C\overline{4,2}$, $C\overline{4,2,3}$, C3PAse
Extrinsic activating enzymes:	Trypsin, thrombin, plasmin, lysosomal enzymes, bacterial enzymes, tissue proteases, Nurse shark serum factor, Agkistrodon, and other snake venoms
Components activated:	C1s, C2, C3, C4, C5, C3PA, HSF

Activation by Unknown Mechanisms

Activators:	C-reactive protein C-polysaccharide complex, lipid A of lipopolysaccharide

undergone some physiochemical change. Under these conditions a much stronger complex results. Thus, efficient activation of C1 requires a change in immunoglobulin molecules such as occurs on aggregation or binding to antigen, and firm, functionally significant, complexing of C6 to C5 occurs only when the C5 has been previously activated.

Following binding to the various activators, reactive sites are generated or uncovered in the component molecules which permit the activated components to interact with and activate the next component in the reaction sequence. These sites, presumably formed by conformational processes, may be specific acceptors for the next component in the sequence. For example, activated C5, C6 and C7 provide binding sites for C8 (Kolb et al., 1972). Alternatively, the newly formed sites may be enzymatically active, as in the case of $C\overline{1}s$ activity which follows binding of C1 to immunoglobulin.

B. Enzymatic Processes

Enzymatic processes are important in the activation of most of the early-reacting components of the classical, and insofar as investigated, the alternate pathway (Table I). Activation may be induced by intrinsic complement enzymes which are formed from inactive precursor molecules by allosteric modifications following binding (see above) or the action of other complement enzymes. Thus, $C\overline{1}r$ activates C1s (Naff and Ratnoff, 1968), $C\overline{1}s$ activates C4 and C2 (Müller-Eberhard et al., 1967; Haines and Lepow, 1964; Budzko and Müller-Eberhard, 1970; Polley and Müller-Eberhard, 1968), $C\overline{4,2}$ activates C3 (Cochrane and Müller-Eberhard, 1968; Müller-Eberhard, 1969; Shin and Mayer, 1968), $C\overline{4,2,3}$ activates C5 (Shin et al., 1971; Cochrane and Müller-Eberhard, 1968), and C3PAse activates C3PA (Müller-Eberhard and Götze, 1972). Many of these components may also be activated by extrinsic or noncomplement enzymes such as trypsin (C1, C4, C2, C3, C5, C3PA), plasmin (C1, C3, C5), lysosomal enzymes (C1, C3, C5), and bacterial enzymes (C3, C5) (Ratnoff and Naff, 1967; Bokisch et al., 1969; Cochrane and Müller-Eberhard, 1968; Cooper, 1971; Donaldson, 1968; Taubman and Lepow, 1971; Chapitis et al., 1971; Lepow, 1971). Activation of C1 by these enzymes and of C5 by trypsin and plasmin leads to activation of the subsequent components and initiation of complement action with these components (Arroyave, 1972). Attacks on C4, C3PA, C2, C3, and C5 by the other extrinsic enzymes are accompanied by cleavage and release of biologically active peptide fragments, but the conditions for activation of subsequently reacting components are not met.

Following enzymatic activation, a portion of the activated molecules become bound. In the case of C2, C3, C4, and C5, the binding reaction is quite inefficient, ranging under comparable conditions from 1–2% of input for C5 to 15–20% of input for C3 (Müller-Eberhard et al., 1966; Cooper and Müller-

Eberhard, 1968, 1970; Cooper *et al.*, 1970, 1971). In addition, it has been found that binding may occur only during a brief period of time following activation. In fact, an appropriate acceptor (which may be a membrane, another component, or an immunoglobulin molecule) must be present at the time of activation in order for binding to occur (Müller-Eberhard, 1969). Neither C2, C3, C4, nor C5 binds to its corresponding activating enzymes; C2 normally complexes with C4, while C3, C4, and C5 bind primarily to membranes although other binding sites may also be utilized. Therefore, transfer from the site of activation to the acceptor site must occur, a process which is presumably governed by diffusion. These observations have led to the postulation that a labile binding site is uncovered in the component molecule following enzymatic activation which enables the component to bind on encountering an appropriate acceptor site (Müller-Eberhard, 1969). It should be emphasized that specific binding sites have not been directly identified. Furthermore, the nature of the physical and/or chemical changes which account for decay are completely unknown.

C1s, which is also enzymatically activated, is an exception in that binding sites for C1q and C1r are present in the native, nonactivated, form of the molecule. The reaction mechanism of C1s is also different in that C1s exists normally complexed with its activating enzyme and transfer presumably does not occur following activation.

A second functional site is uncovered or formed on component molecules following enzymatic activation. It is this second site which functions in activating the subsequent component and thus in enabling the complement reaction to continue. As is true in the case of the components activated by binding, this second functional site may be either a specific acceptor for a complement molecule or a new enzyme. Thus, following activation, C4 serves as a specific acceptor for activated C2 (Müller-Eberhard *et al.*, 1967), and C5 serves as a specific acceptor for C6 and probably C7 (Arroyave, 1972; Kolb *et al.*, 1972; Lachmann and Thompson, 1970), and activated C4 and C2 in complex constitute a new enzyme, C3 convertase (Müller-Eberhard *et al.*, 1967).

The functionally active protein—protein complexes of the various components and the phlogistically active by-products of complement activation may be demonstrated on activation of the complement system either in free solution or on the surface of cells. Complement entirely activated in free solution is not, however, cytolytically active. Cytotoxicity requires completion of the later portion of the complement sequence, beginning with the reaction step involving C5 on the surface of the target cell (Götze and Müller-Eberhard, 1970). For this reason, the reaction steps involving C5—C9 have been termed the attack mechanism of complement. Several enzymes have been found which can initiate the attack mechanism; these are C$\overline{4,2,3}$, an enzyme composed of C3PA and C3, trypsin, and plasmin (Fig. 1) (Arroyave, 1972). These enzymes need not be located on the surface of the target cell, but may be present in free solution or even on the surface of another cell. Thus complement activation initiated at one location may be spread to more distant sites.

C. Other Processes

Complement is also activated by a nonimmune complex of the acute phase protein C-reactive protein with pneumococcal C-polysaccharide (Kaplan and Volanakis, 1971) and by isolated lipid A of lipopolysaccharides derived from *Salmonella* and *E. coli* (Galanos *et al.,* 1971). The mechanism of activation by these substances is not known.

In summary, some complement components are activated by complexing specifically or nonspecifically with component molecules, membranes, or certain other substances. Binding is followed by the generation of new sites which enable the component to function as an activator of the subsequent component. These new sites, which are apparently formed by allosteric effects, may be either acceptors for subsequent-reacting complement components or new indigenous complement enzymes. Other components, representing the early portion of the reaction sequence, are activated by intrinsic complement enzymes or extrinsic enzymes. Enzymatic attack results in the formation of two sites in the component molecule which is being activated; one is used for binding and the other is a functional site which enables the molecules or complex to activate subsequent components. The second type of site may be an acceptor or a new complement enzyme.

IV. ACTIVATION OF THE COMPONENTS OF THE CLASSICAL PATHWAY

A. C1

Binding and activation of C1 are independent processes, as evidenced by the observations that C1 fixation may occur in the absence of activation, and conversely, C1 may be activated under certain circumstances in free solution. The best known and possibly the most important activator of C1 is the immunoglobulin or antibody molecule. Not only is antibody an efficient activator of C1 and thus of the classical pathway, but, in addition, antibody initiates complement activation in proximity to antigen thus providing an element of specificity for the cytopathic and phlogistic activities of the complement system.

The acceptor site for $\overline{C1}$ is present and accessible in the monomeric state of the immunoglobulin molecule, as shown first by Müller-Eberhard and Calcott (1966). In these studies, complex formation between monomeric γG and γM and the C1q subunit of $\overline{C1}$ was observed in the analytical ultracentrifuge. C1q and γG, which have sedimentation coefficients of $11S$ and $7S$, respectively, formed a complex, the extent of which was dependent on the concentration of the reactants and the γG subclass. At full saturation the sedimentation coefficient of the complex was $15S$ and the valence of C1q for γG was 5–6. In recent studies, Augener et al. (1971) found that freshly-deaggregated monomeric γG and γM immunoglobulin preparations also were able to bind macromolecular $C\bar{1}$ (Table II).

These studies appear to conflict with earlier work which indicated that a doublet of γG molecules in close proximity is necessary to initiate complement fixation either in the fluid phase or on the surface of cells (Borsos and Rapp, 1965; K. Ishizaka et al., 1962). Similar studies indicate that a single molecule of γM on the surface of a cell initiates $C\bar{1}$ fixation while an aggregate of γM is required in free solution (Borsos and Rapp, 1965; T. Ishizaka et al., 1968; T. Ishizaka et al., 1967; Plaut et al., 1971). However, it may be that in free solution monomeric γG and γM molecules are cross-linked by $C\bar{1}$ through several of its valences to form doublets and other small aggregates necessary for $C\bar{1}$ binding. The extreme inefficiency of $C\bar{1}$ binding observed in the studies of Augener et al. (1971) supports this hypothesis. This inefficiency and perhaps also a species difference probably explains the failure of other workers to observe $C\bar{1}$ binding by monomeric immunoglobulins (T. Ishizaka et al., 1967; Hyslop et al., 1970).

The affinity of the $C\bar{1}$-binding reaction was greatly increased on aggregation of the immunoglobulin molecules. Furthermore, the enhanced $C\bar{1}$ fixation was related to the extent of aggregation. Thus, γM, which contains five $7S$ subunits, gave 15 times better $C\bar{1}$ binding on a weight basis than either the $7S$ γM subunit or monomeric γG1. Similarly, 27–$35S$ γM polymers were four times more efficient, and $>35S$ polymers eight times more efficient than monomeric γM in binding $C\bar{1}$ (Table II).

The mechanism by which aggregation enhances $C\bar{1}$ binding is not known. The studies of Augener et al. (1971) suggest that aggregation augments $C\bar{1}$

Table II. $C\bar{1}$ Binding Capacity of Immunoglobulin Preparations*

Fragments		Monomers		Aggregates	
Fc(γG1)	18	γG3	9	γM	4
F(ab')$_2$(γG1)	>1000	$7S\gamma M_s$	58	γM polymers	0.5
		γG1	60	Aggregated γG1	0.7
		γG2	370		
		γG4	>1000		
		γA	>1000		
		γD	>1000		
		γE	>1000		

* Data adapted from Augener et al. (1971). Values are expressed as the micrograms of immunoglobulin required to bind 50% of a limited amount of $C\bar{1}$.

binding by increasing the number and proximity of $\overline{C1}$-binding sites. Alternatively, it is possible that the marked conformational changes or structural rearrangements which occur within the Fc region on aggregation reveal additional $\overline{C1}$-binding sites or render the existing $\overline{C1}$-fixing sites more efficient (K. Ishizaka, 1963; T. Ishizaka et al., 1967). New antigenic sites appear secondary to conformational changes which accompany aggregation (Henney and Ishizaka, 1968); furthermore, recent data of Plaut et al. (1971) indicate that many $\overline{C1}$-binding sites are masked in intact γM. Further study is needed to resolve the nature of the $\overline{C1}$-binding site.

The complement system is activated on incubation of serum with a protein obtained from the cell wall of Staphylococcus aureus, termed protein A. This protein aggregates immunoglobulin through the Fc region of the molecule (Forsgren and Sjoquist, 1966). Immunoglobulin aggregated via complexing with protein A efficiently activates complement through C1 (Sjoquist and Stalenheim, 1969; Kronvall and Gewurz, 1970).

C1q- and $\overline{C1}$-binding studies have localized the C1-binding site to the Fc region of the molecule (Müller-Eberhard et al., 1971; Augener et al., 1971; Plaut et al., 1971), a finding entirely in accord with the earlier demonstrations that the Fc portion of the immunoglobulin molecule contains the predominant complement-activating site (Amiraian and Leikhim, 1961; Taranta and Franklin, 1961; K. Ishizaka et al., 1962). Attempts to further localize the $\overline{C1}$-binding site in the immunoglobulin molecule have been reported by Kehoe and Fougereau (1970). Augener and coworkers (1971), however, were not able to find $\overline{C1}$-binding activity in similar preparations.

Immunoglobulins exhibit considerable specificity in binding C1q and $\overline{C1}$, with γG3 being most efficient followed by γG1 (Müller-Eberhard and Calcott, 1966; Augener et al., 1971) (Table II). γG2 is far less active, while γG4 does not bind $\overline{C1}$. The same rank order is observed with γG subclasses, whether they are studied as monomers or in the aggregated form (T. Ishizaka et al., 1967; Augener et al., 1971). γM also complexes with $\overline{C1}$, while γA, γD1, and γE do not (T. Ishizaka et al., 1967; Augener et al., 1971).

Although activation of C1 is initiated by attachment of C1 to the immunoglobulin molecule, activation is a separate process which occurs subsequent to binding, at a rate which is dependent on temperature. Although the isolation of nonactivated C1 has not been reported, Borsos and coworkers (1964) clearly showed that binding and activation were distinct processes. In their studies, immune complexes incubated in serum fixed C1 in a nonactivated state, activation followed at a slower rate. Subsequent work showed differences in the rate of activation between γG and γM immunoglobulins, with γM being more efficient in activating bound C1 (Colten et al., 1969). Much remains to be learned about the role of antibody in the activation of C1. It is not known whether the γG subgroups show identical rates of activation, or, alternatively, whether γG3, in addition to binding C1 more avidly than γG1 and γG2, also activates it more efficiently. This is not unlikely since C1 activation probably results from intramolecular changes which occur within the molecule following fixation. The demonstrated differences in C1 binding may indicate that the various immunoglobulins and aggregates thereof provide different numbers or types of C1-binding sites. These sites may induce the allosteric changes in C1 necessary for activation with varying degrees of efficiency.

Aside from the immunoglobulins, a number of other substances interact with C1q and C1 (Table III). These include anions such as double- and single-stranded DNA, RNA, polyribonucleotides, trinitrophenylated (TNP) bovine serum albumin, dextran sulfate, and carrageenin (Agnello *et al.,* 1969, 1970; Yachnin *et al.,* 1964*a,b*; Borsos *et al.,* 1965). These interactions may be quite firm, in fact, several of these anions are able to precipitate C1q from serum. Agnello and coworkers (1970) have taken advantage of the C1q-precipitating activity of DNA in elaborating a method for C1q purification. The mechanism of complex formation of these anions with C1q is probably ionic, for C1q is one of the most basic proteins of serum.

Several of the anions enumerated in Table III activate C1. In particular, double-stranded DNA leads to a loss of C2 and C4 hemolytic activity, and to a lesser extent, C3, C5, and C8 activity, on addition to serum (Cooper, 1972*b*), as shown in Fig. 3. This pattern of component consumption is diagnostic of C1

Table III. Substances Which Interact with C1

Immunoglobulins
    γG3, γG1, γG2, γM

Anions
    Single- and double-stranded DNA
    RNA
    Polyinosinic, polyguanilic and polyuridilic acids
    TNP-bovine serum albumin
    Dextran sulfate
    Carrageenin

Enzymes
    Trypsin
    Plasmin
    Lysosomal enzymes

Miscellaneous
    Endotoxins
    Lymphocyte membranes
    Enveloped viruses
    Low-ionic-strength conditions

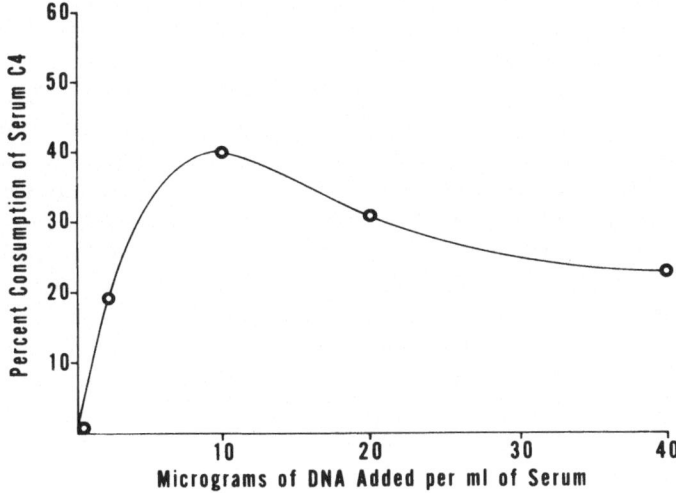

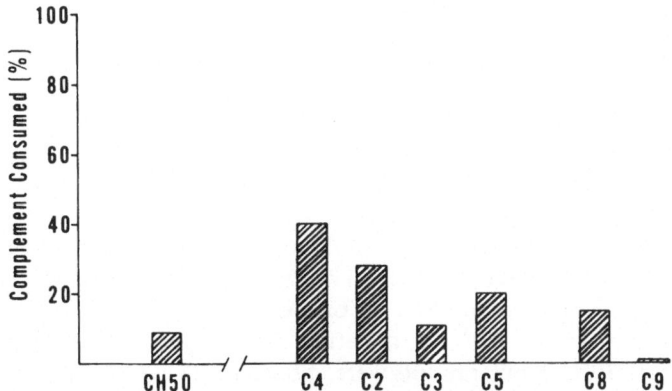

Figure 3. Activation of the classical pathway by double-stranded DNA. The upper panel shows the consumption of serum C4 observed as a function of the amount of DNA added to serum. The lower panel shows a profile of complement consumption on addition of 10 μg DNA/ml serum. The serum–DNA mixtures were incubated for 1 hour prior to performing the titrations.

activation. In this study, the optimal concentration of DNA for C1 activation was 10 μg/ml serum (Fig. 3). Polyinosinic acid also activates serum C1, as shown first by Yachnin *et al.* (1964*a*) and Yachnin and Ruthenberg (1965). In addition, normal erythrocytes in serum are lysed on addition of polyinosinic acid (Yachnin and Ruthenberg, 1965). Presumably this lytic reaction is initiated by activation of serum C1 by the polyribonucleotide. C$\overline{1}$ in turn may activate C4 and C2 and generate a few $C\overline{4,2}$ sites on the erythrocyte surface which interact with C3–C9 and thus produce lysis. Alternatively, $C\overline{4,2,3}$ formed in free solution following C1, C4 and C2 activation may mediate the attachment of cytolytically active C5–C9 to the cell surface (Götze and Müller-Eberhard, 1970). Although originally postulated to be the mechanism of lysis of PNH (paroxysmal nocturnal hemoglobinuria) cells (Yachnin, 1965; Rosse and Dacie, 1966), it is now clear that PNH cell lysis is mediated by the alternate pathway (see below). Yachnin and Ruthenberg (1965) also observed that dextran sulfate induced lysis of normal erythrocytes in serum. While not yet investigated, it is probable that this polysaccharide acts in an analogous fashion to activate serum C1.

Carrageenin, a sulfated polysaccharide, probably does not activate C1. Although a marked loss of hemolytic activity on addition of carrageenin to serum was observed by Davies (1963). The studies of Borsos *et al.* (1965) indicate that the reduction of complement activity is due to precipitation and removal of C1 from serum. These workers failed to find a loss in serum C4 activity which would be expected if carrageenin led to C1 activation.

Several other substances complex with C1 (Table III). The interaction with endotoxin is sufficiently strong to cause precipitation of C1q (Müller-Eberhard *et al.*, 1970). It is not known if the interaction with C1q correlates with the anticomplementary activity which certain lipopolysaccharides possess (Galanos *et al.*, 1971). It is unlikely that the binding of C1q leads to significant activation of the classical complement system, for addition of numerous endotoxins failed to produce significant consumption of C2 and C4 on addition to serum (Gewurz *et al.*, 1968). Endotoxins, however, clearly activate the alternate pathway (see below).

Membranes of lymphocytes in continuous culture have a marked ability to bind and to activate C1 (Cooper, 1972*b*) (Fig. 4). In studies with virus-transformed murine lymphocytes (YCAB), extremely rapid $C\overline{1}$ binding was observed, with $1-2 \times 10^3$ C1 molecules bound per cell in 10 minutes of incubation at 30°C. Similar results were obtained with the WIL-2 and 8866 lines of human lymphocytes in culture. Binding of C1 was followed by activation of the molecule, since C2 and C4 and also the later components were inactivated in the fluid phase on addition of normal serum to the cultured lymphocytes (Lerner *et al.*, 1971) (Fig. 4). C3, C5, and C8 also became bound to the lymphocyte surface. These reactions are apparently not antibody mediated, as the complement-activating property is unaffected by multiple absorptions of the serum with lymphocytes. The mechanism of this reaction is not known. It may be related to the presence of immunoglobulin molecules on the cell surface of these cells. Alternatively, it may be a property of the membrane itself.

The viral envelope of certain RNA viruses, including the Moloney virus and vesicular stomatitis virus, also have the ability to activate C1 in the apparent absence of antibody (Cooper and Oldstone, 1972). Finally, the capsid of the

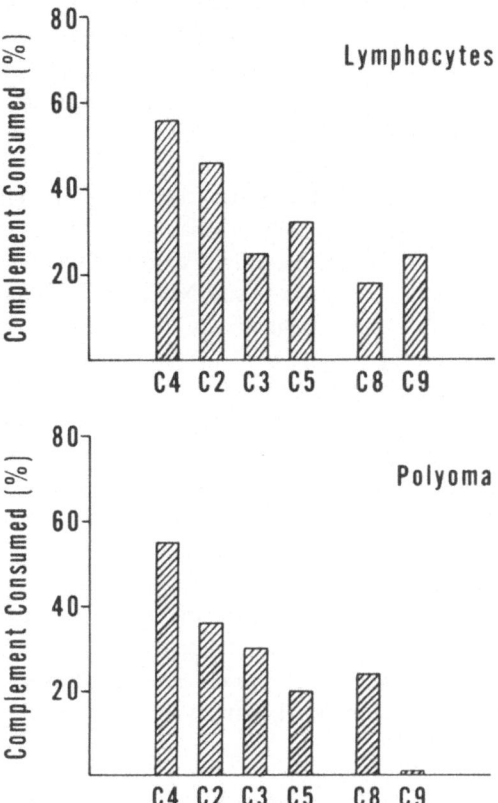

Figure 4. Pattern of loss of complement-component hemolytic activity on addition of virus-transformed murine lymphocytes (*top*) or isolated polyoma virus (*bottom*) to normal human serum.

DNA virus polyoma also activates C1 (Fig. 4). The biological significance of these interactions is unknown.

Low-ionic-strength conditions appear to lead to C1 activation. Complement activity is reduced in the fluid phase on lowering the ionic strength. For example, C4 and C3 may attach to membranes of cells exposed to serum under low-ionic-strength conditions (Mollison and Polley, 1964; Jenkins *et al.,* 1967).

Attachment of the C1 complex via C1q to immunoglobulins or other substances initiates an intramolecular process involving all three subunits which results in activation of the C1s enzyme. Conformational changes undoubtedly occur on attachment of the large C1 molecule to antibody, especially when multiple valences of the molecule are utilized. Different conformational forms of

C1q have been visualized in electron microscopy studies of isolated C1q (Polley, 1971). Colten *et al.* (1970) have demonstrated an antigenic difference between cell-bound and soluble C1. Loos *et al.* (1972), through the use of several inhibitors, have obtained suggestive evidence for changes in the C1 molecule subsequent to cellular binding but prior to the appearance of C1 activity. The nature of these conformational changes is not known.

The final event in the internal activation of C1, i.e., generation of the C1s enzyme, is undoubtedly enzymatically mediated by the C1r subunit. Earlier studies have shown that C1s could be directly activated by trypsin, plasmin, and lysosomal enzymes (Table III) (Ratnoff and Naff, 1967; Taubman and Lepow, 1971). Furthermore, C1s is physicochemically distinguishable from C1s (Nagaki and Stroud, 1970), a finding suggestive of proteolytic attack. Finally, Naff and Ratnoff (1968) observed that partially purified preparations of C1r had enzymatic activity for synthetic substrates; these preparations were also able to directly activate C1s in free solution. Since the enzymatic activity and the C1s-activating properties were similarly affected by alterations in *p*H, ionic strength, and temperature, and by incubation with natural and chemical C1r inhibitors, it is highly probable that C1r activates C1s enzymatically. While the preparations of C1r isolated by Naff and Ratnoff were in an activated form, the functional state of C1r in the C1 macromolecule is not known. If C1s is present with C1 as an activated enzyme, it must be protected from the action of C1r until C1 has become bound. More likely, C1r is present in a precursor state in C1 and activation results from conformational changes following binding.

EFFECT OF C1s ON C2

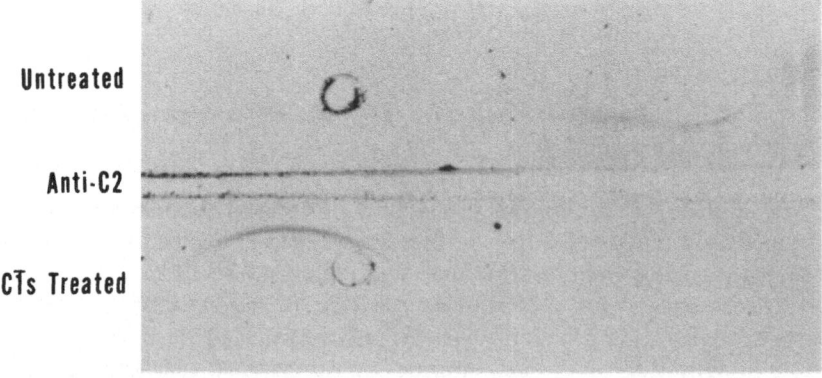

Figure 5. Immunoelectrophoretic analysis of untreated C2 and C2 activated by treatment with C1s. The marked alteration in charge of activated C2 is apparent. The anode is to the right; anti-C1 is in the trough.

B. C$\overline{4,2}$, C3, C5

The second phase of the classical pathway, formation of C$\overline{4,2}$ or C3 convertase, is mediated by the enzymatic properties of C$\overline{1}$. C$\overline{1s}$, an enzyme which is able to cleave a number of synthetic esters, first catalyzes the cleavage and activation of C4 (Müller-Eberhard *et al.*, 1967; Budzko and Müller-Eberhard, 1970). C$\overline{1s}$ next activates C2, a process which is also associated with fragmentation of the molecule (Fig. 5) (Mayer and Miller, 1965; Stroud *et al.*, 1966; Polley and Müller-Eberhard, 1968). In this process, a stable acceptor site for C2 is exposed or created in the C4 molecule and a receptor site is formed in C2 which permits complexing of C4 and C2. Allosteric interactions are important in the assembly of this complex, as shown by the studies of Gigli and Austen (1969*a,b*). They found that C4 was required in order to enable C$\overline{1}$ to activate C2. Further study revealed that C$\overline{1r}$ inhibited activation of C2 by isolated C$\overline{1s}$. This inhibition, however, could be reversed on addition of C4. It may be that C$\overline{1s}$ has a binding site for C2 distinct from the catalytic site which is obscured in the C1 macromolecule. In this interpretation C4 could restore the ability to cleave C2 by interacting with C$\overline{1r}$ or C$\overline{1s}$ to uncover the C2-binding site. Alternatively, C1r and also C4 may allosterically modify C$\overline{1s}$ specificity. Several other possible interpretations indicate cooperative effects between C$\overline{1r}$, C$\overline{1s}$, C4, and C2 in the formation of C$\overline{4,2}$.

A number of enzymes are able to cleave and inactivate C2 and/or C4, including trypsin, bacterial enzymes, snake venoms, and a factor from Nurse shark serum (Table IV) (Müller-Eberhard, 1969; Birdsey *et al.*, 1971; Goldlust *et al.*, 1968; Jensen, 1969; Budzko and Müller-Eberhard, 1970). As yet, none of these agents have been carefully investigated for the ability to jointly activate C2 and C4 to form C$\overline{4,2}$.

Previous studies which suggest that the locus of enzymatic activity of C$\overline{4,2}$ residues in the C2 molecule include those showing (1) the dependence of C3

Table IV. Activators of Individual Components (Nonsustained Activation)

C2:	Trypsin, *Agkistrodon* and other snake venoms, *Clostridium histolyticum* proteinase
C4:	Trypsin, *Agkistrodon* and other snake venoms, nurse shark serum factor
C3:	Trypsin, plasmin, thrombin, tissue proteases, lysosomal enzymes, *Serratia* proteinase, *Agkistrodon* and other snake venoms, hydroxylamine
C5:	Trypsin, lysosomal enzymes, streptococcal proteinase
C3PA:	Trypsin

convertase activity on the amount of C2, (2) the loss of activity on dissociation of C2 from the $\overline{C4,2}$ complex, and (3) the increase in C3 convertase activity following chemical treatment of C2 (Müller-Eberhard *et al.*, 1966, 1967; Polley and Müller-Eberhard, 1967). Recent studies show that the C2 molecule possesses enzymatic activity for synthetic substrates containing basic amino acid residues (Cooper, 1971, 1972*a*). This hydrolytic activity is greatly increased following activation of C2 by $\overline{C1s}$ (Fig. 6). Activated C2, however, does not cleave C3 unless it is complexed with C4. Thus, C4 endows the C2 enzyme with the ability to cleave C3. This could be via allosteric modification of C2 enzymatic specificity. Alternatively, it may be that secondary binding sites are necessary to allow cleavage of the large C3 molecule by C2; these could be provided by C4 or induced by C4 in the C2 molecule.

C3 activation by $\overline{C4,2}$ is associated with cleavage of the molecule into C3a, a peptide of molecular weight 7200 which has anaphylatoxic and chemotactic activities (Dias da Silva *et al.*, 1967; Cochrane and Müller-Eberhard, 1968; Bokisch *et al.*, 1969; Budzko *et al.*, 1971), and into C3b, which has an approximate molecular weight of 180,000. Cleavage of the molecule apparently occurs in the N-terminal region of C3; available evidence indicates that a single

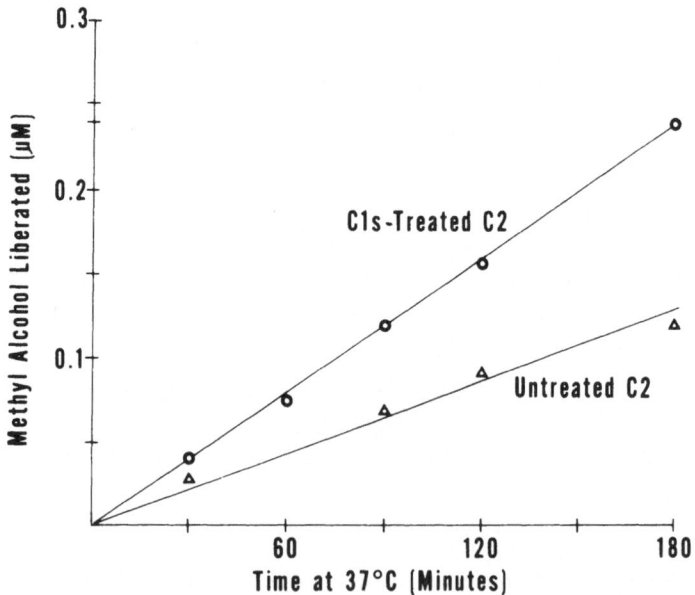

Figure 6. Cleavage of the amino acid ester acetyl glycyl lysine methyl ester by C2 and $\overline{C1s}$-activated C2. Following activation of C2, $\overline{C1s}$ in the reaction mixture was inactivated with DFP. Hydrolysis is expressed as methyl alcohol liberated as a function of time. Increased enzymatic activity is observed on activation of C2.

bond is cleaved in this process (Budzko *et al.*, 1971). For a brief period of time following cleavage, C3b acquires the ability to bind to membranes. In addition to C$\overline{4,2}$, a number of other enzymes, including trypsin, plasmin, thrombin, tissue proteases, lysosomal enzymes, bacterial proteinases, and a chemical, hydroxylamine, have the ability to cleave C3 and liberate biologically active C3a (Table IV) (Dias da Silva *et al.*, 1967; Ward, 1967; Cochrane and Müller-Eberhard, 1968; Bokisch *et al.*, 1969; Hill and Ward, 1971; Lepow, 1971; Budzko *et al.*, 1971). Another enzyme, C3 proactivator, also has this activity; this key enzyme of the alternate pathway will be considered later. Insofar as investigated, the fragments are physicochemically and biologically similar, although the number of amino acids and the C-terminal amino acid may vary slightly depending on the method of formation. Thus, the molecular weight and amino acid composition indicate that the hydroxylamine-derived fragment (7800) is somewhat larger than that produced by C$\overline{4,2}$ (7200) (Budzko *et al.*, 1971).

Cleavage and activation of C3 are necessary events for formation of a new enzyme which requires C$\overline{4,2}$ and C3 for its activity. This enzyme, which is able to activate C5 and the attack mechanism of complement (see below), may be formed on the surface of cells or in free solution. The extent of generation of the C$\overline{4,2,3}$ enzyme is directly dependent on the number of C$\overline{4,2}$ and C3 molecules present in the reaction mixture (Cooper and Müller-Eberhard, 1970). In earlier studies, cells bearing C$\overline{4,2}$ and C3 were found to be able to cleave the synthetic peptide glycyl-L-tyrosine in a manner which suggested enzymatic mediation (Cooper and Becker, 1967). Generation of this activity was dependent on the joint presence of C$\overline{4,2}$ and C3. Hydrolysis of the peptide was directly dependent on the number of C3 molecules per cell, but only at very low levels of C3 input (Cooper and Müller-Eberhard, 1967). These observations suggested that a critical relationship of bound C3 molecules to a C$\overline{4,2}$ site was necessary for the generation of the enzyme. Although the interactions between C$\overline{4,2}$ and C3 in the formation of C$\overline{4,2,3}$ are not clear, it is probable that C3 acts to modify the specificity of the C$\overline{4,2}$ enzyme. This might be via allosteric modification of the enzymatic site enabling the C$\overline{4,2}$ catalytic center to attack C5, or it could be by provision of binding sites which immobilize C5 during the activation process.

C5 is cleaved during activation into a peptide which has anaphylatoxic and chemotactic activities and into a major fragment which possesses a receptor for membranes. C5 is the first reacting member of the membrane attack system; it will be considered in that section.

V. ACTIVATION OF THE ALTERNATE PATHWAY

A. Early-Reacting Factors

Much remains to be learned about the proteins of the alternate pathway and their mechanism of action (Fig. 1). Three of the factors, C3PAse, HSFa, and

C3PA, have thus far been isolated. C3PAse is a 3S normal serum protein of a-globulin mobility which is able to effect conversion of C3 proactivator in the presence of HSFa and metal ions (Müller-Eberhard and Götze, 1972). It is not known whether this protein is enzymatically active in normal serum. HSFa appears to be a fragment derived from C3, closely resembling, if not identical to C3b (Müller-Eberhard and Götze, 1972). Thus, HSF and C3 correlate in distribution on various separatory media, and highly purified C3 possesses HSF activity. Anti-HSFa is reactive only with C3 in native serum, and isolated HSFa gives a reaction of partial identity with anti-C3. Nevertheless, conclusive proof must await comparative chemical studies of HSF and HSFa with C3 and C3b. If HSFa proves to be C3b, the alternate pathway would be secondarily activated on triggering of the classical pathway. Also to be pointed out is the fact that HSFa may well be a product of activation of the alternate pathway. If true, the first few molecules of HSFa formed would allow C3PAse to activate C3PA, cleave C3, and form more HSFa, and a cyclical amplyifying or autocatalytic system would be established.

Numerous substances are able to effect conversion of C3PA in serum (Table V). These include complex polysaccharides such as inulin, yeast cell walls, endotoxin and agar, and aggregates of γG1, γG2, γG3, γA1, γA2, and γE (Götze and Müller-Eberhard, 1971; Spiegelberg et al., 1972; T. Ishizaka et al., 1972). The reactive site of human immunoglobulins is located in the Fc region, while in guinea pig and rabbit immunoglobulins it is present in the F(ab$'$)$_2$ region of the molecule (Sandberg et al., 1971a,b; Spiegelberg et al., 1972). Neither C3PA nor C3 is cleaved on addition of inulin to a mixture of C3PAse, C3PA, C3, and metal ions (Müller-Eberhard and Götze, 1972). Apparently, therefore, at least one additional serum factor is required for triggering by inulin and possibly the

Table V. Activation of the Alternate Pathway

Immunoglobulins
    γG1, γG2, γG3, γG4b
    γA1, γA2
    γD($\pm$)
    γE

Polysaccharides
    Inulin
    Agar
    Endotoxin
    Yeast cell walls

Miscellaneous
    Cobra venom factor
    Trypsin

other substances. The mechanism of entry of this additional factor, or factors, into the C3PAse, HSFa, C3PA, C3 sequence is not known; the most likely possibilities would be that this factor either activates C3PAse or forms HSFa from C3.

B. C3PA

C3PA is a heat-labile 5.5S β-pseudoglobulin with a molecular weight of 80,000 (Götze and Müller-Eberhard, 1971). The protein, or more correctly, the major cleavage product, C3 activator, is antigenically identical to β_2-glycoprotein Type II, first isolated by Haupt and Heide (1965). It is also antigenically related to the protein isolated by Boenisch and Alper (1970) termed glycine-rich β-glycoprotein. C3PA is an integral member of the alternate pathway of complement activation which appears to be identical with the properdin system described some years ago by Pillemer et al. (1954, 1955, 1956). The properdin system functions in bactericidal reactions, neutralization of some viruses, and lysis of erythrocytes from patients with paroxysmal nocturnal hemoglobinuria (PNH) (Pillemer et al., 1954, 1955, 1956; Hinz et al., 1956; Wedgwood et al., 1956). C3PA is undoubtedly identical to factor B of the properdin system for the following reasons: (1) Removal of the protein from serum gives diminished bacteriolysis (Götze and Müller-Eberhard, 1971). (2) The protein participates in the lysis of PNH erythrocytes (Götze and Müller-Eberhard 1972). (3) The isolated protein substitutes for factor B in functional assays for this factor (Götze and Müller-Eberhard, 1971; Goodkofsky and Lepow, 1971). (4) It has the same physicochemical characteristics as factor B.

Activation of C3PA by C3PAse and HSFa is characterized by cleavage of the molecule into a major, 4.5S, 60,000-molecular-weight fragment and a minor, 2.6S, 20,000-molecular-weight fragment (Götze and Müller-Eberhard, 1971). Cleavage of the molecule in serum is readily assessed on performing immunoelectrophoretic analyses in agar containing EDTA. The native protein has β mobility, while the cleavage product has the mobility of a γ-globulin. The other cleavage product, which is negatively charged is not detected with most antisera. C3-cleaving activity is a property of the major fragment. For this reason, it is called the C3 activator.

C3PA shares numerous physicochemical and functional properties with C2; in addition, C3PA has the ability to cleave synthetic esters containing basic amino acids (Cooper, 1971). Activation of the molecule is accompanied by increased enzymatic activity directed toward synthetic esters (Cooper, 1972b); in this regard also, the protein behaves in a manner analogous to C2. The hydrolytic activity is a property of the positively charged treatment. C3PA may also be activated by mild treatment with trypsin. This treatment produces cleavage of C3PA (Fig. 7) and increased enzymatic activity for synthetic sub-

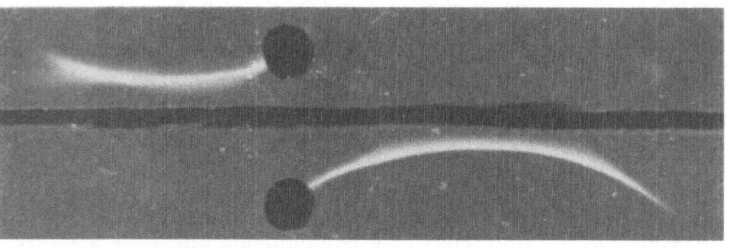

Trypsin
Treated

Anti-C3PA

Untreated

Figure 7. Activation of C3 proactivator by treatment with trypsin. C3PA was treated with 1% trypsin for 5 minutes at 37°C. An immunoelectrophoretic analysis in agar is shown; the anode is to the right.

strates (Cooper, 1972b). In this case, the enzymatic activity is associated with the fragment having γ-globulin mobility.

An isolated protein from cobra venom (Naja naja) leads to marked depletion of C3–C9 without significant consumption of C1, C4, and C2 on addition to serum (Shin *et al.*, 1969; Pickering *et al.*, 1969). Activation of serum complement at the C3 step by this factor has been found to be a property of an 8.5–9S complex of the 7S cobra venom factor (CVF) with a normal serum protein subsequently identified as the C3 proactivator (Müller-Eberhard and Fjellström, 1971; Nelson, 1966; Cochrane *et al.*, 1970). Recent sucrose gradient ultracentrifugation studies of mixtures of cobra venom factor with C3PA in serum or in isolated form clearly show that the C3-activating complex contains both C3PA and cobra venom factor (Cooper, 1972b). However, an additional serum factor is required to generate a firm complex of C3PA with cobra venom factor (Cooper, 1972b) and to endow this complex with the ability to cleave C3 (Hunsicker *et al.*, 1972; Cooper, 1972b). Although the accessory factor shares physicochemical properties with C3PAse, it has not yet been conclusively identified as the same enzyme. The mechanism of action of this factor in engendering a complex of cobra venom factor with C3PA which is able to activate C3 is not yet known.

C. C3

Activation of C3 by C3PA or by the C3PA–CVF complex produces cleavage of C3 and formation of C3 anaphylatoxin (Cochrane and Müller-Eberhard, 1968; Götze and Müller-Eberhard, 1971). Nevertheless, it is not known whether the same bond in C3 is cleaved by the $\overline{C4,2}$ and C3PA enzymes. Indeed, recent evidence indicates that products of C3 derived from alternate-pathway activation inhibit the cytolytic activity of the classical pathway (Koethe *et al.*, 1972). If confirmed, these data would indicate that the cleavage products of C3 produced by the two pathways are not identical. C5 is also consumed and activated and anaphylatoxin is generated on addition of cobra venom factor (Shin *et al.*, 1969; Jensen, 1967), inulin (Fig. 2), or endotoxin (Gewurz *et al.*, 1968; Jensen, 1967) to serum. Apparaently, therefore, C3PA must activate C3 and then interact with it to form an enzyme able to activate C5 in a manner analogous to the formation of $C\overline{4,2,3}$ on addition of C3 to $C\overline{4,2}$.

VI. ACTIVATION OF THE MEMBRANE ATTACK MECHANISM

The membrane attack mechanism, which consists of C5, C6, C7, C8, and C9, is activated by the action of $C\overline{4,2,3}$ or by an analogous enzyme composed of C3PA and C3 (Fig. 1, Table VI). Recently, Arroyave (1972) showed that activation of the attack system may also be induced by the noncomplement enzymes, trypsin and plasmin. Thus the cytolytic properties as well as the phlogistic activities of complement may be initiated by non-complement-dependent pathways. It is not unlikely that other trypsinlike enzymes derived from tissue or lysosomal extracts or serum will be found to be able to activate the attack system.

The activating enzyme need not be present on the target cell membrane. It may be located in free solution or even on the surface of another cell (Götze and Müller-Eberhard, 1970). However, as would be expected, cytolysis is facilitated when the components of the attack system are activated in proximity to the target cell membrane. This is because binding of the components of the attack mechanism is a prerequisite for the production of cell membrane changes and/or cytolysis.

The initial target (C5) is cleaved by activating enzymes to produce C5a which has anaphylatoxic and chemotactic activities (Jensen, 1967; Cochrane and Müller-Eberhard, 1968; Ward, 1968). C5 is also effectively cleaved by lysosomal enzymes and bacterial proteinases (Ward and Hill, 1970; Lepow, 1971). These latter enzymes have not been examined for ability to initiate the complement reaction at the C5 step.

Several lines of evidence point to the existence of two reaction mechanisms for C5, C6, and C7. By inference, there may well be two modes of activation of these components. First, C5 may bind in the active form to EAC1,4,2,3 in the absence of C6 and C7 (Cooper and Müller-Eberhard, 1970; Nilsson and Müller-Eberhard, 1967). In the presence of C6 and C7, C5 binds more efficiently to EAC1,4,2,3, suggesting that a C5,6,7 complex binds as a functional unit (Cooper and Müller-Eberhard, 1970; Arroyave, 1972; Nilsson and Müller-Eberhard, 1967; Götze and Müller-Eberhard, 1970). Additional evidence suggest-

Table VI. Activators of the Membrane Attack Mechanism

Intrinsic activating enzymes:	C4,2,3, C3PA + C3
Extrinsic activating enzymes:	Trypsin, plasmin

ing a dual mechanism of action of C5, C6, and C7 is found in the work of Polley and Müller-Eberhard (1973) who showed that EAC1,4,2,3, prepared with reduced and alkylated C3 bound C5 as well as cells prepared with native C3. However, the cells prepared with treated C3 were unable to mediate the enhanced binding of C5 which normally occurs on simultaneous addition of C5, C6, and C7 to EAC1,4,2,3. C5 present in the supernatant fluid following reaction with EAC1,4,2,3 prepared with normal C3 was unable to bind again to EAC1,4,2,3 alone or in the presence of C6 and C7. C5 following incubation with EAC1,4,2,3 bearing reduced and alkylated C3 was also unable to bind to EAC1,4,2,3. However, this C5 could bind to cells in the presence of C6 and C7. These studies suggest that C5 possesses two binding sites, one of which involves binding of isolated C5, and the other of which functions in binding of C5 complexed with C6 and C7. They further show that chemical modification of a component of the activating enzyme alters the mode of activation of C5, C6 and C7.

Sequential reactivity of C5, C6, and C7 can be demonstrated on activation of these components with EAC1,4,2,3, although binding as a functional unit is the predominant mode of action. Only unit binding of C5, C6 and C7 occurs on activation with C3PA and C3, with fluid phase C$\overline{4,2,3}$, or with trypsin (Götze and Müller-Eberhard, 1970; Arroyave, 1972; Lachmann and Thompson, 1970).

Recent evidence indicates that C8 and C9 bind to the C5,6,7 complex to form a large multimolecular complex consisting of C5, C6, C7, C8, and C9 in a molar ratio of 1:1:1:1:6 (Kolb et al., 1972; Haxby and Kolb, 1972; Kolb and Haxby, 1972; Arroyave, 1972). These deductions are based on fluid-phase complexing and cellular binding studies with isolated radiolabeled components and also on cytolysis-inhibition studies with specific antisera. The geometric arrangement may be visualized as a basic triangular complex of C5, C6, and C7, each molecule of which is in contact with the cell surface and with each other. C8 is thought to bind in the central region of this triangle to form a tetrahedron; the six molecules of C9 in turn are postulated to bind to C8 as two triplets.

These components exhibit various physicochemical interactions with each other in the absence of activation, thus C6 and C7 can be shown to form a loose complex with each other in free solution (Nilsson and Müller-Eberhard, 1967; Arroyave, 1972) and C8 similarly complexes in free solution with C9 (Haxby and Kolb, 1972). These components therefore exhibit an affinity for each other in native form which is increased and intensified following activation of the attack system.

Activation of the attack system, as discussed above, follows catalytic enzyme attack on C5, C6, and possibly C7. It is not difficult to conceive of these components forming a firm complex following activation and simultaneously acquiring the ability to bind, as this is a situation analogous to the formation of C4,2 which has the capacity to bind to membranes on activation of C4 and C2.

Details of the enzymatically-mediated C5, C6 activation process are, however, not yet clear. In particular, the location and identification of the binding sites in the components for membranes and for each other is not known, nor is it known whether the activating enzymes confine their attack to C5 or also affect C6. C7 is not necessary for the formation of the activated C5,6 complex and thus must not be a substrate of the activating enzymes. The mechanism by which isolated activated C5,6 is enabled to bind following incubation with C7 and the nature and location of the cellular binding site also remains to be determined.

The absence of inactivation of either C8 or C9, the high binding efficiency of each component, and the independence of C8 and C9 uptake on changes in pH, ionic strength, and temperature makes enzymatic activation of these components highly unlikely (Kolb et al., 1972; Haxby and Kolb, 1972; Haxby et al., 1972; Kolb and Haxby, 1972). Instead, the binding appears to be adsorptive. This type of mechanism requires that a binding acceptor site for C8 is uncovered in C5, C6, or C7 following formation of the trimolecular complex and that the acceptor sites for C9 be created in the C8 molecule following its attachment.

The question concerning the mechanism by which the attack system alters membranes is presently unanswered. Ultrastructural lesions are evident in erythrocyte membranes after activation of C5 (Polley et al., 1971); there is also membrane swelling (Polley, 1971). These lesions appear to be functionally inconsequential as the integrity of the membrane is unaltered and there is no loss of small ions (Polley et al., 1971; Polley, 1971). However, the lesions may become damaging on subsequent addition of C6 to C9. Similar lesions are produced in erythrocyte membranes by saponin (Bangham and Horne, 1964; Lucy and Glauert, 1964) and the antibiotic filipin (Kinsky et al., 1967), and in lipopolysaccharide films (Bladen et al., 1967), bacterial cell walls (Bladen et al., 1966), and artificial phospholipid membranes (Lachmann et al., 1970) on reaction with complement. The artificial phospholipid membranes (liposomes) are also lysed by the activated complement system (Knudson et al., 1971; Haxby et al., 1969; Lachmann et al., 1970; Kataoka et al., 1971). The nature of the final lytic event is not clear. Enzymatic attack has been implicated in the studies of several groups (Smith and Becker, 1968). However, other studies have not shown evidence of enzymatic processes (Inoue and Kinsky, 1970; Humphrey et al., 1967). The studies of complement with artificial phospholipid membranes (Haxby et al., 1969; Knudson and Bing, 1971) and the studies of membrane alterations produced by the polyene antibiotics suggest that hydrophobic alterations of membrane lipids may play a major role in complement induced lysis (Kinsky et al., 1967).

VIII. CONCLUSIONS

The various mechanisms of activation of the complement components have been considered in this chapter. Included among the various activators are a number of substances and enzymes which are able to trigger the complement system in the absence of antigen and specific antibody. Some of the complement components are activated on forming a complex with other component molecules, membranes, or other substances. Following binding, a functional site is generated in the complement component molecule, presumably by conformational processes, which enables it to activate the next reacting component in the sequence. This site may be an acceptor for another complement component, alternatively, it may be enzymatically active. Most of the complement components reacting early in the sequence are activated following enzymatic attack by intrinsic complement enzymes. Enzymatic activation is manifested in most instances by limited proteolytic attack and release of a small fragment which may have biological activity. Simultaneously two reactive sites are formed on the major cleavage product. One of these sites is a receptor which allows the activated component to bind to membranes or to an appropriate acceptor site located on another component. The second site is a functional site which enables the complement molecule to activate the next component; this functional site may be an acceptor or it may represent a newly formed complement enzyme.

During activation, molecules of complement components become attached to each other and to membranes, a process which is often associated with cytotoxic damage to the cells. In addition, reactive sites located in the bound complement molecules may trigger other cellular effector systems. Small fragments released from components during enzymatic activation interact with cell membranes and stimulate histamine release. These same fragments induce migration of leukocytes to an area of complement activation. Thus it is clear that the biological activity of the complement system requires an extensive series of activation events.

ACKNOWLEDGMENTS

This is publication No. 615 from the Department of Experimental Pathology, Scripps Clinic and Research Foundation, La Jolla, California 92037. This work was supported by the United States Public Health Service Grant No. AI-07007.

REFERENCES

Agnello, V., Carr, R. I., Koffler, D., and Kunkel, H. G. (1969). *Federation Proc.* 28: 696.
Agnello, V., Winchester, R. J., and Kunkel, H. G. (1970). *Immunology* 19: 909.
Amiraian, K., and Leikhim, E. J. (1961). *Proc. Soc. Exp. Biol. Med.* 108: 454.
Arroyave, C. M. (1972). *Federation Proc.* 31: 659.

Augener, W., Grey, H. M., Cooper, N. R., and Müller-Eberhard, H. J. (1971). *Immuno-chemistry* 8: 1011.
Bangham, A. D., and Horne, R. W. (1964). *J. Mol. Biol.* 8: 660.
Becker, E. L. (1956). *J. Immunol.* 77: 469.
Bianco, C., Patrick, R., and Nussenzweig, V. (1970). *J. Exp. Med.* 132: 702.
Birdsey, V., Lindorfer, J., and Gewurz, H. (1971). *Immunology* 21: 299.
Bladen, H. A., Evans, R. T., and Mergenhagen, S. E. (1966). *J. Bacteriol.* 91: 2377.
Bladen, H. A., Gewurz, H., and Mergenhagen, S. E. (1967). *J. Exp. Med.* 125: 767.
Boenisch, T., and Alper, C. A. (1970). *Biochim. Biophys. Acta* 221: 559.
Bokisch, V. A., Müller-Eberhard, H. J., and Cochrane, C. G. (1969). *J. Exp. Med.* 129: 1109.
Borsos, T., and Rapp, H. J. (1965). *Science* 150: 505.
Borsos, T., Rapp, H. J., and Walz, U. L. (1964). *J. Immunol.* 92: 108.
Borsos, T., Rapp, H. J., and Crisler, C. (1965). *J. Immunol.* 94: 662.
Budzko, D. B., and Müller-Eberhard, H. J. (1970). *Immunochemistry* 7: 227.
Budzko, D. B., Bokisch, V. A., and Müller-Eberhard, H. J. (1971). *Biochemistry* 10: 1166.
Chapitis, J.. Ward, P. A., and Lepow, I. H. (1971). *J. Immunol.* 107: 317.
Cochrane, C. G., and Müller-Eberhard, H. J. (1968). *J. Exp. Med.* 127: 371.
Cochrane, C. G., Müller-Eberhard, H. J., and Aikin, B. S. (1970). *J. Immunol.* 105: 55.
Colten, H. R., Borsos, T., and Rapp, H. J. (1969). *Immunochemistry* 6: 461.
Colten, H. R., Borsos, T., and Rapp, H. J. (1970). *J. Immunol.* 104: 1048.
Cooper, N. R. (1971). In Amos, B. D. (ed.), *Progress in Immunology,* Academic Press, New York, p. 567.
Cooper, N. R. (1972*a*). In *Biological Activities of Complement,* Karger, Basel, p. 158.
Cooper, N. R. (1972*b*). (unpublished data)
Cooper, N. R. (1972*c*). *Prog. Transfusion Transplantation* AABB: 191.
Cooper, N. R., and Becker, E. L. (1967). *J. Immunol.* 98: 119.
Cooper, N. R., and Müller-Eberhard, H. J. (1967). *Federation Proc.* 26: 361.
Cooper, N. R., and Müller-Eberhard, H. J. (1968). *Immunochemistry* 5: 155.
Cooper, N. R., and Müller-Eberhard, H. J. (1970). *J. Exp. Med.* 132: 775.
Cooper, N. R., and Oldstone, M. B. A. (1972). (unpublished observations)
Cooper, N. R., Polley, M. J., and Müller-Eberhard, H. J. (1970). *Immunochemistry* 7: 341.
Cooper, N. R., Polley, M. J., and Müller-Eberhard, H. J. (1971). In Samter, M. (ed.), *Immunological Diseases,* Vol. I, Second Edition, Little, Brown and Co., Boston, p. 289.
Davies, G. E. (1963). *Immunology* 6: 561.
Dias da Silva, W., Eisele, J. W., and Lepow, I. H. (1967). *J. Exp. Med.* 126: 1027.
Donaldson, V. H. (1968). *J. Exp. Med.* 127: 411.
Forsgren, A., and Sjoquist, J. (1966). *J. Immunol.* 97: 822.
Frank, M. M., May, J., Gaither, T., and Ellman, L. (1971). *J. Exp. Med.* 134: 176.
Galanos, C., Rietschel, E. T., Lüderitz, O., and Westphal, O. (1971). *European J. Biochem.* 19: 143.
Gewurz, H., Shin, H. S., and Mergenhagen, S. E. (1968). *J. Exp. Med.* 128: 1049.
Gigli, I., and Austen, K. F. (1969*a*). *J. Exp. Med.* 129: 679.
Gigli, I., and Austen, K. F. (1969*b*). *J. Exp. Med.* 130: 833.
Goldlust, M. B., Luzzatti, A., and Levine, L. (1968). *J. Bacteriol.* 96: 1961.
Goodkofsky, I., and Lepow, I. H. (1971). *J. Immunol.* 107: 1200.
Götze, O., and Müller-Eberhard, H. J. (1970). *J. Exp. Med.* 132: 898.
Götze, O., and Müller-Eberhard, H. J. (1971). *J. Exp. Med.* 134: 90s.
Götze, O., and Müller-Eberhard, H. J. (1972). *New Engl. J. Med.* 286: 180.
Haines, A. L., and Lepow, I. H. (1964). *J. Immunol.* 92: 468.
Haupt, H., and Heide, K. (1965). *Clin. Chim. Acta* 12: 419.
Haxby, J. A., and Kolb, W. P. (1972). *Federation Proc.* 31: 740.
Haxby, J. A., Götze, O., Müller-Eberhard, H. J., and Kinsky, S. C. (1969). *Proc. Natl. Acad. Sci. U.S.* 64: 290.
Haxby, J. A., Manni, J. A., Kolb, W. P., and Müller-Eberhard, H. J. (1972). (in preparation)
Henney, C. S., and Ishizaka, K. (1968). *J. Immunol.* 100: 718.

Hill, J. H., and Ward, P. A. (1971). *J. Exp. Med.* **133**: 885.

Hinz, C. F., Jordan, W. S., and Pillemer, L. (1956). *J. Clin. Invest.* **35**: 453.

Humphrey, J. H., Dourmashkin, R. R., and Payne S. N. (1967). *Immunopathol. Intern. Symp. 5th (1965)* **5**: 209.

Hunsicker, L. G., Ruddy, S., and Austen, K. F. (1972). *Federation Proc.* **31**: 788.

Hyslop, N. E., Dourmashkin, R. R., Green, N. M., and Porter, R. R. (1970). *J. Exp. Med.* **131**: 783.

Inoue, K., and Kinsky, S. C. (1970). *Biochemistry* **9**: 4767.

Ishizaka, K. (1963). *Prog. Allergy* **7**: 32.

Ishizaka, K., Ishizaka, T., and Sugahara, T. (1962). *J. Immunol.* **88**: 690.

Ishizaka, T., Ishizaka, K., Salmon, S., and Fudenberg, H. (1967). *J. Immunol.* **99**: 82.

Ishizaka, T., Tada, T., and Ishizaka, K. (1968). *J. Immunol.* **100**: 1145.

Ishizaka, T., Sian, C. M., and Ishizaka, K. (1972). *J. Immunol.* **108**: 848.

Jenkins, D. E., Hartmann, R. C., and Kerns, A. L. (1967). *J. Clin. Invest.* **46**: 753.

Jensen, J. A. (1967). *Science* **155**: 1122.

Jensen, J. A. (1969). *J. Exp. Med.* **130**: 217.

Kaplan, M. H., and Volanakis, J. E. (1971). *Federation Proc.* **30**: 471.

Kataoka, T., Inoue, K., Lüderitz, O., and Kinsky, S. C. (1971). *Eurpean J. Biochem.* **21**: 80.

Kehoe, J. M., and Fougereau, M. (1970). *Nature* **224**: 1212.

Kinsky, S. C., Luse, S. A., Zopf, D., van Deenen, L. L. M., and Haxby, J. A. (1967). *Biochim. Biophys. Acta* **135**: 844.

Klein, P. G., and Wellensiek, H. (1965). *Immunology* **8**: 590.

Knudson, K. C., Bing, D. H., and Kater, L. (1971). *J. Immunol.* **106**: 258.

Koethe, S., Gigli, I., and Austen, K. F. (1972). *Federation Proc.* **31**: 787.

Kolb, W. P., and Haxby, J. A. (1972). *Federation Proc.* **31**: 659.

Kolb, W. P., Haxby, J. A., Arroyave, C. M., and Müller-Eberhard, H. J. (1972). *J. Exp. Med.* **135**: 549.

Kronvall, G., and Gewurz, H. (1970). *Clin. Exp. Immunol.* **7**: 211.

Lachmann, P. J., and Thompson, R. A. (1970). *J. Exp. Med.* **131**: 643.

Lachmann, P. J., Munn, E. A., and Weissmann, G. (1970). *Immunology* **19**: 983.

Lepow, I. H. (1971). In Amos, B. D. (ed.), *Progress in Immunology,* Academic Press, New York, p. 578.

Lepow, I. H., Ratnoff, O. D., Rosen, F. S., and Pillemer, L. (1956). *Proc. Soc. Exp. Biol. Med.* **92**: 32.

Lerner, R. A., Oldstone, M. B. A., and Cooper, N. R. (1971). *Proc. Natl. Acad. Sci. U.S.* **68**: 2584.

Loos, M., Borsos, T., and Rapp, H. J. (1972). *J. Immunol.* **108**: 683.

Lucy, J. A., and Glauert, A. M. (1964). *J. Mol. Biol.* **8**: 727.

Mayer, M. M., and Miller, J. A. (1965). *Immunochemistry* **2**: 71.

Mollison, P. L., and Polley, M. J. (1964). *Nature* **203**: 535.

Müller-Eberhard, H. J. (1969). *Ann. Rev. Biochem.* **38**: 389.

Müller-Eberhard, H. J., and Calcott, M. A. (1966). *Immunochemistry* **3**: 500.

Müller-Eberhard, H. J., and Fjellström, K. E. (1971). *J. Immunol.* **107**: 1666.

Müller-Eberhard, H. J., and Götze, O. (1972). *J. Exp. Med.* **135**: 1003.

Müller-Eberhard, H. J., Dalmasso, A. P., and Calcott, M. A. (1966). *J. Exp. Med.* **123**: 33.

Müller-Eberhard, H. J., Polley, M. J., and Calcott, M. A. (1967). *J. Exp. Med.* **125**: 359.

Müller-Eberhard, H. J., Bokisch, V. A., and Budzko, D. B. (1970). *Immunopathol. VI Intern. Symp. 6th*, Grune and Stratton, New York, p. 191.

Müller-Eberhard, H. J., Calcott, M. A., and Grey, H. M. (1971). (unpublished data).

Naff, G. B., and Ratnoff O. D. (1968). *J. Exp. Med.* **128**: 571.

Nagaki, K., and Stroud, R. M. (1970). *J. Immunol.* **105**: 162.

Nelson, R. A. (1966). *Surv. Ophthal.* **11**: 498.

Nilsson, U. R., and Müller-Eberhard, H. J. (1967). *Immunology* **13**: 101.

Pickering, R. J. Wolfson, M. R., Good, R. A., and Gewurz, H. (1969). *Proc. Natl. Acad. Sci. U.S.* **62**: 521.

Pillemer, L., Blum, L., Lepow, I. H., Ross, O. A., Todd, E. W., and Wardlaw, A. C. (1954). *Science* **120**: 279.

Pillemer, L., Schoenberg, M. D., Blum, L., and Wurz, L. (1955). *Science* 122: 545.
Pillemer, L., Blum, L., Lepow, I. H., Wurz, L., and Todd, E. W. (1956). *J. Exp. Med.* 103: 1.
Plaut, G., Cohen, S., and Tomasi, T. B. (1971). *Science* 176: 55.
Polley, M. J. (1971). In Amos, B. D. (ed.), *Progress in Immunology*, Academic Press, New York, p. 597.
Polley, M. J., and Müller-Eberhard, H. J. (1967). *J. Exp. Med.* 126: 1013.
Polley, M. J., and Müller-Eberhard, H. J. (1968). *J. Exp. Med.* 128: 533.
Polley, M. J., and Müller-Eberhard, H. J. (1973). (in preparation).
Polley, M. J., Müller-Eberhard, H. J., and Feldman, J. D. (1971). *J. Exp. Med.* 133: 53.
Ratnoff, O. D., and Naff, G. B. (1967). *J. Exp. Med.* 125: 337.
Rosse, W. F., and Dacie, J. V. (1966). *J. Clin. Invest.* 45: 736.
Sandberg, A. L., Osler, A. G., Shin, H. S., and Oliveira, B. (1970). *J. Immunol.* 104: 329.
Sandberg, A. L., Oliveira, B., and Osler, A. G. (1971a). *J. Immunol.* 106: 282.
Sandberg, A. L., Götze, O., Müller-Eberhard, H. J., and Osler, A. G. (1971b). *J. Immunol.* 107: 920.
Shin, H. S., and Mayer, M. M. (1968). *Biochemistry* 7: 2997.
Shin, H. S., Snyderman, R., Friedman, E., Mellors, A., and Mayer, M. M. (1968). *Science* 162: 361.
Shin, H. S., Gewurz, H., and Synderman, R. (1969). *Proc. Soc. Exp. Biol. Med.* 131: 203.
Shin, H. S., Pickering, R. J., and Mayer, M. M. (1971). *J. Immunol.* 106: 473.
Sjoquist, J., and Stalenheim, G. (1969). *J. Immunol.* 103: 467.
Smith, J. K., and Becker, E. L. (1968). *J. Immunol.* 100: 459.
Spiegelberg, H. L., Götze, O., and Müller-Eberhard, H. J. (1972). *Federation Proc.* 31: 655.
Stroud, R. M., Mayer, M. M., Miller, J. A., and McKenzie, A. T. (1966). *Immunochemistry* 3: 163.
Taranta, A., and Franklin, E. C. (1961). *Science* 134: 1981.
Taubman, S. B., and Lepow, I. H. (1971). *Immunochemistry* 8: 951.
Ward, P. A. (1967). *J. Exp. Med.* 126: 189.
Ward, P. A. (1968). *J. Immunol.* 101: 818.
Ward, P. A., and Hill, J. H. (1970). *J. Immunol.* 104: 535.
Ward, P. A., and Newman, L. J. (1969). *J. Immunol.* 102: 93.
Wedgwood, R. L., Ginsberg, H. S., and Pillemer, L. (1956). *J. Exp. Med.* 104: 707.
Yachnin, S. (1963). *J. Clin. Invest.* 42: 1947.
Yachnin, S. (1965). *J. Clin. Invest.* 44: 1534.
Yachnin, S., and Ruthenberg, J. M. (1965). *J. Clin. Invest.* 44: 518.
Yachnin, S., Rosenblum, D., and Chatman, D. (1964a). *J. Immunol.* 93: 540.
Yachnin, S., Rosenblum, D., and Chatman, D. (1964b). *J. Immunol.* 93: 549.

Chapter 8

HL-A Antigens, Antibody, and Complement in the Lymphocytotoxic Reaction

S. Ferrone* and M. A. Pellegrino

Department of Experimental Pathology
Scripps Clinic and Research Foundation
La Jolla, California

I. INTRODUCTION

Histocompatibility antigens are genetically segregating allotypic substances which are associated with or included in the membrane of cells of some, but not all, members of a species. Tissues or cells in suspension that carry such antigens induce an immune response when introduced into another member of the homologous species. This immunity can be measured in several ways, such as: (1) by detection of antibodies in the serum of a patient who has received a transplant from an incompatible donor, (2) by accelerated rejection of a second graft from the same donor, or (3) by demonstration of increased immunological reactivity in the lymphoid cells of the recipient. In man, the major histocompatibility system is controlled by genes at the HL-A locus (human leukocyte locus A).

The history of the HL-A system is relatively short. Since the first leukocyte antigen, Mac, was described in 1958 by Dausset, the joint efforts of teams of investigators from Europe and from the United States have amassed a large amount of data which accelerated characterization of HL-A antigens and understanding of their roles in biology and medicine. The HL-A system is controlled by an autosomal region which consists of two closely linked segregant series, LA and Four, each of which contains a rather large and still unknown number of mutually exclusive alleles (Ceppellini *et al.,* 1967; Singal *et al.,* 1968; Dausset *et al.,* 1969; Kissmeyer-Nielsen *et al.,* 1970).

* Dr. Ferrone is a visiting scientist from the University of Milan, Italy.

Results of experimental skin grafts (van Rood *et al.*, 1964; Amos *et al.*, 1966; Ceppellini *et al.*, 1966; Dausset *et al.*, 1966; van Rood *et al.*, 1966; Walford *et al.*, 1969) as well as of kidney transplants (van Rood *et al.*, 1967; Terasaki *et al.*, 1967; Dausset *et al.*, 1968*a*; Payne *et al.*, 1968; Singal *et al.*, 1969) indicate that at least among siblings the HL-A system plays a major role in determining the survival of grafts. In reactions to grafts between unrelated individuals, the primary function of HL-A antigens in this regard is questioned (Mickey *et al.*, 1971), since other factors such as immunologic responsiveness of the recipient seem to be important in determining the destiny of the transplanted organ (van Rood, 1971; Opelz *et al.*, 1972).

A number of clinical investigations suggest association between the HL-A type of individuals and hematologic (Amiel *et al.*, 1967; Forbes and Morris, 1970; Walford *et al.*, 1970; Zervas *et al.*), autoimmune (Grumet *et al.*, 1971), or renal diseases (Patel *et al.*, 1969; Mickey *et al.*, 1970). The subject has been recently reviewed by Walford *et al.* (1971).

A whole array of procedures such as application of detergents (Metzgar *et al.*, 1967), proteolytic enzymes (Davies, 1968; Mann *et al.*, 1968; Sanderson and Batchelor, 1968), low-frequency sound (Kahan *et al.*, 1968; Reisfeld *et al.*, 1970), and salt extraction (Mann and Fahey, 1971*b*; Reisfeld *et al.*, 1971) have been utilized to solubilize HL-A antigen cell surface membranes in an attempt to characterize the chemical nature of these antigens. The data thus far available indicate that HL-A antigens are essentially protein in composition and apparently consist of single polypeptide chains with a molecular weight of 31,000 (Reisfeld and Kahan, 1972). During the past 15 years many assays to evaluate histocompatibility antigens have been devised which fall into two broad categories, i.e., biological and serological. Biological tests evaluate either (1) the fates of tissue grafts on a sensitized animal, (2) the production of humoral antibodies, (3) the induction of a state of delayed hypersensitivity to injected antigens, or (4) the response of lymphocytes when confronted in tissue culture with allogeneic cells. Although biological tests are the only meaningful way to study immunogenicity, they are usually complex, time consuming, and cumbersome. On the other hand, serological assays, which measure the extent to which an antibody can form a specific complex with its alloantigenic determinants, are simple and rapid. Therefore, these assays have been the most useful tool for the characterization of histocompatibility antigens.

Leukoagglutination proved effective in delineating the first 10 well-defined HL-A antigens. This initial success was based on the fact that this test is relatively insensitive; thus, many alloantisera reacted as if they were monospecific. In the ensuing years, other serological techniques have included complement fixation (Aster *et al.*, 1964; Shulman *et al.*, 1964; Colombani *et al.*, 1967), antiglobulin consumption (Colombani *et al.*, 1964), mixed agglutination (Milgrom *et al.*, 1964), immune adherence (Melief *et al.*, 1967; Miyakawa *et al.*, 1971), and cytotoxicity (Terasaki and McClelland, 1964; Walford *et al.*, 1964;

Engelfriet and Britten, 1965; Amos, 1966). Currently, the lymphocytotoxic test is by far the most widely used, especially since miniaturization of the method by Terasaki and McClelland (1964). The microlymphocytotoxic test has proved to be most efficient for extensive study of the HL-A system since it requires only minute quantitites of alloantisera and low numbers of target cells. Since the sensitivity of this method is inversely proportional to the number of target cells employed (Jensen and Stetson, 1961; Boyse *et al.*, 1962; Wigzell, 1965), sensitivity is increased appreciably by using 1000—2000 cells. Cytotoxic reactions can be performed with small amounts of alloantisera, e.g., 1 μl, thus minimizing the problems of limited supplies of these reagents and, in addition, making possible the international exchange of antisera.

The reaction system consists of (1) human peripheral lymphocytes or cultured lymphoid cells as target cells, (2) HL-A alloantisera or heteroantisera as source of antibodies, and (3) fresh serum as the source of complement. The cytotoxic test relies upon alterations in permeability of the cell membrane induced by the action of complement on target lymphocytes which have been exposed to cytotoxic antibody.

Information from scanning and transmission electron microscopy has been used to characterize the lesions induced on lymphocytes by HL-A antibodies and complement (Walford *et al.*, 1966; Claesson *et al.*, 1971; Lambertenghi-Deliliers *et al.*, 1971). Under the scanning electron microscope, these target lymphocytes have abnormal shapes and irregular craters with cracked surfaces. By using transmission electron microscopy, severe degenerative changes in the nucleus and in the cytoplasm can be detected. The nucleus is round in shape with a predominantly heterochromatin substance condensed into compact masses; in the interchromatinic areas numerous interchromatin granules, and in some cells bundles of fibers, are seen. The perinuclear space is dilated and occasionally expanded into large sacs, but the perinuclear membrane is without perforations and seems fairly well preserved, even in the most advanced stages of lysis. Advanced lymphoid cell decay also is manifested in the cytoplasm by hydropic swelling and numerous intracellular vacuoles. The cytoplasm is electron-transparent because of the almost complete absence of ribosomes, whereas the mitochondria are swollen and their cristae fragmented. Rough endoplasmic reticulum profiles are not observed. In the majority of degenerated lymphocytes, small electron-dense bodies lie in close contact with the membranous systems. The cytoplasmic membrane has no projections and presents some gaps; the perforations of the lymphocyte membrane seem to be relatively large (100—300 Å) as compared with those in sheep red blood cell membranes exposed to antibody and complement described by Borsos *et al.* (1964).

It is noteworthy that all these lesions, which may be considered to represent a pyknotic type of cell necrosis, are not characteristic of the damage induced by HL-A antibody and complement. They have in fact also been observed in nonimmunologic conditions (Zucker-Franklin, 1965; Walford *et al.*, 1966; Lucas and Peakman, 1969), and thus they may actually represent a general consequence of cytoplasmic membrane injury rather than a specific effect of cytotoxic HL-A alloantibody (Glick et al., 1970; Claesson et al., 1971).

Of several indicator systems to measure cell death, one of the most widely applied is the use of supravital dyes, such as eosin (Terasaki et al., 1967) or trypan blue (Walford et al., 1964; Amos, 1966), which penetrate the membranes and stain dead cells but are excluded by viable cells. Morphologic studies (Terasaki and McClelland, 1964) are based on the loss of refractibility of dead lymphocytes when examined under phase-contact microscopy. Whereas living cells have poorly resolved nuclei in the cytoplasm, killed cells are dark, slightly enlarged, and exhibit a clearly distinguishable nucleus within the cytoplasm. Still another indicator system, introduced by Rotman and Papermaster (1966), has been used for the study of HL-A antigens by several investigators (Bodmer et al., 1967; Celada and Rotman, 1967; Tosi et al., 1967; Takasugi, 1971). In this test, viable cells preincubated with fluoresceindiacetate appear fluorescent under polarized light since fluorescein accumulates after the esterase-catalyzed hydrolysis of acetate. In contrast, dead cells show no fluorescence since they rapidly lose the fluorescing material. The cytotoxic action of alloantisera can also be detected by the loss of intracellular isotopic markers from dead cells. Thus, in the radiochromium technique (Rogentine, 1967; Sanderson and Batchelor, 1967) lymphocytes labeled with sodium dicromate (^{51}Cr) are exposed to antibodies and complement, and the amount of chromium released in the supernatant is measured.

The aim of this assay is to critically evaluate some aspects of the lymphocytotoxic reaction by which HL-A antigens are defined under a variety of conditions. Rather than review the extensive literature on this subject, we have focused on the problems encountered when (1) classifying HL-A types of cultured human lymphoid cells, (2) evaluating the serologic activity of soluble HL-A antigens, (3) utilizing HL-A heteroantisera as a source of antibodies, and (4) studying the activation of the complement component system.

II. HL-A ANTIGENS ON CULTURED HUMAN LYMPHOID CELLS

HL-A antigens are present on cultured human lymphoid cells even after long-term tissue culture (Papermaster et al., 1969; Rogentine and Gerber, 1969; Rogentine and Gerber, 1970). These cells possess a higher density of HL-A determinants than that found on autologous peripheral lymphocytes (Rogentine and Gerber, 1970; Pellegrino et al., 1972a). This higher density is reflected by increased titer with HL-A alloantisera in the direct cytotoxic test (Bernoco et al., 1969) and by the greater lytic efficiency of human complement (Ferrone et al., 1971b) (Fig. 1) which is usually poorly effective in the cytotoxic test with peripheral lymphocytes. In this regard, the density of HL-A determinants on cultured lymphoid cells might actually be sufficient to fix an IgG doublet

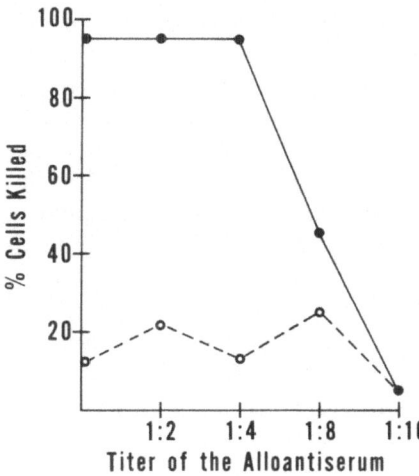

Figure 1. Efficiency of human complement in the cytotoxic reaction with human cultured cells or with peripheral lymphocytes. Alloantiserum   TO-11-03   (anti-HL-A2): (o----o) peripheral lymphocytes (B.P.); (•————•) cultured human lymphoid cells RPMI 1788 derived from the peripheral lymphocytes of donor B.P.

resulting in complement-mediated cytolysis, without the need for the natural antibody present in the rabbit complement (Ferrone *et al.*, 1971*b*). Data from quantitative absorption studies indicate that the ratio of the absorbing capacity between human cultured lymphoid cells and peripheral lymphocytes ranges from 2 to 5.2 (Rogentine and Gerber, 1970; Pellegrino *et al.*, 1972*a*). The difference in antigen expression in two cells of the same morphological series but with varying degrees of maturity is not characteristic of the lymphoid tissue, since reticulocytes have been reported to contain HL-A antigens whereas mature erythocytes lack them altogether (Harris and Zervas, 1969; Silvestre *et al.*, 1970). The mechanism responsible for the expression of varying densities of HL-A determinants on cultured cells and peripheral lymphocytes is presently unknown. Perhaps steric differences at the cell surface affect availability of antigenic determinants for absorption. Should this prove to be the case, then the antigenic content in these cells may not really differ. Alternatively, tissue-cultured lymphoblasts and mature lymphocytes may have differing control mechanisms for the content of HL-A antigens on the surface membrane, e.g., mature lymphocytes may more readily shed HL-A antigens. The difference in the density of HL-A determinants between cultured human lymphoid cells and peripheral lymphocytes must be taken into account when one compares the results of typing cultured human lymphoid cells and peripheral lymphocytes. In this regard there have been several reports (Dick and Steel, 1971; MacKintosh *et al.*, 1971; Dick *et al.*, 1972; Moore and Woods, 1972) of additional HL-A determinants acquired by human lymphoid cells following either short- or long-term tissue culture. The clinical counterpart of this observation might be the demonstrable changes in HL-A determinants on peripheral lymphocytes of some patients with acute leukemia (Pegrum *et al.*, 1971): new HL-A antigens appear during the acute phase of the disease, disappear during remission, and reappear during relapse. However, these investigations have only made use of the direct cytotoxic test which does not permit one to exclude discrepancies observed in the HL-A phenotypes between cultured human lymphoid cells and peripheral lymphocytes that are an expression of CYNAP (cytotoxicity negative, absorption positive reactions) (Ferrone et al., 1967). In fact, when both the direct cytotoxic test and the absorption test were employed, no qualitative differences should be detected with HL-A antigen content of either cultured human lymphoid cells or peripheral lymphocytes from the same donor (Rogentine and Gerber, 1970; Pellegrino et al., 1972a). Whenever the peripheral lymphocytes appeared to be negative and the cultured lymphoid cells positive upon direct cytotoxicity typing, the peripheral lymphocytes could absorb the alloantibody, although a large number of peripheral lymphocytes were needed to remove the antibody activity from the serum, suggesting a low density of HL-A determinants on the cell surface (Table I). The low density of HL-A determinants on the cell surface might explain the negative result in the direct lymphocytotoxic test; in fact, complement–antibody-mediated lysis of cells requires a

Table I. Reactivity in the Lymphocytotoxic Test and Absorbing Capacity for HL-A Alloantisera of Peripheral Lymphocytes and Cultured Lymphoid Cells Derived from the Same Donor

Donor	Cell type	Test	HL-A			
			2	3	5	7
B.P.	P.L.[a]	Direct Cytotoxicity	+	–	–	+
		Absorption	2,800[c]	>50,000	>50,000	3,800
	C.L.[b]	Direct Cytotoxicity	+	+	–	+
		Absorption	825	>50,000	>50,000	1,800
D.O.	P.L.	Direct Cytotoxicity	+	–	–	–
		Absorption	3,200	>50,000	>50,000	23,000
	C.L.	Direct Cytotoxicity	+	+	–	+
		Absorption	800	>50,000	>50,000	3,500

[a] Peripheral leukocytes.
[b] Cultured human lymphoid cells.
[c] Number of cells required to reduce by 50% the lymphocytotoxic activity of HL-A alloantisera (AD_{50}).

critical concentration of complement at the cell surface which cannot be reached, even with a large excess of antibody and complement, should the density of antigen receptors be very low.

There may be other reasons for discrepancies between the HL-A phenotypes of cultured human lymphoid cells and peripheral lymphocytes from the same donor. Alloantisera routinely employed for HL-A typing are usually derived from multiparous women or transfused subjects and are only operationally monospecific (Walford et al., 1967). Most of these antisera contain additional weak anti-HL-A antibodies which can be clearly demonstrated by increasing the sensitivity of the cytotoxic system such as by treatment of target cells with proteolytic enzymes (Grothaus et al., 1971b; Braun et al., 1972; Gibofsky and Terasaki, 1972) or with the sulfhydryl compound 2-aminoethylisotiouromium bromide (AET) (Sirchia and Ferrone, 1970). The same phenomenon occurs when the sensitivity of the lymphocytotoxic reaction is enhanced by addition of sublytic amounts of rabbit anti-human lymphocyte serum to the rabbit complement (Ting, Ferrone, and Terasaki, unpublished observations). Since cultured human cells are more sensitive in the cytotoxic test than peripheral lymphocytes, the former can react with the weak anti-HL-A antibodies present in the typing sera which have been characterized on the basis of their reactivity with peripheral lymphocytes. During typing of cultured human lymphoid cells (Ferrone et al., 1972a), it was observed that some cells possessed more than two HL-A determinants within each segregant series: specifically, cells RPMI 1788 had the phenotype HL-A2,3,10,7,W14 and cells RPMI 7249 had HL-A1,2,3,7,8. In order to rule out the possibility that some positive reactions between cultured human lymphoid cells and operationally-monospecific HL-A antisera were triggered by additional HL-A antibodies, direct typing was cross-checked by absorption typing. In some instances the cells could not absorb the typing antibodies from the serum, although they could react positively in the direct cytotoxic test, suggesting that positive reactions were caused by anti-HL-A antibodies other than those already defined. In fact, typing by absorption resulted in: RPMI 1788, HL-A2+,10+,7+, W14+ and RPMI, HL-A1+,2+,7+,8+.

Cultured cells possess some receptors which are not present in significant amounts on peripheral lymphocytes from the majority of normal subjects, including the donors from whom the lines were derived. These antigens have been designated as "lymphoblast in vitro antigens" (Bernoco et al., 1969), and do not seem to be related to the HL-A system or to correspond to a new genetic polymorphism. Antibodies reacting with these determinants are present both in HL-A alloantisera and in normal human sera. Although the exact nature of these antigens is still poorly understood, they represent another source of variability to be taken into account when analyzing the reactivity of cultured cells with HL-A alloantisera. HL-A antigens persist on cultured human lymphoid cells even after many years of continued growth in tissue culture. Hence these cells offer an opportunity to study biosynthesis and cell surface expression of HL-A antigens and also represent an excellent source for the extraction of soluble HL-A antigens (Mann *et al.*, 1968; Reisfeld *et al.*, 1970; Mann and Fahey, 1971*a*; Reisfeld and Kahan, 1972). The organs of single donors yield only limited amounts of HL-A antigens, making any meaningful comparisons between various preparations an impossible task (Kahan *et al.*, 1968). These cultured cells represent in the HL-A field what inbred animal lines offer for the study of histocompatibility antigens of other species. The long-term, continuous availability of the source from which soluble HL-A antigen is extracted permits integration of new knowledge into a controlled study. However, the recent finding of some Epstein-Barr viral genomes even in cultured cells derived from normal donors (zur Hausen *et al.*, 1972) has somewhat impaired the usefulness of these calls as a source of soluble antigens for biological studies.

Cultured cells also are highly useful once chromosomal abnormalities can be induced which induce a qualitative change in antigen content thus facilitating the chromosomal localization of HL-A antigens. Furthermore, qualitative and quantitative changes of HL-A antigens may be followed after a variety of manipulations *in vitro,* such as exposure to known chemicals, viral carcinogens, radiation, and differing hormonal environments. Since histocompatibility antigens appear to be a central part of a cellular recognition system, such experiments may yield important clues concerning the processes of cellular immunity and neoplasia.

The mechanism of biosynthesis of HL-A antigens is being studied by using several inhibitors of macromolecular synthesis effecting cell surface expression of HL-A determinants (Ferrone *et al.*, 1972*c*). Actinomycin D does not affect the cell surface expression of HL-A antigens in logarithmically-growing cells, thus suggesting that the messenger-RNA coding for HL-A antigens is relatively long-lived. In contrast, Cikes and Klein (1972) reported that actinomycin D could enhance the expression of H-2 antigens in cultured murine cells and this superinductive effect was blocked by puromycin and cycloheximide. The discrepancy between his report and our data might reflect the different experimental conditions used; Cikes and Klein (1972) utilized Moloney-leukemia-virus-induced murine tumor cells to study the expression of H-2 antigens, while in our experiment, cells were derived from a subject free of malignancy.

Several lines of evidence suggest an influence of malignancy on the expression of histocompatibility antigens. Decrease of H-2 antigens has been documented in H-2 homozygous murine tumor cells (Amos, 1956; Hoecker and Hauschka, 1956) and irreversible loss of antigens controlled from one of the two H-2 alleles have been observed in H-2 heterozygous tumors (see Hellström and Möller, 1965 for review). In murine leukemia cells induced by dimethylbenzanthracene, some H-2 specificities are decreased while others are increased (Bruley and Motta, 1971). In TL leukemia, an inverse relationship was found between the quantitative expression of tumor-specific cell surface antigens and normal H-2 antigens: the phenotypic expression of TL antigens reduces the demonstrable amount of certain H-2 determinants on cell surface (Boyse *et al.*, 1967), while the decrease of TL antigens caused by a modulation phenomenon evokes a compensatory increase in H-2 antigen expression (Old *et al.*, 1968). Parallel observations have been made in humans; decrease or loss of HL-A antigens have been reported in course of malignancy (Bertrams *et al.*, 1971; Seigler *et al.*, 1971; van Rood and van Leeuwen, 1971), while in other cases there has been an increased reactivity of leukemic cells with some anti-HL-A alloantisera, probably reflecting a heightened expression of HL-A antigens (Walford *et al.*, 1971). Finally, changes in the HL-A profile of some patients with acute leukemia have been reported in parallel with the activity of the disease; new HL-A antigens which appear during the acute phase of the disease, disappear during remission, and then appear upon relapse (Pegrum *et al.*, 1971).

5-Bromodeoxyuridine, ethidium bromide, rifampicin, and chloramphenicol did not affect the expression of HL-A antigens on cell surfaces during periods of up to 18–24 hours of incubation at 37°C. On the contrary, puromycin reduced the capacity of WIL$_2$ cells to absorb specifically anti-HL-A alloantisera directed against antigenic determinants of the first and second segregant series. The effects of this drug on the expression of HL-A antigens as well as on the amount of ^{3}H-labeled leucine incorporated into protein depended on the duration of incubation as well as on the dose (Fig. 2). The effects of puromycin on the expression of HL-A antigens were reversible; in fact, cells depleted of HL-A antigens by treatment with puromycin, once washed and incubated in fresh medium, again acquired a full expression of HL-A antigens within 5 hours.

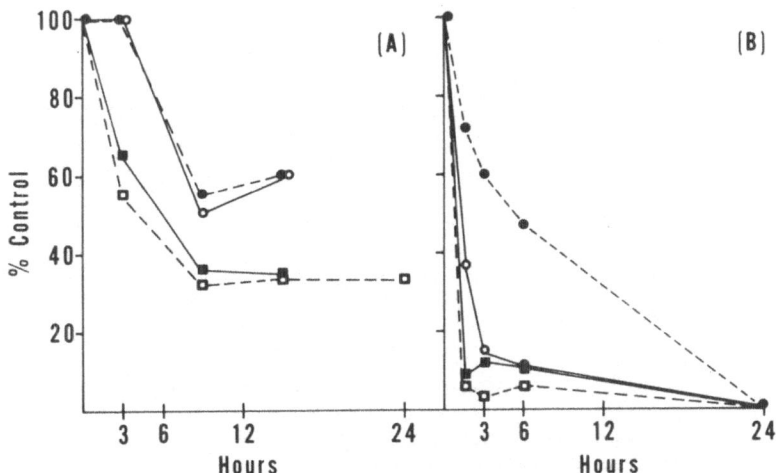

Figure 2. Effect of different doses of puromycin on (A) the cell surface expression of HL-A antigens and on (B) incorporation of ^{3}H-labeled leucine. ●---● 1μg/ml, ○——○ 5 μg/ml, ■——■ 25 μg/ml; □---□ 50 μg/ml.

Actinomycin D did not affect the reexpression of HL-A antigens which, in turn, was blocked by puromycin (Fig. 3). These results are in accord with the recent report (Turner *et al.,* 1972) that human peripheral lymphocytes from which HL-A2 determinants had been removed *in vitro* by treatment with papain again expressed these HL-A determinants within 6 hours of incubation in a nutritive medium. Once puromycin was added to these cultures, expression of HL-A2 determinants was completely inhibited, yet actinomycin D did not show this inhibitory affect.

Cycloheximide, like puromycin, interferes with the normal function of the translational complex, but by a different mechanism. Thus, puromycin, an analog of amino-acyl-tRNA, accepts a growing polypeptide chain and then dissociates from the polyribosome, whereas cycloheximide inhibits peptide chain initiation as well as elongation. This drug, although inhibiting the incorporation of ^{3}H-labeled leucine into protein by at least 95% (i.e., at a level similar to that obtained with puromycin) did not significantly change the capacity of cultured cells to absorb anti-HL-A alloantisera for periods up to 24 hours. The different effects of puromycin and cycloheximide suggest that the mechanism for the biosynthesis of HL-A antigens is similar to that of protein synthesis in mitochon-

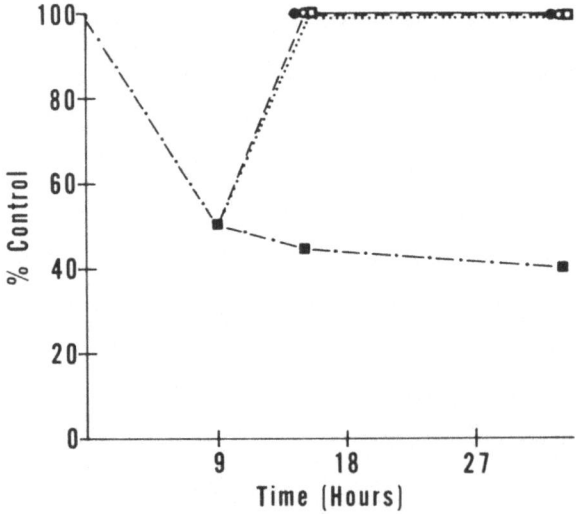

Figure 3. Effect of actinomycin D, puromycin, and cycloheximide on the expression of HL-A antigens on cultured
human lymphoid cells WIL$_2$ initially treated with puromycin
(50 mg/ml) for 9 hours (■----■). Cells were thoroughly
washed and then reincubated in medium (1) without any
further addition of inhibitors (●---●); (2) with puromycin (50
mg/ml) (■----■); (3) with actinomycin D (5 mg/ml) (○---○);
and (4) with cycloheximide (100 mg/ml (□·····□).

dria, especially since Galper and Darnell (1971) have shown that protein synthesis in the mitochondrial fractions of HeLa cells is sensitive to puromycin, but not to cycloheximide. Ashwell and Work (1968) have found that this insensitivity is not the result of a permeability barrier. The hypothesis that the mechanism for the biosynthesis of HL-A antigens is similar to that of protein synthesis in mitochondria is attractive to explain the differences observed in cells treated with puromycin or with cycloheximide. However, the possibility that these differences may be the result of secondary effects of these drugs cannot be ignored. Whatever the mechanism of action of these inhibitors, understanding of the control of HL-A antigenic expression may be of considerable importance since it may provide a completely novel approach to the problem of allograft rejection. Furthermore, since the extensive polymorphism of the HL-A system may be important to the host's defense against viral infections (Ceppellini *et al.*, 1967), regulation of this expression may be useful for treatment of diseases heretofore resistant to common drug regimens.

III. DISTRIBUTION OF HL-A ANTIGENS ON THE SURFACES OF LYMPHOID CELLS

Few investigations have been performed on the distribution of HL-A antigens on the surface of lymphoid cells, and results have been divergent probably due to the utilization of different methods, among which are direct and indirect immunofluorescence and ferritin-conjugated antibody techniques. By indirect tests, the HL-A antigens on the membrane of peripheral lymphocytes (Kourilsky *et al.*, 1971) and of cultured lymphoid cells (Pellegrino *et al.*, 1972e) are discontinuously distributed, forming patches without periodicity, separated by intervals free of any staining. The labeling of cultured lymphoid cells is more intense than that of peripheral lymphocytes and probably reflects the already-mentioned higher density of HL-A determinants (Fig. 4). These observations have been recently confirmed and extended by Neauport-Sautes *et al.* (1972) by means of a more sophisticated technique in which hybrid antibodies bind electron-dense particles to anti-HL-A antibodies. These investigators also showed by double radiolabeling experiments that HL-A antigens are not renewed at a detectable level during the labeling procedure in those areas of the cell surface which are not primarily labeled with ferritin—anti-IgG—anti-HL-A complexes. A discontinuous pattern was also observed for mouse H-2 antigens (Aoki *et al.*, 1969), for virus-associated membrane antigens at the surfaces of mouse (Aoki *et al.*, 1970) and human cells (Silvestre *et al.*, 1969), for antigens of the Rh system, and for some autoantigens in human hemolytic anemia (Davis *et al.*, 1968). These observations are contrary to reports describing the almost-continuous labeling pattern on erthrocyte membranes with anti-A antisera (Lee and Feldman, 1964).

However, with an indirect, elaborate, sandwich labeling technique, Willing-

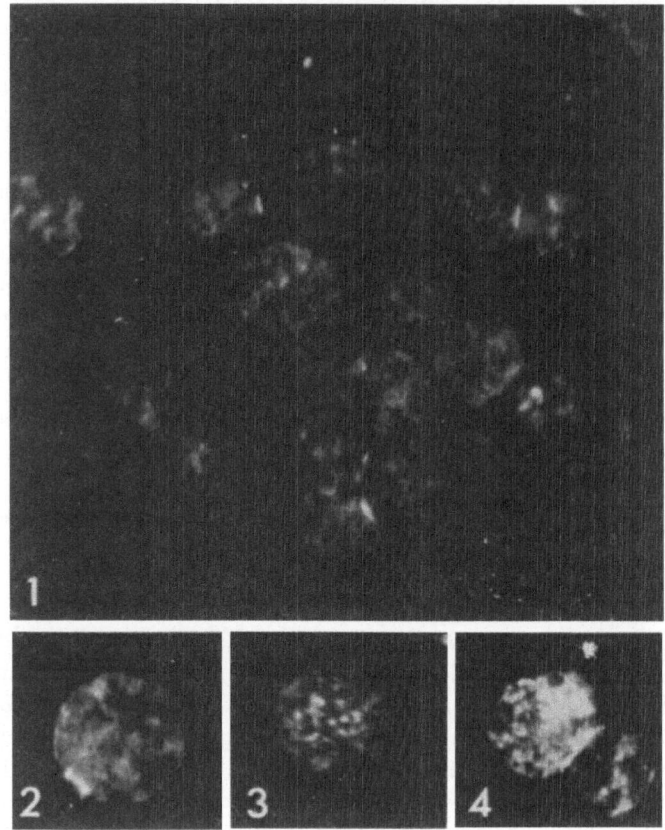

Figure 4. Cellular surface distribution of HL-A determinants on cultured lymphoid cells WIL$_2$ (HL-A1,2,5, Te57). The cells were reacted with the alloantiserum Pena (anti-HL-A2) in the indirect immunofluorescence test.

ham *et al.* (1971) found evidence for continuous distribution of HL-A antigens. In addition, Davis *et al.* (1971) have shown that the distribution of histocompatibility antigens appears continuous when examined by the direct ferritin-conjugated antibody technique, and discontinuous when studied by the indirect technique. The possibility exists, therefore, that the patchy distribution of HL-A antigens is an artifact. Some possible causes of this phenomenon have been suggested by Davis *et al.* (1971) and Davis (1972) to be the following: (1) gamma globulins that are not conjugated with ferritin may block part of the cell surface (Aoki *et al.*, 1969), (2) regions of the cell surface which may be inaccessible to antibody because of membrane folding during labeling, (3) the natural outer coat of cells causes steric hindrance and prevents binding of the anti-globulin antibodies to the alloantibodies attached to the cell surface (Willingham *et al.*, 1971), and (4) histocompatibility antigens as well as other components of cell membranes may not have fixed positions on the cell membrane which undergoes continuous renewal (Frye and Edidin, 1970; Singer and Nicolson, 1972). Absorption of antibody to the cell surface may cause modifications in the distribution of HL-A antigen structures on the cell membrane, such as clustering of fluorescein-labeled anti-HL-A antibodies after their absorption on the membrane of human lymphocytes (Kourilsky *et al.*, 1972) and of Ig determinants on lymphocytes (Taylor *et al.*, 1971). HL-A antigens on cell surfaces renew continuously since cells coated with HL-A alloantisera lose their susceptibility to complement-dependent lysis after incubation for some hours at 37°C (Miyajima *et al.*, 1972). The refractoriness of sensitized cells to lysis is not a consequence of the modulation phenomenon described by Old *et al.* (1968) for thymus leukemia antigens since the addition of fresh aliquots of the antiserum used for sensitization kills the target cells. Actually, active turnover of some areas of the cell membrane is suggested by the fact that inhibitors of cell metabolism such as actinomycin D and puromycin inhibit the escape of antibody-coated cells from sensitization. It has not yet been established whether the lymphocytes coated with antibody catabolize the HL-A antibody thereby minimizing complement fixation, or release antibodies or antigen–antibody complexes from their membranes.

IV. CELL SURFACE EXPRESSION OF HL-A ANTIGENS DURING THE GROWTH CYCLE

The composition of the cell membrane, as well as the turnover rate of its components, changes during the cell growth cycle (Warren and Glick, 1968), as revealed by cell surface markers such as blood groups H and AB (Kuhns and Bramson, 1968; Kuhns *et al.*, 1969) and virus receptors or the ability of a cell to accommodate attached virus particles on its surface (Cikes, 1970; Lerner *et al.*, 1971). Interest in the cell surface expression of histocompatibility antigens during the growth cycle is both theoretical and practical. Aside from accumulating knowledge of the metabolism of histocompatibility antigen, it is important to determine whether variability of the HL-A typing (Rogentine and Gerber, 1969; Ferrone and Pellegrino, unpublished observations) result from technical reasons or from variable expressions of HL-A antigens during the cell growth cycle. Furthermore, since cultured cells are a major source from which soluble histocompatibility antigens are extracted, thorough knowledge of the expression of these antigens during the cell growth cycle determines experimental conditions for optimal yields.

After the first report by Bjaring *et al.* (1969) that histocompatibility antigens in mouse lymphoma varied cyclically in tissue cultures, Cikes and Friberg (1971) reported differential expression of H-2 surface antigens during the growth cycle of murine lymphoma cells (JVS-V-9) induced by Moloney leukemia virus. H-2 antigens were maximally expressed during the G_1 period of the cell cycle, as judged by the sensitivity of the cells in the lymphocytotoxic test, by their absorbing capacities as well as by indirect immunofluorescence tests. Results were similar when cultured human lymphoid cells derived from Burkitt lymphoma were reacted with polyspecific anti-HL-A alloantisera in an indirect immunofluorescence test (Cikes, 1971). However, when cultured lymphoid cells WIL_2 derived from a donor free of malignancy were examined (Ferrone et al., 1972b; Pellegrino et al., 1972c), their sensitivities to operationally-monospecific anti-HL-A alloantisera were unchanged throughout the cell cycle, both when human or rabbit (Fig. 5) serum were used as sources of complement (Ferrone et al., 1972b). Thus, the expression of HL-A determinants and of antigenic determinants against which the natural antibodies present in rabbit complement are directed appears constant throughout the cell cycle. In addition, sensitivity of the cell membrane to the lytic action of complement remains equal throughout. Specifically, the uptake of labeled complement components by cells coated with anti-HL-A antibodies do not vary significantly during the cell growth cycle (Ferrone et al., 1972b). The percentage of antigen-positive cells in the indirect immunofluorescence test seems to be the same in G_1 and S phases, although quantitation is difficult with this technique because the

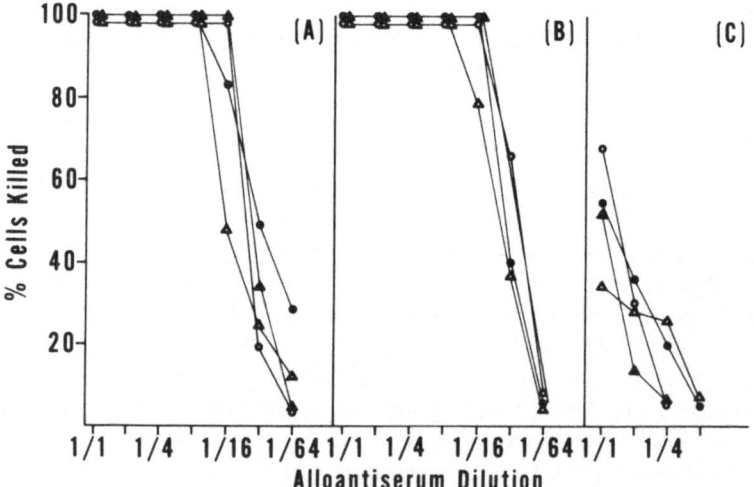

Figure 5. Relationship between phases of the growth cycle and susceptibility to lysis of cultured human lymphoid cells WIL_2 by HL-A alloantisera and complement. The source of complement is a mixture of fresh rabbit and human sera. (A) Alloantiserum Pinquette (anti HL-A2), (B) alloantiserum Victor (anti-HL-A5), (C) alloantiserum Gillespie (anti-HL-A1). (●————●) log phase; (▲————▲) resting phase; (○————○) G_1 phase; (△————△) S phase.

number and intensity of fluorescent patches on positive cells vary greatly (Pellegrino *et al.,* 1972e). The absorbing capacity of the cells alters during the cell cycle, as cells in G_1 phase absorb less than half the amount of HL-A antisera as those in S phase and slightly more than cells in G_0 (Fig. 6) (Pellegrino *et al.,* 1972e). However, if these values are corrected for volume changes, then there is essentially an equal number of determinants available to react with HL-A antibodies per cell volume during the different phases of the growth cycle. These different behaviors of normal cells and tumor cells do not reflect a technical artifact: results similar to those described by Cikes (1971) and by Karb and Goldstein (1971) were obtained in this laboratory, when the same techniques utilized for human cultured lymphoid cells derived from a donor free of malignancy were applied to investigate the cell surface expression of H-2 antigens on cultured leukemia cells (Götze *et al.,* 1972b). It is indeed possible that the differential expression of histocompatibility antigens on tumor cells during the growth cycle may reflect a specific defect of these cells in the regulation of either synthesis or expression of cell surface antigen. In this regard, it has been reported that methylcholanthrene- and virus-induced tumor cells and TL(+) leukemia cells in mice show an inverse relationship between the quantitative expressions of tumor-specific cell surface antigens and H-2 histocompatibility antigens (Boyse *et al.,* 1967; Haywood and McKhann, 1971; Ting and Herberman, 1971). Alternatively, should histocompatibility antigens be involved in cellular growth regulation, their cyclic fluctuations may denote a disturbed or

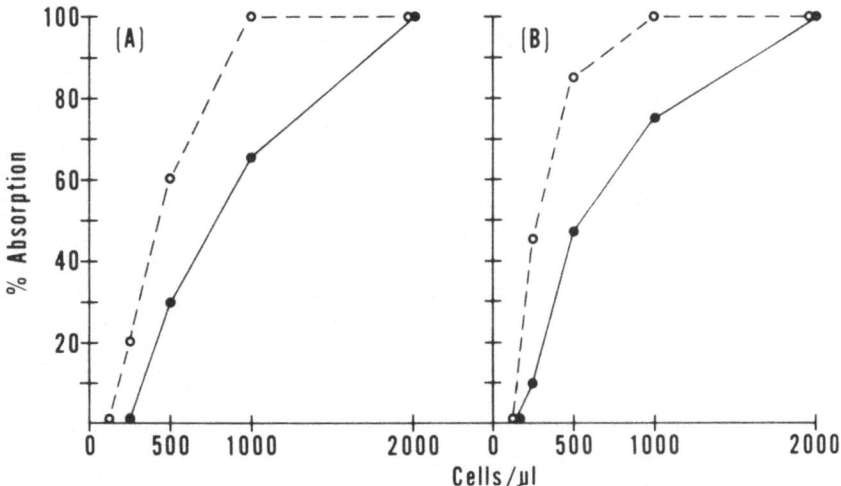

Figure 6. Influence of growth phase on absorbing capacity of nonsynchronized cultured cells. S phase (o---o); G_1 phase (●————●). The alloantisera used for absorption were (A) Perry (anti-HL-A5) and (B) Pena (anti-HL-A2).

defective feedback mechanism, normally controlled by histocompatibility antigens, but nonresponse in tumor cells. This could lead to an accumulation of histocompatibility antigens during log phase.

Although the cell surface expression of HL-A antigens on cultured cells derived from donors free of lymphoid malignancy does not change during the cell cycle, the yield of soluble HL-A antigen from cultured cells as judged by the amount of extractable protein and by the specific serologic activity of the preparation varies during the different phases of cell growth (Table II). Thus, preparations from cultures in the late log phase or in resting phase are more active than those in early log phase (Pellegrino *et al.*, 1972*c*). When the cells are kept in resting phase for several days, a marked increase in the dead cells and a dramatic decrease in the immunologic potency of the soluble antigen is observed. Density of HL-A determinants apparently does not contribute to the yield *per se*, since these determinants remain essentially equal throughout the cell growth cycle (Ferrone *et al.*, 1972*b*; Pellegrino *et al.*, 1972*e*). The viability of the cells cannot account for the difference in antigen yield between cultures in early log phase and those in resting phase, since the percentage of dead cells, as determined by trypan blue uptake, was negligible in both cases. On the contrary, the marked increase of dead cells in the cultures kept in resting phase for several days can, at least in part, cause a reduction in the amount of HL-A antigens extracted; dead cells are a poor antigenic source whenever 3 M KCl is utilized for extraction (Reisfeld *et al.*, 1971).

Serological data suggest that not all histocompatibility determinants on the cell surface are equally reactive with alloantibody, as some are apparently masked. Thus, treatment of human normal lymphocytes with enzymes (Grothaus *et al.*, 1971*b*; Gibofsky and Terasaki, 1972) or with sulfhydryl compounds (Sirchia and Ferrone, 1970) renders the cells more reactive in the cytotoxic reaction *in vitro*. Variation in the amount of "masking substance," e.g., mucopolysaccharide, and/or in its spatial relationship on the cell surface with HL-A antigens might make the latter more or less available to the extraction procedure. The composition of the cell membrane changes, and the turnover of its components is low in log phase and high in resting phase of the cell growth cycle (Warren and Glick, 1968). Cell metabolism may also exert an influence, since yields of soluble HL-A antigens from the spent medium of cultures at different stages of the cell growth cycle are invariable (Pellegrino *et al.*, 1972*c*). In this case, the HL-A determinants are attached to nonmetabolizing cell fragments (Pellegrino *et al.*, 1972*g*). However, it should be pointed out that the fluctuating yields of soluble HL-A antigens from cultured cells may depend on other variables such as the possible presence of pools of HL-A antigens inside the cells. If so, these pools may vary in size or availability during the cell growth cycle.

The continuous expression of HL-A antigens throughout the growth cycle of cultured cells and their persistence on cells after several years of tissue culture suggest that these antigens are either a part of the cytoarchitecture *per se* or play

Table II. Solubilization of HL-A Antigens from Cultured Lymphoid Cells (WIL$_2$) in Different Stages of Cell Growth

Cells/ml (×10^6)	Cell growth stage	AD$_{50}$ units[a]		Protein, mg (10^9 cells)	ID$_{50}$ units[b]		HL-A2 specificity ratio[c]	% Recovery[d]	
		HL-A2	HL-A5		HL-A2	HL-A5		HL-A2	HL-A5
0.80	early log	2.0×10^6	1.1×10^6	50	2.5×10^5	1.0×10^5	100	12.5	9
1.90	late log	1.0×10^6	0.6×10^6	20	1.0×10^6	0.5×10^6	190	100	83
2.46	resting	1.0×10^6	0.6×10^6	20	1.0×10^6	0.5×10^6	200	100	83
1.8[e]	late resting	6.2×10^6	3.7×10^5	19	3.1×10^4	4.0×10^3	50	5	1

[a] AD$_{50}$ (number of cells required to reduce by 50% the lymphocytotoxic activity of HL-A alloantisera) per 10^9 cells.

[b] Number of ID$_{50}$ (µg of soluble HL-A alloantigen required to halve the cytotoxicity of HL-A alloantisera per mg protein) obtained from 10^9 viable cells.

[c] Ratio between the reciprocal of amount of the soluble antigen inhibiting the indifferent antiserum Cutten (anti-HL-A7) and that required for the inhibition of the homologous antiserum Eriksson (anti-HL-A2).

[d] Recovery is equal to (ID$_{50}$/AD$_{50}$)×100 and represents the percent of the absorbing capacity of cells recovered as soluble antigen.

[e] In the late resting phase there was 50% dead cells whereas in all other stages there was full cell viability.

an important role in the mediation of transport and contact phenomena which are crucial to cell survival. This view is reinforced by the observation that human diploid fibroblasts, which have a finite life span *in vitro*, show metabolic, functional, and morpologic changes during the senescence process, but retain the cell surface expression of HL-A antigens practically unchanged throughout their *in vitro* lifetime (Brautbar *et al.*, 1972*a,b*). Furthermore, the attempts to produce variants of murine tumor cells which had completely lost their H-2 determinants have been unsuccessful (Hellström and Möller, 1965).

V. INCREASED REACTIVITY OF LYMPHOCYTES

Human peripheral lymphocytes can be rendered more reactive in the lymphocytotoxic reaction *in vitro* by treatment with enzymes or sulfhydryl compounds such as that used in the manifestation of reactions with red cells (Morton and Pickles, 1947; Unger, 1951; Yachnin *et al.*, 1961; Sirchia *et al.*, 1965; Mittal *et al.*, 1968; Mittal *et al.*, 1969; Sirchia and Ferrone, 1970; Yunis *et al.*, 1970; Grothaus *et al.*, 1971*b*; Mercuriali *et al.*, 1971; Gibofsky and Terasaki, 1972). Following such treatment, the increased reactivity of altered lymphocytes is indicated by the higher titer of cytotoxic alloantisera and the higher percentage of "killed" cells in cytotoxic reactions. The frequency of reactivity of operationally-monospecific HL-A alloantisera with a panel of treated lymphocytes is increased. In some cases, these extra positive reactions are due to cross-reacting antibodies that are CYNAP for normal lymphocytes (Mercuriali *et al.*, 1971; Braun *et al.*, 1972), whereas in other instances they reflect the activity of weak antibodies which contaminate the operationally-monospecific HL-A alloantisera and are present in amounts which are sublytic for normal lymphocytes. The increased reactivity of treated lymphocytes is also indicated by the finding that the lymphocytotoxic reaction can be accomplished in a shorter time (Mittal *et al.*, 1969; Mercuriali *et al.*, 1971) with less complement than necessary

Table III. Lysis of Normal and AET-Treated Lymphocytes from the
Same Subject at Different Concentrations of Human
Complement[a]

Complement (vol)	10	8	6	4	3	2	1	0
Hanks (vol)	0	2	4	6	7	8	9	10
Normal lymphocytes	95	95	95	60	0[b]	0	0	0
AET-treated lymphocytes	95	95	95	95	95	50	0	0

[a] Lymphocytes were sensitized with HL-A alloantisera. Numbers indicate the percentage of stained cells.

[b] 0 = negative reaction.

for the reaction with untreated cells (Sirchia and Ferrone, 1970; Mercuriali *et al.*, 1971) (Table III). Finally, fresh human serum, which is a poor source of complement when reacted with normal lymphocytes, is much more effective with treated cells (Sirchia and Ferrone, 1970; Mercuriali *et al.*, 1971). Studies by transmission and scanning electron microscopy revealed a morphological basis for the increased reactivity of AET-treated lymphocytes exposed to anti-HL-A antibodies and complement in the lymphocytotoxic test (Lambertenghi-Deliliers *et al.*, 1971). Thus, the alterations of AET-treated lymphocytes exposed to the action of anti-HL-A antibodies and complement are pronounced on single cells and affect a large proportion of the cell population. The scanning electron microscope revealed that a large number of AET-treated lymphocytes treated with anti-HL-A antibodies and complement were clumped to such an extent that their surface was hidden by amorphous materials, making evaluation of their abnormalities quite difficult. Nonclumped cells showed alterations ranging from craters and cracking on the surface to gross deformation and collapse of the cell. Analysis by transmission electron microscopy revealed damage from anti-HL-A antibodies and complement that produced alterations of the cell membrane, cytoplasm, and nucleus, including chromatin condensation, appearance of intranuclear fibers, dilation of the perinuclear space, absence of ribosomes and of mitochondria, presence of small electron-dense bodies close to the membranes, and fragmentation of the cytoplasmic membrane.

Although the increased sensitivity of either enzyme- or sulfhydryl-compound-treated cells in the cytotoxic test may be shown with antisera directed against various specificities, the HL-A antigens of the two segregant series seem to reach different levels of sensitivity. In fact, by treatment with trypsin, antigens of the second segregant series were unmasked *in vitro* more frequently than those of the first series (Gibofsky and Terasaki, 1972). The lesion caused by altering compounds is reversible; i.e., lymphocytes treated with neuraminidase lose their increased reactivity in the cytotoxic test after 2–6 days in tissue culture (Grothaus *et al.*, 1971*b*).

Relatively little is known about the mechanism by which the altering compounds cause the increased reactivity of lymphocytes in the cytotoxic test, since cells treated with neuraminidase, trypsin (Fig, 7), or AET (Ferrone and Pellegrino, unpublished results) do not possess greater absorbing capacity than unmasked cells. Therefore, the abnormal reactivity of treated lymphocytes is caused by increased sensitivity of altered membrane to the lytic action of complement similar to that observed on human red cells treated with AET (Sirchia and Dacie, 1967). This explains the increased number of positive reactions observed with treated lymphocytes. In the lymphocytotoxic reaction, complement plays a crucial role. Any factor lowering the ratio of complement to antigen and/or antibody, such as an excessive number of target cells or anti-complementary activity of the reaction mixture, etc., can prevent lysis of the lymphocytes (Ferrone *et al.*, 1967). Consequently, increase in this ratio through

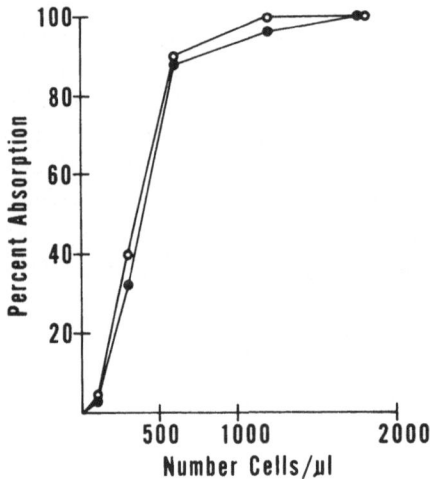

Figure 7. Absorbing capacity of normal (•————•) and trypsin-treated (o-----o) cultured human lymphoid cells WIL₂ (HL-A1,2,5 Te57) for alloantiserum Pinquette (anti-HL-A2).

a rise in sensitivity of the cell membrane makes false negative results less likely to occur.

Treated human lymphocytes may be important to transplantation immunology; for example, it has been shown that hyperacute rejection of a renal transplant resulted when the transplant recipient's serum contained cytotoxic antibodies directed against the donor's lymphocytes (Terasaki *et al.,* 1965; Kissmeyer-Nielsen *et al.,* 1966; Patel and Terasaki, 1969). While studying hyperacute rejection of a kidney transplant, Braun *et al.* (1972) found that serum from the graft recipient contained cytotoxic antibodies against the donor's lymphocytes which were, however, only detectable after trypinization of the cells. The use of lymphocytes rendered more reactive in the cytotoxic test then may improve the chances to detect positive cross-matches.

VI. SEROLOGIC EVALUATION OF SOLUBLE HL-A ANTIGENS

In recent years, a growing interest in soluble HL-A antigens has arisen from the finding of Medawar (1963) that murine, nonparticulate, subcellular, antigenic preparations are more favorable for the induction of prolonged allograft survival than intact cells for several reasons: (1) cells tend to produce a sensitization, (2) cells raise the specter of runt disease, and (3) cells are capable of recolonizaton and competition with host cells.

To detect these soluble antigens and to evaluate their immunologic potency *in vitro,* the serological assay has been widely used (Kahan *et al.,* 1968; Mann *et al.,* 1968; Sanderson, 1968; Pellegrino *et al.,* 1972*b,d*). This assay is based on the ability of soluble HL-A antigen to inhibit the cytotoxic potency of operationally-monospecific alloantisera against target cells in the lymphocytotoxic test (Fig. 8). This method is simple, rapid, reprodicible, and sensitive, since amounts of antigen as small as 0.001 µg can be detected. The validity of the test is underscored by the fact that antigenic preparations which are inactive in the serologic assay also fail to elicit production of cytotoxic heteroantibodies (Pellegrino *et al.*, 1972*d*). Of several parameters which have been adopted in an attempt to standardize the serological evaluation of HL-A antigens (Pellegrino *et al.*, 1972*b*), it seems worthwhile to mention two: (1) inhibition dosage (ID_{50}), i.e., the amount of soluble HL-A antigen required to inhibit by 50% the cytotoxicity of an operationally-monospecific alloantiserum directed against an HL-A specificity present on the cell used as source for the extraction of the antigen and (2) specificity ratio (Sanderson, 1968; Kahan *et al.*, 1971), i.e., the ratio between the concentration of antigen required to obtain 50% inhibition of the cytotoxic effect of an alloantiserum directed against an HL-A specificity not present in the phenotype of the antigenic source and the concentration required to inhibit an alloantiserum directed against a determinant present in the phenotype of the antigenic source. Whereas ID_{50} expresses the immunologic potency of the soluble HL-A antigen, the specificity ratio is an expression of its immunologic specificity.

The extensive use of the inhibition assay for the evaluation of soluble HL-A antigens has brought up some interesting problems in HL-A serology. An array

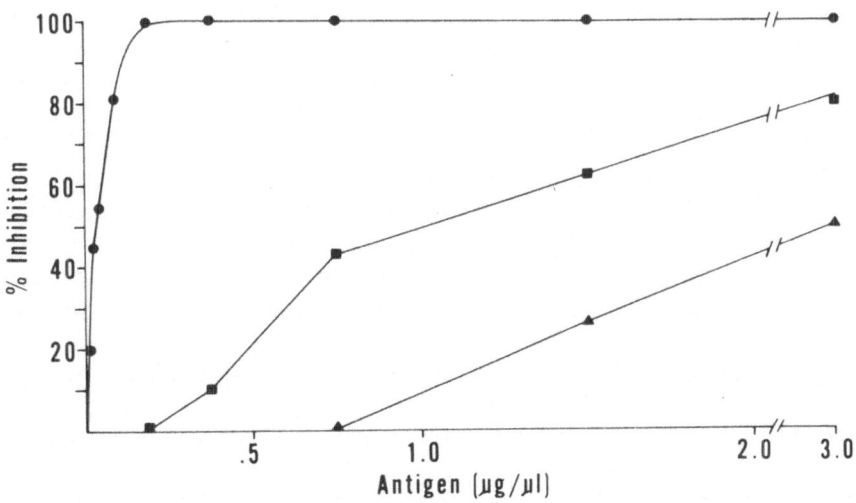

Figure 8. Inhibition of cytotoxic activity of alloantisera TO-11-03 (anti-HL-A2) (●————●); Grubisch, 2-65-0-02-25-01 (anti-HL-A9) (■————■); and D66-6222-IV (anti-HL-A5) (▲————▲) by soluble HL-A antigen RPMI 1788 (HL-A2,10,7,W14). Alloantisera were employed at zero cytotoxic units.

of operationally-monospecific alloantisera directed against HL-A specificity differ in their susceptibility to inhibition by the same preparation of a soluble HL-A alloantigen, even when used at the same functional level and with the same target cells (Pellegrino et al., 1972b). This variability, which does not seem to correlate with the titer of alloantisera, may be caused by the different affinity of the alloantibody for soluble HL-A antigen; i.e., if the antibody has a low affinity for the soluble antigen, the antigen–antibody complex can be readily broken when target cells are added to the reaction mixture, and the antibody thus released can kill the cells, resulting in a decrease of ID_{50}. This hypothesis is supported by the observation that cytotoxic alloantisera which kill a low percentage of target cells in a two-stage cytotoxic procedure were inhibited by a larger amount of soluble alloantigen in the blocking test. However, another possible mechanism underlying this phenomenon may be additional antibodies directed against different HL-A determinants present at a sublytic concentration in operationally-monospecific alloantisera. Since synergism of several HL-A antibodies with differing specificities has been shown in the cytotoxic reaction (Ivascová et al., 1969; Svejgaard, 1969), less antigen is necessary to block the cytotoxic antibody from lysing target cells, thus resulting in lower ID_{50} values. An alternative explanation for the variable efficiency of HL-A alloantisera in the blocking test is the interaction of various components of human sera (aside from HL-A alloantibodies) with rabbit complement; in fact, human and rabbit complement components are incompatible (Cooper, N.R., unpublished observations) and human IgM inhibits natural rabbit antibodies (Herberman, 1970) which play a crucial role in the lymphocytotoxic reaction (Ferrone et al., 1971b). The different level of residual human complement components and the variable amount of IgM present in HL-A alloantisera can differently influence the lymphocytotoxic test, thus affecting the serological detection of soluble HL-A alloantigens.

The target cell can greatly influence the values of ID_{50} in several ways (Etheredge et al., 1971; Kahan et al., 1971; Ferrone et al., 1972d; Pellegrino et al., 1972b,d). It is known that there is quantitative variation in the cytotoxic effect of operationally-monospecific alloantisera against target lymphocytes from different individuals bearing the same HL-A specificity. The reason for this variability has not yet been determined; however, it might reflect a difference in the number of antigen determinants present on the cell surface. Thus, when the density of HL-A determinants was evaluated on the peripheral lymphocytes from different subjects, a twofold variation was observed in the number of antigenic sites available to react with antibodies (Pellegrino et al., 1972a). Decreased numbers of antigenic receptors on the cells caused a marked increase in the amount of antibody needed to form a given number of cells coated by antibody and C1 (Linscott, 1970). Additional sources of target-cell variability might be (1) qualitative differences of HL-A antigenic determinants, (2) interference of some HL-A specificities with the expression of others, and (3) differences in sensitivity of the cell membrane to the lytic action of complement or (4) in the amount or relationship with HL-A determinants of the antigen against which the natural antibodies present in the rabbit complement are directed. Whatever the mechanism of the different reactivities of various target cells against one operationally-monospecific alloantiserum, it causes significant variation in ID_{50} values. Thus, if the titer of the alloantiserum with a given target cell is high (i.e., the amount of antibody required to cause the cytotoxic effect on the target cell is low), with the sera being used at the 95%-lytic end point, then the amount of antibody present in the reaction mixture is low. Consequently, the quantity of soluble antigen required to block the antibody is also comparatively low. The target cells also seem to affect the value of ID_{50} through other means; although some alloantisera display equivalent titers with different target cells bearing the same HL-A specificity, the specific combination of alloantisera and target cells can influence ID_{50} values. This observation may possibly reflect greater avidity of the alloantibody for the cell-bound antigen than for the soluble antigen, or alternatively indicate a latent heterospecificity of the alloantisera.

Soluble HL-A antigens, when used at relatively high concentrations, can inhibit the cytotoxic activity of operationally-monospecific, indifferent alloantisera, i.e., sera directed against HL-A determinants not present and not cross-reacting with those detected on the cells used as a source for antigen extraction. As already mentioned, the ratio between the amount of antigen required to obtain 50% inhibition of the cytotoxic effect of an indifferent antiserum and the amount required to inhibit an alloantiserum directed against an HL-A specificity present in the phenotype of the antigen source is the specificity ratio and is considered a good measure of immunologic specificity of soluble HL-A antigen. The reason why the cytotoxic activity of indifferent antisera is inhibited by soluble HL-A antigens remains undetermined. Although this could simply be an example of an expression of a nonimmunological interaction, other more interesting explanations may be considered. For example, highly-concentrated antigenic preparations might become anticomplementary. Since the cytotoxic reaction is complement-dependent, inhibition of the indifferent serum could be caused not by a reaction of the soluble antigen with the cytotoxic alloantiserum, but by a decreased activity of rabbit complement for an interaction of soluble antigen with complement components and natural antibodies present in rabbit serum. The antigenic preparation could interfere with the absorption of alloantibody on the target cells; many components have been reported to inhibit the lymphocytotoxic reaction, probably because antigenic sites on the target cells become covered (Hirata and Terasaki, 1972). However, the mechanisms of the inhibition seem to be different in the two blocking tests. In fact, due to binding and covering of antigenic sites on the lymphocytes, inhibition of the different compounds tested becomes much more effective after they are incubated with target cells rather than with alloantibody. On the other hand, since these antigens interact with antibody, the inhibition of indifferent sera by soluble HL-A antigens is equally effective whether they are incubated with target cells or alloantisera (Pellegrino *et al.*, 1972*d*). Soluble HL-A antigens may fail to interact with target cells as suggested by the observation that lymphocytes lacking an HL-A specificity, e.g., HL-A3, do not acquire any sensitivity to anti-HL-A3 in the lymphocytotoxic reaction (Mittal, Ferrone, and Pellegrino, unpublished results) when incubated with large amounts of soluble HL-A3 antigen. Cross-reactivity is very common in the HL-A system (Dausset *et al.*, 1968*b*; Svejgaard and Kissmeyer-Nielsen, 1968; Mittal and Terasaki, 1972; Mittal *et al.*, 1972*a*; Pellegrino *et al.*, 1972*f*) and may be another explanation. Thus, an indifferent serum could be inhibited if the antigenic preparation shares determinants in common with the HL-A specificity against which the alloantibody is directed. Finally, inhibition of the indifferent alloantiserum could be an expression of HL-A determinants present in the antigenic preparation and recognized by the alloantiserum but not by typing of the cell source (Kahan *et al.*, 1968; Mann and Fahey, 1971*a*).

VII. CROSS-REACTIVITY

Cross-reactivity is a well-known phenomenon within the ABO system. Antibodies in some group-O sera cross-react with the blood-group antigens A and B; some antibodies absorbed from group-O sera by either A or B erythrocytes and subsequently recovered by elution can agglutinate both A and B cells. The mechanism of cross-reactivity is unknown, and many hypotheses have been advanced to explain it (Race and Sanger, 1958). Cross-reactivity occurs also within the HL-A system as indicated by *in vitro* and *in vivo* experiments (Table IV). Extensive serological investigations have shown that human lymphocytes (Svejgaard and Kissmeyer-Nielsen, 1968; Thorsby *et al.*, 1970), human cultured lymphoid cells (Pellegrino *et al.*, 1972*f*), or platelets (Dausset *et al.*, 1968*b*; Svejgaard and Kissmeyer-Nielsen, 1968; Colombani *et al.*, 1970; Mittal and

Table IV. Schematic Representation of Cross-Reactivity Among HL-A Specificities*

First segregant series	HL-A1, HL-A3, HL-A10, HL-A11, Te59 (W32), Te63 (W29), Te66 (W31)
	HL-A2, HL-A9, Te40 (W28)
Second segregant series	HL-A5, HL-A12, Te50 (W5), Te55 (W15), Te57 (W17), Te58 (W18)
	HL-A7, HL-A13, Te51 (W22), Te52 (W27), Te60 (W10)
	HL-A8, Te54 (W14)

*Cross-reactivity may occur among all specificities within one segregant series.

Teraski, 1972, Mittal *et al.*, 1972*a*) bearing a given HL-A specificity can absorb from operationally-monospecific alloantisera antibodies to other HL-A determinants, even though these antibodies cannot be detected by direct cytotoxic tests. Simiarly, HL-A antigens solubilized from human cultured lymphoid cells can specifically inhibit operationally-monospecific anti-HL-A alloantisera directed against determinants cross-reacting with those present 0n the cells used for the extraction (Ferrone *et al.*, 1972*d*). In this case, the amount of soluble HL-A antigen is greater than that required to inhibit an homologous HL-A alloantiserum, but significantly less than that necessary to inhibit indifferent antisera (Table V). Multiparous women (Thorsby *et al.*, 1970) or subjects immunized by transfusions (Legrand *et al.*, 1971; Thorsby and Kissmeyer-Nielsen, 1970) or skin allografts (Legrand *et al.*, 1971) may produce antibodies against antigens not present on the husband's or donor's cells, but against cross-reacting HL-A specificities. Similar observations were made in this laboraoty in experiments with heteroimmunization. For example, rabbits immunized with soluble HL-A antigens (HL-A2,10,7, W14) produced cytotoxic antibodies correlating with HL-A determinants present on the soluble immunogen and antibodies directed against cross-reacting specificities as well (Ferrone *et al.*, 1972*e*). This cross-reactivity seems to be of clinical relevance since skin grafts (Dausset *et al.*, 1970; Dausset, 1971) and kidney transplants (Dausset, 1971) have longer survivals when incompatibility is within a group of cross-reacting antigens rather than between different groups.

The data thus far clearly indicate that cross-reactivity occurs only between allelic gene products of a single HL-A segregant series, and not between those of the two different series (Svejgaard and Kissmeyer-Nielsen, 1968; Colombani *et al.*, 1970; Mittal and Terasaki, 1972). According to some investigators, it is possible to identify within each segregant series, groups or families of cross-reacting HL-A specificities (Colombani *et al.*, 1970; Dausset and Hors, 1971), while others have found that cross-reacting groups do not form isolated clusters but are interconnected (Mittal and Terasaki, 1972). Cross-reactivity may be unidirectional or bidirectional, and is exhibited only by some antisera of a given specificity as well as only by some cells possessing cross-reacting antigens (Colombani *et al.*, 1970; Dausset, 1971; Ferrone *et al.*, 1972*d*; Mittal and Terasaki, 1972; Pellegrino *et al.*, 1972*f*).

The reactivity of cells with cross-reacting antisera does not depend exclusively on the density of HL-A determinants on their surfaces, since in some cases cells with low densities effectively cross-absorb whereas cells with high densities do not. It is tempting to speculate that antigenic determinants considered identical on the basis of serological tests may actually possess subtle structural differences detected by these cross-absorptions. Furthermore, the differences in HL-A phenotype of the cells used for cross-absorption experiments may play a role in cross-reactivity, as different HL-A determinants can interfere to various extents with the absorbing capacity of cells. The importance of spatial distribu-

Table V. ID$_{50}$ ($\mu g/\mu l$) of Soluble HL-A Antigens for Different HL-A Specificities

Soluble HL-A antigens	HL-A specificities								
	First segregant series					Second segregant series			
	HL-A1	HL-A2	HL-A3	HL-A9	HL-A10	HL-A5	HL-A7	HL-A8	W14
127-103[a] RPMI 1788 (HL-A2,10,7, W14)	3.0	0.025	3.0	1.0	1.5	2.5	0.09	1.2	0.15
155-103[a] RPMI 4098 (HL-A3, Te63)	3.0	3.0	0.01	3.0	3.0	3.0	3.0	3.0	3.0
179-103[a] WIL$_2$ (HL-A1,2,5, Te57)	0.2	0.016	1.0	1.0	5.0	0.047	4.8	4.5	5.0
107-103[a] RPMI 7249 (HL-A1,2,7,8)	0.1	0.1	10.0	1.0	10.0	10.0	1.0	0.1	10.0

[a]Each number denotes a single preparation of soluble alloantigen.

tion of HL-A determinants for absorbing capacity has been shown by the fact that cells presenting HL-A determinants governed by genes in *trans* or *cis* position display a different absorbing capacity (Legrand and Dausset, 1971). Conversely, the lack of reactivity with cross-reacting HL-A determinants of some antisera that have the identical HL-A specificities suggests certain heterogeneity of antibody molecules and limited combination of these with cross-reacting antigens.

These data suggest that the serology of the HL-A system is extremely complex, and the delineation of antigens is uncertain. In the study of cross-reactivity, the choice of antibodies and cells used to unravel cross-reactions are of primary importance as they greatly influence the results and may account for the discrepancies among data reported from different laboratories.

Several explanations of cross-reactivity have been given, but they can essentially be summarized as follows: the phenomenon might occur because of structural similarities between several separate HL-A antigens or because some HL-A specificities have antigenic structures in common against which the cross-reacting antibodies are directed. The possibility that cross-reactions are caused by contamination with an antibody of low avidity in the operationally-monospecific alloantisera seems somewhat unlikely, because cross-reactivity does not occur with a variety of groups in a random fashion, but with only specific antigens. In addition, cross-reactivity can be shown when the alloantisera are used at relatively high dilutions, which increase the specificity of the anti-HL-A alloantisera (Ferrone *et al.*, 1972*d*; Pellegrino *et al.*, 1972*f*). The same experiment has shown that the number of cells required to absorb cross-reacting antibodies is significantly higher than that needed for cells bearing the specificity against which the antiserum is directed, suggesting that relatively small numbers of available determinants react with cross-reacting antibodies (Table VI) and might thus account for the incapability of F(ab)$_2$ fragments from cross-reacting antisera to block the activity of homologous alloantisera in the cytotoxic test (Carbonara *et al.*, 1972). The same phenomenon could explain why cells give a CYNAP reaction with most cross-reacting antisera in the direct cytotoxic test. In fact, should the density of antigenic receptors be low, the critical concentration of complement on the cell surface required to effect cell lysis is not reached even with a large excess of antibody and complement. This observation is in agreement with the fact that antisera with a given specificity can react in the direct cytotoxic test with cells bearing a cross-reacting specificity provided that the amount of natural antibodies present in the rabbit complement is increased in the reaction mixture (Ting, Ferrone, and Terasaki, unpublished observations). Similarly, when the reactivity of the cells is increased *in vitro* by treatment with proteolytic enzymes or with the sulfhydryl compound AET, the cells react in the direct cytotoxic test with antisera directed against cross-reacting specificities (Mercuriali *et al.*, 1971; Braun *et al.*, 1972).

Table VI. AD_{50}[a] of Human Cultured Lymphoid Cells for Different HL-A Specificities

Cells	HL-A phenotype[b]	First segregant series					Second segregant series			
		HL-A1	HL-A2	HL-A3	HL-A9	HL-A10	HL-A5	HL-A7	HL-A8	W14
RPMI 1788	2,10,7,W14	50,000	800	50,000	15,000	6,000	50,000	1,800	N.d.[c]	800
RPMI 4098	3,Te63	50,000	50,000	600	50,000	50,000	50,000	50,000	50,000	50,000
RPMI 7249	1,2,7,8	500	800	50,000	N.d.	N.d.	50,000	3,500	N.d.	N.d.
RPMI 6237	2,3,7	50,000	1,000	2,000	18,000	50,000	50,000	400	50,000	50,000
RPMI 8866	2,3,7,12	50,000	500	1,000	24,000	50,000	50,000	400	50,000	50,000
WIL$_2$	1,2,5,Te57	800	400	8,000	3,200	50,000	1,000	50,000	50,000	50,000
PG-1P-11	2,3,7,12	50,000	1,600	1,000	50,000	50,000	20,000	2,400	50,000	50,000
PF-170	3,10,5	50,000	50,000	600	50,000	1,600	1,000	50,000	50,000	50,000
PG-LC-42-F	3,10,5	50,000	50,000	300	50,000	4,000	2,500	50,000	50,000	50,000
PG-1P-7	3,10,5	50,000	50,000	600	50,000	1,600	3,000	50,000	50,000	50,000

[a]Number of cells required to reduce by 50% the cytotoxicity of HL-A alloantisera.
[b]Determined by direct cytotoxicity.
[c]Not done.

HL-A antigens have been shown to cross-react with streptococcal antigens. M1 proteins are able to inhibit the cytotoxicity of histocompatibility-typing sera directed against different HL-A specificities (Hirata and Terasaki, 1970), and human isoimmune antisera can be absorbed by streptococci (Amos, 1966). These data have been confirmed by studying the DNA synthesis of human lymphocytes stimulated by M1 preparations in short-term culture (Pellegrino *et al.*, 1972*h*) (Fig. 9). The M1 stimulation was markedly inhibited by anti-HL-A alloantisera of different specificity (Table VII), probably by a masking of the mitogenic site on the M1 protein in such a way as to prevent interaction between M1 and the specific lymphocyte receptors necessary for induction of the proliferative response. Cross-reactivity between HL-A antigens and M1 protein seems to be unidirectional, since anti-M1 antibodies present in human sera or induced in immunized rabbits do not show any activity against human lympho- cytes in the cytotoxic test (Fox and Peterson, 1970; Hirata *et al.*, 1970). Cross-reactivity between HL-A determinants and bacterial antigens is of great clinical interest and might be a key to understanding susceptibility to some diseases. Antigens shared between man and bacteria might favor the parasite, as the host is unable to respond immunologically against the shared antigens. If this is the case, the polymorphism of the HL-A system might be a safeguard to preserve the human species.

Cross-reactions between antigens within the HL-A system have recently been shown to extend to isoantigens of other species, as reported between rabbits and mice (Abeyounis and Milgrom, 1969) and mice and rats (Sachs *et al.*, 1971). The sharing of antigens between HL-A and ChL-A, the histocompatibility system in chimpanzees, is apparent (Balner *et al.*, 1971). Chimpanzee lympho-

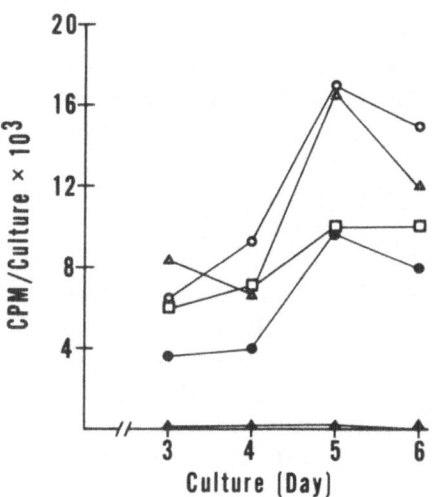

Figure 9. Kinetics and dose effect of M1 stimulation of lymphocyte transformation. (▲———▲) control (●————●)5 mg M1/100 μl culture; (□-------□) 10 mg M1; (△———△) 20 mg M1; (○————○) 40 mg M1.

Table VII. Inhibition of Lymphocyte Transformation by HL-A Alloantisera and Heteroantisera

		Lymphocyte transformation indices						
		Anti-HL-A alloantisera					Anti-HL-A heteroantisera[b]	
M1[a] (μg)	Control	HL-A1	HL-A2	HL-A7	HL-A8	To-2	H1	H2
10	5.3	1.0	0.92	1.0	1.0	1.1	1.0	0.72
20	6.7	2.4	0.90	1.0	1.7	2.0	1.1	0.73

[a]Added per 50,000 target cells L. W. (HL-A3,7).

[b]Rabbit anti-HL-A antiserum prepared against soluble HL-A alloantigen RPMI 1788 (HL-A2,10,7, W14) from 2 different rabbits, H1 and H2.

cytes can be typed with anti-HL-A alloantisera (Shulman et al., 1966; Metzgar and Zmijewski, 1966) and human sera absorbed with chimpanzee cells (Balner et al., 1967). Conversely, sera from chimpanzees immunized by skin grafts (Dorf and Metzgar, 1970) and chimpanzee leukocytes (Metzgar et al., 1965; Dorf and Metzgar, 1970) discriminate clearly when tested against a panel of related or unrelated human subjects. A close similarity was found between chimpanzee and HL-A specificities; chimpanzee alloantisera can specifically detect HL-A1, HL-A11, 4a, and 4b in the human population, and human HL-A1, HL-A11, 4a, and 4b antisera give like reaction patterns with chimpanzee antisera in the chimpanzee population. (Metzgar and Seigler, 1972). Detailed data on this subject are available in the issue of *Transplantation Proceedings* (Vol. 4, No. 1, 1972) which reports the results of the First Workshop on Transplantation Genetics of Primates held in Rijswijk (Netherlands) in September, 1971.

The HL-A system has also been shown to cross-react with the mouse histocompatibility system. Sera from rabbits, immunized with soluble HL-A antigens extracted from human lymphoid cells by 3 M KCl, reacted in the cytotoxic test not only with human lymphocytes but also with murine lymphocytes from different strains (Götze et al., 1972a). Although the same immunogen was used in all the animals, some rabbits produced antibodies reacting with a broad panel of cells from many mouse strains, while others produced antibodies reacting only with cells of certain mouse strains (Table VIII). This variability may also be due to similarities between human and rabbit histocompatibility antigens (Albert et al., 1969). H-2 antigen solubilized from murine lymphoid cells L1210 (H-2^d) by the 3 M KCl method could specifically inhibit the cytotoxic activity of anti-HL-A rabbit heteroantisera with a level of activity like that in the inhibition test with monospecific H-2 alloantisera. The specificity of the reaction is indicated by the lack of inhibitory activity of antigen solubilized

Table VIII. Cytotoxic Reactivity of Sera from Rabbits Immunized with HL-A Antigen Solubilized from Cultured Human Lymphoid Cells RPMI 1788 (HL-A2,10,7, W14) Against Lymphoid Cells of Three Mouse Strains

Rabbit No.	Antigen[a]	Adjuvant[b]	Route[c]	Cytotoxic activity[d] of rabbit anti-HL-A sera against			
				Human lymphocytes	Mouse spleen cells		
					B10/D2	B10/BR	C_{57} Bl/10
8095	10^9 cells	CFA	FP	1:16000	1:25	1:32	1:32
8103	saa	–	IV	1:32	1:32	1:4	1:32
8101	saa	–	PL	1:64	1:4	1:2	n.t.[e]
8099	saa	CFA	PL	1:128	1:4	1:2	1:2
8633	saa	P(UA)	PL	1:8	1:4	1:1	1:4
8092	saa	P(UA)	FP	1:128	1:8	1:4	n.t.
7666	saa	CFA	FP	1:64	1:4	1:2	n.t.
8634	saa	–	FP	1:8	1:4	1:1	0
8094	10^9 cells	CFA	FP	1:16000	1:32	–	n.t.
8398	saa	–	PL	1:32	1:6	0	1:10
7667	saa	CFA	FP	1:512	1:12	0	1:8
8098	saa	CFA	PL	1:64	1:8	0	0
8635	saa	–	FP	1:2	0	0	0
8632	saa	P(UA)	PL	1:32	1:4	0	
7325	sia	–	PL	0	0	0	n.t.
8114	sia	CFA	PL	0	0	0	n.t.
7327	FCS	CFA	PL	0	0	0	n.t.
7328	FCS	CFA	FP	0	0	0	n.t.

[a] Cells:cultured human lymphoid cells RPMI 1788; saa = serologic active antigen; sia = serologic inactive antigen; FCS = 0.2 ml fetal calf serum dil. 1:5.
[b] CFA = complete Freund's adjuvant; P(UA) = polyuridine–polyadenin.
[c] FP = foot pad; IV = intravenous; PL = popliteal lymph node.
[d] Titers of the serum five weeks after the antigen injection.
[e] n.t. = not tested.

from murine lymphoid cells which do not react with the immune rabbit serum either in the direct cytotoxic test or in the absorption test. These results appear to contrast only with the findings by Einstein *et al.* (1971*a*), who could not show any activity in the lymphocytotoxic test of sera from rabbits immunized with partially-purified, papain-solubilized cell membrane components bearing HL-A activity against murine lymphoid cells. The cultured lymphoid cells used as a source for extraction of soluble HL-A antigen had a different phenotype from those used in the experiments of Einstein *et al.* (1971*a*) and the immune rabbit sera were tested only against cells of one mouse strain. The specific cross-reactivity between HL-A and H-2 could very well explain the negative findings by Einstein *et al.* (1971*a*).

Cross-reactivity between the HL-A and H-2 systems cannot be tested by reacting operationally-monospecific anti-HL-A alloantisera against murine lymphoid cells because of the high, nonspecific cytotoxic titer of human sera against murine cells. When human sera from 8 healthy subjects were tested against murine spleen cells from 3 strains with different H-2 type, the nonspecific cytotoxic titers ranged between 1:100 and 1:500. Thus, the absorbing capacities of murine lymphoid cells for operationally-monospecific alloantisera directed against different HL-A specificities were evaluated. Cultured murine lymphoid cells L1210 (H-2^d) and splenic lymphocytes from 4 mouse strains with different H-2 type seem to be able to absorb specifically some anti-HL-A alloantisera. Furthermore, antigen solubilized from cultured murine lymphoid cells L1210 (H-2^d) can specifically inhibit HL-A alloantisera directed against the specificities HL-A1,3, and 5, but not against the specificities HL-A2,9,7, and 8. Conversely, H-2 monospecific alloantisera are active in the cytotoxic test against human lymphocytes and are absorbed by cultured human lymphoid cells with a different HL-A phenotype. The specificity of these reactions is under investigation.

Study of the cross-reactivity between HL-A system and histocompatibility systems of other species is of both theoretical and practical interest, as it may provide insight into the phylogeny of histocompatibility antigens in many species. With this knowledge, animals can be selected for the production of heterologous antisera that are specific for HL-A alloantigenic determinants, and HL-A antisera can be acquired without resorting to the potentially hazardous isoimmunization of human volunteers. This approach is under investigation in our laboratory. Based on the knowledge of cross-reactivity of human and murine histocompatibility system, mice from different strains have been selected for immunization with soluble HL-A alloantigen extracted from cultured lymphoid cells RPMI 1788 with the phenotype HL-A2,10,7, W14. Preliminary results suggest that the strain B10/D2 produces anti-HL-A antibodies of more restricted specificity than the strain B10/BR. More complete knowledge of cross-reactions of histocompatibility antigens from different species may be of great help in selecting donors of xenografts from other species for transplantation into humans.

VIII. ANTIBODIES

Most anti-HL-A antisera are obtained from women with a history of multiple pregnancies or from individuals having received multiple blood transfusions. In some cases, immunization of human volunteers with skin grafts or buffy coats has been performed and has occasionally yielded antibodies of rarer specificities. However, these antisera are usually of low titer and in limited supply. The availability of suitable typing sera is limited by the low incidence of lymphocytotoxic antibody among pregnant women, i.e., about 20% (Ferrone et al., 1968). Only one out of 517 sera from pregnant women is monospecific (van der Weerdt et al., 1970). Moreover, lymphocytotoxic antibodies tend to persist for a short time in the circulation so that only a few bleedings can be performed. In the case of immunization of healthy subjects, ethical aspects must be emphasized; sensitization of human volunteers to strong transplantation antigens might jeopardize the success of subsequent allografts if required. In addition, there is always the problem of introducing infections, particularly infectious hepatitis.

To overcome these problems, alternative nonhuman sources of antisera are sought for production of heteroantibodies by immunizing different species with whole human cells or with soluble HL-A antigens. HL-A antibodies produced in other species may have a higher resolution capacity than the average human antiserum (van Rood et al., 1972). In fact, in man, cellular immunity may be innate against all but one's own HL-A antigens which, in turn, may "confuse" the production of anti-HL-A antibodies during the immunization process.

HL-A antigens solubilized from lymphoid cells are used as immunogen for the production of cytotoxic heteroantisera. The first attempts have been rather discouraging as only species-specific antibodies were obtained even after absorption (Batchelor, 1969). Recent results, however, seem to be much more promising. Einstein et al. (1971b) produced cytotoxic antibodies in rabbits immunized with papain-solubilized human lymphoid membrane components bearing HL-A antigens. No correlation of cytotoxic activity with the HL-A type of normal random donor cells was noted for the unabsorbed antisera. However, these heteroantisera acquired correlation with HL-A specificities after absorption with cultured human lymphoid cells, although cytotoxic antibody titers decreased two orders of magnitude. In our laboratory, an extensive program is in progress to evaluate production of anti-HL-A heteroantisera by immunizing different species with soluble HL-A alloantigen extracted from human cultured lymphoid cells by the 3 M KCl method.

Rabbits were injected with HL-A antigens solubilized from cell line RPMI 1788 (HL-A2,10,7, W14) with the schedules reported in Table IX (Ferrone et al., 1972e). These HL-A antigens appeared immunogenic also when injected intravenously without adjuvant. No marked differences in titer or in specificity of cytotoxic antibodies present in the sera from rabbits immunized with differ-

Table IX. Immunization Schedule of 35 Rabbits with HL-A Antigen
Solubilized from Cultured Lymphoid Cells RPMI 1788
(HL-A2,10,7,W14)

Antigen dose (mg protein)	Route	Adjuvant
1.0	Intravenous	None
1.0	Foot pad	None P(UA)[a] CFA[b]
0.1	Popliteal lymph node	None P(UA) CFA

[a] Polyuridine–polyadenine

[b] Complete Freund's adjuvant

ent schedules were detected. However, when antigen was administered in the foot pad without adjuvant, the titer of antibodies was lower, indicating the importance of the route of immunization in inducing cytotoxic antibodies (Fig. 10). The specificity of the antibodies was studied by testing the serum from each bleeding, undiluted or at several dilutions, against a panel of at least 80 unrelated donors. Although most of the sera contained multiple anti-HL-A antibodies, the specificities of the cytotoxic antibodies produced by immunized rabbits correlated closely with HL-A determinants present on the soluble HL-A alloantigen used for immunization. Some antisera, however, also contained antibodies against determinants not present in the immunogen. The occurrence of these additional antibodies can be explained, at least in part, by the known cross-reactivity of HL-A determinants. In our experiments the possibility has to be considered that immunization of rabbits with soluble HL-A antigens also may increase the titer of rabbit natural antibodies cross-reacting with HL-A determinants.

In order to obtain monospecific HL-A antisera from rabbit heteroantisera, four approaches have been attempted: (1) dilution of immune rabbit sera, (2) absorption of immune rabbit sera with cultured human lymphoid cells, (3) decrease of the sensitivity of the test by using a poor source of complement (i.e., fresh human serum), and (4) elution from murine cultured lymphoid cells used for absorptions of immune rabbit HL-A antisera (Ferrone *et al.*, 1972*f*).

When sera obtained from rabbits at different stages of the immunization procedure were tested at several dilutions against a panel of human lymphocytes, 27 out of 672 samples became monospecific; some of these sera are listed in Table X. In addition, 11 diluted immune rabbit sera were correlated to the specificity Te64; 60 samples reacted with a percentage ranging between 3 and

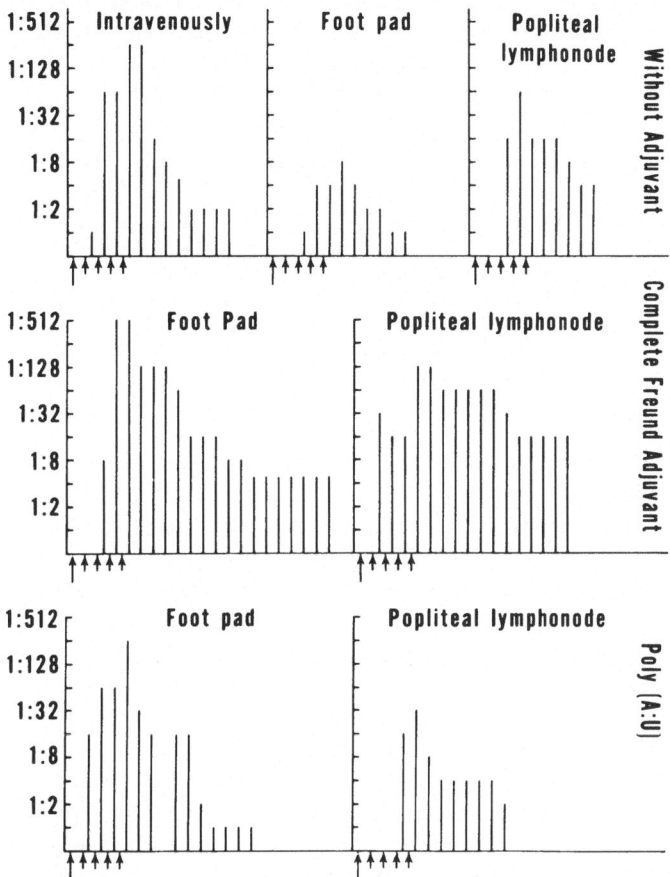

Figure 10. Kinetic of lymphocytotoxic antibodies production in rabbits immunized with HL-A antigen solubilized from cultured lymphoid cells RPMI 1788 ↑ indicates the immunizing stimuli and boosters given. The dose of antigen given is indicated in Table IX.

27% of the panel tested, and did not correlate with any known HL-A specificity. Dilution of the heteroantisera to reduce their polyspecificity is economical and quick; however, since it is effective only shortly after immunization or at a relatively long time interval after the last booster injection, the titer of antibodies is low. Furthermore, their avidity is weak as indicated by the low value of index strength, i.e., mean frequency of strong total kill reactions. Terasaki and Mickey (1971) have pointed out that typing with HL-A alloantisera with low percentages of strong reactions is difficult to reproduce. Therefore, the hetero-

Table X. Specificity of Some Diluted Sera from Rabbits Immunized
with HL-A Antigen Solubilized from Cultured Lymphoid Cells RPMI 1788
(HL-A2,10,7,W14)

Rabbit No.	Bleeding	Dilution	Specificity	Strength index*
7666	18	1:4	Te40 (W28)	27.78
7667	15	1:4	Te52 (W27)	42.86
8092	15	1:1	Te40 (W28)	25.00
8098	8	1:12	Te51 (W22)	44.44
8099	3	1:4	Te52 (W27)	22.73
8102	13	1:4	Te71	34.78
8634	14	1:2	Te59 (W32)	50.00

*Indicates percentage of strong positive reactions.

antisera rendered monospecific by dilution seem to be relatively poor reagents for HL-A typing.

After absorption of immune rabbit sera with human cultured lymphoid cells, 3 out of 133 sera were monospecific, 2 were directed against the specificity W14, and 1 was directed against the specificity Te63. These sera possessed a higher value on the strength-index scale than diluted immune rabbit sera. However, the absorption procedure has its limitations: (1) it requires large numbers of human cultured lymphoid cells, (2) it is time consuming, and (3) the optimal ratio between the number of absorbing cells and the amount of serum is extremely difficult to ascertain. We attempted to calculate the number of absorbing cells on the basis of the titer of the unabsorbed heteroantisera; unfortunately, this approach failed in most cases since at times no further antibody activity could be detected and at other times absorption was incomplete as antibodies of different specificities remained.

Heteroantisera rendered monospecific both by absorption and dilution gave a relatively high number of positive reactions with target cells which were not reactive with alloantisera of the same HL-A specificity. These additional positive reactions might indeed be false. Alternatively, these heteroantisera may react in the direct cytotoxic test with cells which give CYNAP reactions with alloantisera, since the sensitivity of the test is greatly increased. In fact, when human sera are the source of antibodies, incompatibility exists between human and rabbit complement components (Ferrone et al., 1967). In addition, human IgM reacts with the natural antibodies present in the rabbit complement (Herberman, 1970), thus decreasing its efficiency. Alternatively, these extra positive reactions may result from natural antibodies present in the rabbit sera. When 127 normal rabbit sera were tested against a large panel of normal human lymphocytes, some sera reacted with 2–98% of the panel in the lymphocytotoxic test (Mittal et al., 1972b).

When human serum was the source of complement, rabbit immune sera which reacted with 100% of the panel in the regular test gave polymorphic reactions; the specificity of some antibodies is indicated in Table XI (Ferrone *et al.*, 1972*f*). Finally, eluates from cultured murine lymphoid cells L1210 (H-2^b) used for absorption of immune rabbit sera contained antibodies related to HL-A2,10, and cross-reacting specificities (Ferrone *et al.*, 1972*f*).

All these data suggest that a possibility of producing HL-A heteroantisera exists, although optimal experimental conditions have yet to be devised. Experiments are in progress to evaluate induction of unresponsiveness against species-specific antigens in new-born rabbits which can later be challenged with HL-A antigens.

IX. LYMPHOCYTOTOXIC ANTIBODIES IN DISEASE

HL-A antibodies are not detected in the sera of healthy individuals who have no history of previous blood transfusions or pregnancies. Cytotoxic antibodies directed against human lymphocytes have been reported in sera from patients with a variety of diseases such as infectious mononucleosis (Mottironi and Terasaki, 1970), rubella (Mottironi and Terasaki, 1970), measles (Mottironi and Teraski, 1970), multiple myeloma (Kreisler *et al.*, 1971; Waters *et al.*, 1971), benign monoclonal gammopathy (Waters *et al.*, 1971), rheumatoid arthritis (Mittal *et al.*, 1970; Stastny and Ziff, 1971), and systemic lupus erythematosus (Mittal *et al.*, 1970). In the latter, the incidence of lymphocytotoxic antibodies may be as high as 74% (Mittal *et al.*, 1970). Antibodies in the sera of patients suffering from these diseases are usually of low titers (Waters *et al.*, 1971), optimally active in the cold, and principally 19S in nature. Generally speaking, the cytotoxic reactions induced with these sera are less reproducible than those with HL-A immune sera (Waters *et al.*, 1971). Some patients' sera show a clear-cut statistical relationship to defined HL-A specificities on population studies (Mittal *et al.*, 1970; Waters *et al.*, 1971), appear mutually exclusive to

Table XI. Specificity of Immune Rabbit* Sera Tested with Human Complement

Rabbit No.	Bleeding	Dilution	HL-A specificities
8398	5	1:10	Te64 (W16)
8099	5	1:10	HL-A10, HL-A7, Te60 (W10), Te64 (W16)
8634	5	1:10	Te64 (W16)
7665	5	1:10	HL-A8, Te51 (W22)
8632	5	1:20	HL-A10, HL-A7, Te60 (W10), Te64 (W16)
8101	5	1:20	HL-A10, HL-A7, Te64 (W16)

* The sera were obtained from rabbits immunized with HL-A antigen solubilized from cultured lymphoid cells RPMI 1788.

certain existing specificities, or segregate with the HL-A system as judged from family studies (Waters *et al.*, 1971). Some antisera do not correlate with known HL-A factors, and they may represent as yet undiscovered HL-A specificities or, alternatively, detect non-HL-A antigenic factors (Mittal *et al.*, 1970).

At the present time, one can only speculate as to the mechanism of formation of these antibodies. They may be produced in response to infections with viruses or bacteria which possess cross-reacting antigenic determinants structurally similar to HL-A. Crossreactivity between viral or bacterial antigenic determinants and the HL-A system may represent an important selective force in evaluation that explains the extreme polymorphism at the HL-A locus in man (Ceppellini *et al.*, 1967). Pathogenetic mechanisms for the formation of these antibodies can be hypothesized. For example, it is possible that components of the lymphocyte cell membrane become immunogenic as a result of yet-unknown processes during pathological events in disease (Mittal *et al.*, 1970). Alternatively, cytotoxic antibodies may be simple by-products of antibody synthesis against specific antigens. Finally, Jerne's recent theory (Jerne, 1970) of the generation of self-tolerance and antibody diversity may explain production of isoantibodies against histocompatibility antigens from subjects who neither possess them nor have had prior contact with them. Jerne postulates that all immunocompetent cells arise either directly or by mutation from primogenitor cells possessing genes initially coding for histocompatibility factors. Genes coding for "self" are suppressed as such, but may undergo somatic mutation and hence give rise to a diversity of mutant cells from which the selection of useful antibody-forming cell clones can be made. In contrast, cells coding for allogeneic factors may not be specifically stimulated in the normal course of events, but may produce globulins showing detectable HL-A or other isospecificities during pathological processes.

X. COMPLEMENT

Rabbit serum is the most effective source of complement in the lymphocytotoxic reaction (Walford *et al.*, 1964) despite its relatively low titer in the conventional hemolytic test system with sensitized sheep erythrocytes (Nelson and Biro, 1968). It has been reported, but not confirmed (Etheredge *et al.*, 1971), that mixtures of fresh rabbit complement and human complement are more effective than rabbit complement alone (Engelfriet, 1966; Kissmeyer-Nielsen and Thorsby, 1970). In our hands, however, the addition of human complement to rabbit complement greatly decreases the sensitivity of the cytotoxic test, in some cases resulting in false negative reactions (Ferrone *et al.*, 1967).

The inhibitory activity of human serum on rabbit complement is caused by incompatibility between human and rabbit complement (Cooper, N.R., unpublished observations) and by blocking of natural rabbit antibodies by human IgM

(Herberman, 1970). As will be discussed later, natural rabbit antibodies play an important role in the lymphocytotoxic reaction. In addition, soluble HL-A antigens have been detected in human sera (Charlton and Zmijewski, 1970; van Rood et al., 1970a,b; Miyajima et al., 1972; Schultz and Shreffler, 1972). These soluble antigens may interact with anti-HL-A antibodies, so addition of human sera to the reaction mixture does not seem advisable.

When human peripheral lymphocytes are utilized as target cells in lymphocytotoxic testing, rabbit serum which lacks any spontaneous cytotoxic activity must be selected as the source of complement. Whenever cultured human lymphoid cells are chosen as the targets, rabbit sera must be either absorbed (McDonald et al., 1970) or diluted (Rogentine and Gerber, 1969; Ferrone et al., 1971a; Takasugi, 1971) to eliminate their direct cytotoxic effects on these cells. Another peculiarity of the lymphocytotoxic reaction is that even when the number of target cells is low, large amounts of rabbit sera have to be used, with the ratio between antiserum and complement ranging from 2:3 to 1:5.

However, the lymphocytotoxic reaction does not differ from the hemolytic test system as far as the ratio between antigen saturation with antibody and complement requirement is concerned, as more complement is required when the saturation of the antigenic sites is lowered (Table XII) (Ferrone et al., 1967). In addition, the lymphocytotoxic reaction does not differ from the hemolytic reaction insofar as the requirement of complement components is concerned (Ferrone et al., 1971b). Heat inactivation of rabbit complement (56°C for 30 min) or addition of EDTA to a final concentration of 0.01 M renders rabbit serum ineffective as a complement source in the cytotoxic reaction. Serum from rabbits with a genetic deficiency of C6 (sixth component of complement) is not active in the cytotoxic reaction (Ferrone et al., 1971b). However, cytotoxicity is restored on addition of increasing amounts of immunochemically- and functionally-pure human C6 (Fig. 11). When cultured human lymphoid cells are sensitized with anti-HL-A alloantibodies and reacted with C6 deficient rabbit comple-

Table XII. Titration of Complement at Different Antibody Concentrations[a]

Complement	10	8	6	5	4	3	2.5	2.0	1.5	1.25	0
Hanks	0	2	4	5	6	7	7.5	8.0	8.5	8.75	10
Serum 11/38											
1/1	95[b]	95	95	95	95	95	95	95	95	60	5
1/4	95	95	95	95	95	95	95	95	95	73	5
1/16	95	95	95	95	80	44	4	5	5	5	5
1/64	5	5	5	5	5	5	5	5	5	5	5

[a] The incubation mixture was: C' or dilutions of it with Hanks, in the proportions indicated by the top figure, 3 μl; Serum 11/38 or dilutions of it with Hanks, 2 μl; Cell suspension in Hanks, 1 μl.

[b] The figures indicate the percentage of killed cells.

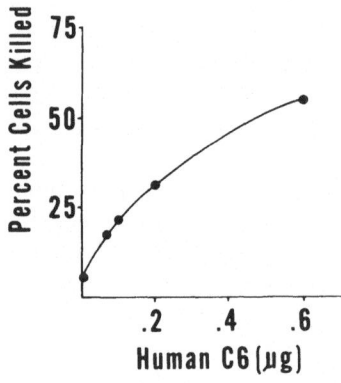

Figure 11. Dependence of sensitized-peripheral-lymphocyte killings upon C6 concentration in the reaction mixture. Peripheral lymphocytes S.F. were sensitized with alloantiserum Pinquette (anti-HL-A2), washed, and then reacted with C6 deficient rabbit C combined with different amounts of human C6.

ment, the cytotoxic reaction is accomplished only by the addition of C6,7,8,9 (Ferrone *et al.*, 1971*b*) (Table XIII). Similar results were obtained when purified human complement components were added sequentially to human cultured lymphoid cells sensitized with anti-HL-A alloantisera (Ferrone *et al.*, 1971*b*). Whereas cells sensitized with antibodies were not killed by the addition of C1,4,2,3, cytotoxicity was observed on addition of the late-acting complement components. These data clearly indicate that the same 9 complement components required for hemolysis of sensitized sheep erythrocytes are also needed to kill target cells in the lymphocytotoxic reaction. Therefore, the superior effectiveness of rabbit serum as source of complement in the lymphocytotoxic reaction depends on more than the supply of complement components. Rabbit serum contains natural antibodies directed against antigenic receptors present on lymphoid cells; these antibodies are complement-dependent, heat-labile, and either 7*S* or 19*S* in size (Ferrone *et al.*, 1971*b*).

As mentioned earlier, complement–antibody-mediated lysis of cells depends on a critical concentration of complement of the cell surface. This level cannot be reached even with a large excess of antibody and complement in situations where the density of antigen receptors is low (Linscott, 1970). The relatively low density of histocompatibility antigens on cell surfaces is probably the cause of insufficient binding of complement for the interaction with anti-HL-A antibodies to ultimately effect cell lysis. Therefore, human complement is poorly cytolytic on peripheral human lymphocytes reacted with anti-HL-A alloantisera. This view is reinforced by the greater efficiency of human complement against cultured human lymphoid cells, which have a higher concentration of HL-A antigens on their surface, than against peripheral lymphocytes (Fig. 1) (Ferrone *et al.*, 1971*b*). On the other hand, rabbit serum contributes to the cytotoxic reaction not only by providing complement, but also by the presence of natural antibodies reacting with antigenic determinants present on lymphoid cells. The latter enhance the binding of complement by HL-A antibodies and increase their

Table XIII. Requirement of Complement
Components in the Cytotoxic Reaction*

Complement components added	Killing of target cells, %
C6, 7, 8, 9	66
C7, 8, 9	23
C8, 9	21
C6	24
C7	28
C8	27
C9	30
None	29

* Cultured human lymphoid cells RPMI 1788 were sensitized with alloantiserum Pinquette (HL-A2) and then reacted with rabbit C with C6 deficiency. The CA-rabbit C1,4,2,3,5 were reacted with different human C components.

cytolytic activity by a synergistic affect. In this regard, Möller and Möller (1962) showed that murine cells which were partially or completely resistant to a single isoantiserum could be made sensitive to humoral isoantibodies provided they were treated with a mixture of antisera of different specificities. Synergism by antibodies of different HL-A specificity has also been described (Ivascová et al., 1969; Svejgaard, 1969; Ahrons and Thorsby, 1970). The role of natural antibodies in the rabbit serum is clearly indicated by the low efficiency of rabbit complement absorbed with peripheral leukocytes or with human cultured lymphoid cells in the cytotoxic reaction. The titer of the alloantiserum is reduced (Fig. 12), and with some alloantisera false negative reactions occur, when rabbit serum absorbed with cultured cells or peripheral lymphocytes is used (Ferrone et al., 1971b). Furthermore, rabbit serum with a low level of natural antibodies is poorly effective as a source of complement in the lymphocytotoxic test. In fact, when the efficiency of sera from 5 rabbits was evaluated as source of complement, the percentage of killed target cells and titers of antisera varied greatly (Fig. 13) (Ferrone, Pellegrino, and Cooper, unpublished observations). Complement titers as determined in the conventional hemolytic test system with sensitized sheep erythrocytes differed among the 5 rabbits, but did not correlate with the efficiency of the sera in the cytotoxic tests, as the rabbit serum with a high complement level had little activity. On the contrary, the efficiency of rabbit sera as source of complement correlated with the cytotoxic activity of the rabbit sera against human cultured lymphoid cells, reflecting the combined action of natural antibodies and complement components (Fig. 13). Further-

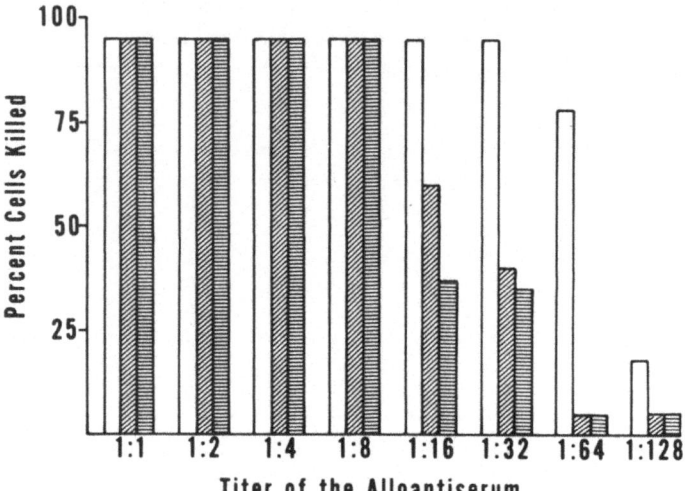

Figure 12. Comparison of the activity in the cytotoxic reaction of unabsorbed selected rabbit complement to that absorbed with human cultured lymphoid cells or with peripheral lymphocytes. Alloantiserum TO-11-03; peripheral lymphocytes B.P. (□ unabsorbed selected rabbit C; ▨ selected rabbit C absorbed with human cultured lymphoid cells; ▤ selected rabbit C absorbed with human peripheral lymphocytes.

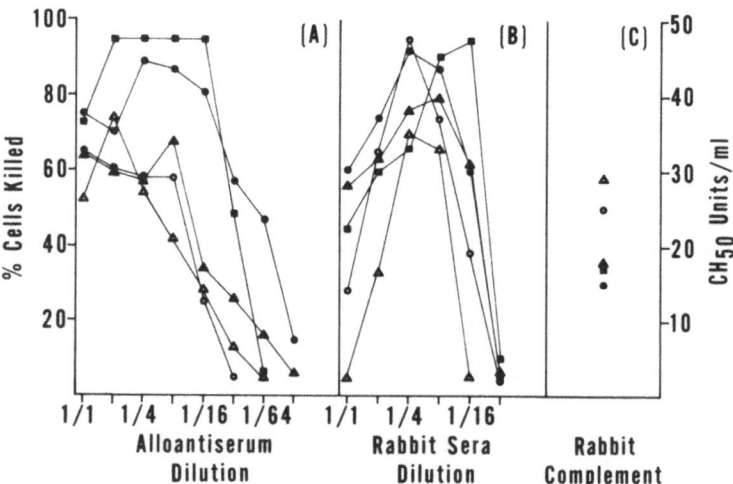

Figure 13. Comparison between the efficiency of rabbit sera as source of complement in the lymphocytotoxic reaction and their spontaneous cytotoxicity against cultured human lymphoid cells. (A) The titer of alloantiserum Pinquette against the target cells #2 utilizing five normal rabbit sera as source of complement. (B) The spontaneous cytotoxicity of normal rabbit sera against cultured human lymphoid cells 8866. (C) The level of complement in the normal rabbit sera as determined in the hemolytic test system. The same symbols are employed in panels A–C.

more, increased quantities of natural rabbit antibodies directed against antigens present in the lymphoid tissue greatly improve the sensitivity of the lymphocytotoxic test. Sublytic amounts of rabbit anti-human lymphocyte serum were added to the rabbit complement since the natural antibodies are labile and present in only small amounts in rabbit sera, and thus it is difficult to isolate sufficient amounts. When this mixture was used in the cytotoxic reaction, the time of incubation could be shortened and the titer of the alloantisera increased (Ting, Ferrone, and Terasaki, unpublished results). Most of the alloantisera react in the direct test with cells bearing cross-reacting specificities (Ting, Ferrone, and Terasaki, unpublished results). As previously discussed, the density of HL-A determinants on the cell surface reacting with cross-reacting antibodies is low, and therefore, the concentration of complement on the cell membrane to effect lysis cannot be reached. An increase of natural antibodies in rabbit serum can overcome this problem and can account for changed reactivity of the cells in the cytotoxic test.

Rabbit serum has been shown to be the most effective source of complement in cytotoxic reactions utilizing many different target cells (Hildemann, 1957; Boyse et al., 1962; Möller and Möller, 1962; Winn, 1965; Haughton and McGehee, 1969; Wood and Morton, 1970; Götze and Ferrone, 1972) and to contain cytotoxic activity or antibody against cells from various species (Kidd and Friedewald, 1942; Hildemann, 1957; Terasaki et al., 1961; Möller and Möller, 1962; Colley and Waksman, 1970). The discussed mechanism of action of rabbit complement in the cytotoxic test with human lymphoid cells could be valid for other cytotoxic systems.

XI. CONCLUSION

In the previous pages, the three components of the lymphocytotoxic reactions, antigen, antibody, and complement, have been discussed separately. It is worthwhile, however, to emphasize that the ultimate result of the lymphocytotoxic reaction, i.e., killing of the target cell, derives from the complex interplay among antigen, antibody, and complement molecules to perform the lytic event on the cell surface. These components influence the reaction at different levels. The participation of antigenic determinants relates to their density and distribution; the density of HL-A determinants with identical specificities on lymphocytes from different subjects seems to vary significantly, a threefold variation having been reported for some HL-A specificies (Pellegrino et al., 1972a). If the fluid mosaic model of membrane structure proposed by Singer and Nicolson (1972) is taken into account, then diffusion of antigen within the cell membrane may be another source of variability. The possible influence of the HL-A profile on the reactivity of each HL-A specificity with antibodies also has to be considered, since cells presenting HL-A determinants governed by genes in *trans* or *cis* position display different absorbing capacities (Legrand and Dausset, 1971). Antibodies influence the reaction by their affinity and ability to activate the complement sequence; HL-A antibodies being mostly 7*S* IgG (Colombani *et al.*, 1964; Walford *et al.*, 1965; Engelfriet, 1966; Metzgar and Seigler, 1967; Ahrons and Glavind-Kristensen, 1971) are poor at complement fixation. It has recently become clear that there are two pathways of activation of complement sequence (Götze and Müller-Eberhard, 1971). The classical pathway proceeds through the action of C1, C4, and C2, whereas in the alternate pathway another group of serum proteins interact to enter the complement sequence at the C3 level. HL-A antibodies of different specificities seem to initiate different pathways; in fact, some activate the classical pathway, while others activate both the classical and the alternate pathways (Ferrone *et al.*, 1972*b*). When both complement sequences have been activated, killing of target cells seems to be more efficient than when only the classical pathway functions; this may explain the different requirements for complement of HL-A determinants with various specificities, false negative reactions occurring more frequently with the HL-A specificity 4b (Ferrone *et al.*, 1967). When rabbit serum is the source of complement, the influence of natural rabbit antibodies directed against determinants present on lymphoid cells also has to be considered; these antibodies have different specificities and titers, and determinants are expressed on lymphocytes from different subjects in variable amounts. The spatial relationships between these determinants and HL-A antigens may also be important. Finally, the nature of the lytic event at the cell surface is completely unknown. The structural and functional conditions of the cell membrane may be important in determining the ability of the cell to repair lesions in the plasma membrane produced by immune cytolysis.

All these factors indicate that the lymphocytotoxic reaction is complex and that immune cytolysis of lymphocytes cannot be regarded as a direct consequence of the reaction of HL-A alloantibodies with target cells. This view is reinforced by the fact that HL-A antibodies, although they activate the late complement components to a similar extent, may show great variability in their cytolytic affects (Ferrone *et al.*, 1972*b*). In the same manner, murine leukemia cells, induced by Moloney virus and sensitized by anti-Moloney virus antibody, activate the complement system at like levels throughout their growth cycles, but are sensitive in the cytotoxic test only in G_1 phase (Lerner *et al.*, 1971). Thus, the complexity of the lymphocytotoxic reaction can account for the massive influence of minor variations in the results. Changes in incubation time, temperature, ionic strength, or antiserum diluents can dramatically alter the results of the test (Grothaus *et al.*, 1971*a*). Certainly, caution should be exercised in analyzing the results of the cytotoxic test which for the present is still the best for histocompatibility antigens.

ACKNOWLEDGMENTS

This is publication No. 623 from the Department of Experimental Pathology, Scripps Clinic and Research Foundation, La Jolla, California. This work was supported by United States Public Health Service grants AI 10180 and CA 10596 from the National Institutes of Health, National Cancer Institute contract 72-2046, and grant IC-5 from the American Cancer Society. We would like to thank Dr. R. A. Reisfeld for his helpful suggestions and criticisms. The critical discussions with Dr. D. Götze during the preparation of the manuscript are acknowledged.

REFERENCES

Abeyounis, C. J., and Milgrom, F. (1969). *Transplant. Proc.* 1: 556.
Ahrons, S., and Glavind-Kristensen, S. (1971). *Tissue Antigens* 1: 129.
Ahrons, S., and Thorsby, E. (1970). *Vox Sanguinis* 18: 323.
Albert, E., Kano, L., Abeyounis, C. J., and Milgrom, F. (1969). *Transplantation* 8: 466.
Amiel, J. L., Mery, A. M., and Mathé, G. (1967). *Congr. Colloq. Univ. Liege* 43: 197.
Amos, D. B. (1956). *Ann. N.Y. Acad. Sci.* 63: 706.
Amos, D. B. (1966). In Amos, D. B., and van Rood, J. J. (eds.), *Histocompatibility Testing*, Williams and Wilkins, Baltimore, p. 175.
Amos, D. B., Hutchin, P., Hattler, B. G., McCloskey, R., and Zmijewski, C. M. (1966). *Lancet* 1: 300.
Aoki, T., Hammerling, U., de Harven, E., Boyse, E. A., and Old, L. J. (1969). *J. Exp. Med.* 130: 979.
Aoki, T., Boyse, E. A., Old, L. J., de Harven, E., Hammerling, U., and Wood, H. A. (1970). *Proc. Natl. Acad. Sci. U.S.* 65: 569.
Ashwell, M. A., and Work, T. S. (1968). *Biochem. Biophys. Res. Commun.* 32: 1006.
Aster, R. H., Cooper, H. E., and Singer, D. L. (1964). *J. Lab. Clin. Med.* 63: 161.
Balner, H., van Leeuwen, A., Dersjant, H., and van Rood, J. J. (1967). *Transplantation* 5: 624.
Balner, H., Gabb, B. W., Dersjant, H., van Vreeswijk, W., van Leeuwen, A., and van Rood, J. J. (1971). In Chiarelli, B. (ed.), *Comparative Genetics in Monkeys, Apes, and Man*, Academic Press, London, p. 97.
Batchelor. J. R. (1969). *Transplantation* 7: 554.
Bernoco, D., Glade, P. R., Broder, S., Miggiano, V. C., Hirschhorn, K., and Ceppellini, R. (1969). *Haematologica* 54: 795.
Bertrams, J., Kuwert, E., Gallmeier, W. M., Reis, H. E., and Schmidt, C. G. (1971). *Tissue Antigens* 1: 105.
Bjaring, B., Klein, G., and Popp, I. (1969). *Transplantation* 8: 38.
Bodmer, W. F., Tripp, M., and Bodmer, J. G. (1967). In Curtoni, E. S., Mattiuz, P. L., and Tosi, R. M. (eds.), *Histocompatibility Testing*, Munksgaard, Copenhagen, p. 341.
Borsos, R., Dowmashkin, R. R., and Humphrey, J. H. (1964). *Nature* 202: 251.
Boyse, E. A., Old, L. J., and Stockert, E. (1962). *Ann. N.Y. Acad. Sci.* 99: 574.
Boyse, E. A., Stockert, E., and Old, L. J. (1967). *Proc. Natl. Acad. Sci. U.S.* 58: 954.
Braun, W. E., Grecek, D. R., and Murphy, J. J. (1972). *Transplantation* 13: 337.
Brautbar, C., Payne, R., and Hayflick, L. (1972a). *Exp. Cell Res.* 75: 31.
Brautbar, C., Pellegrino, M. A., Ferrone, S., Payne, R., Reisfeld, R. A., and Hayflick, L. (1972b). *Exp. Cell Res.* (in press).
Bruley, M., and Motta, R. (1971). Quoted in Walford, R. L., Smith, G. S., and Waters, H. (1972). *Transplant. Rev.* 7: 78.

Carbonara, A. O., Mattiuz, P. L., Richiardi, P., and Ceppellini, R. (1972). *Proc. Intern. Symp. Standardization HL-A Reagents, 1972, Copenhagen* (in press).

Celada, F., and Rotman, B. (1967). *Proc. Natl. Acad. Sci. U.S.* **57**: 630.

Ceppellini, R., Curtoni, E. S., Mattiuz, P. L., Leigheb, G., Visetti, M., and Colombi, A. (1966). *Ann. N.Y. Acad. Sci.* **129**: 421.

Ceppellini, R., Curtoni, E. S., Mattiuz, P. L., Miggiano, V., Scudeller, C., and Serra, A. (1967). In Curtoni, E. S., Mattiuz, P. L., and Tosi, R. M. (eds.), *Histocompatibility Testing*, Munksgaard, Copenhagen, p. 169.

Charlton, R. K., and Zmijewski, C. M. (1970). *Science* **170**: 636.

Cikes, M. (1970). *J. Natl. Cancer Inst.* **45**: 979.

Cikes, M. (1971). *Transplant. Proc.* **3**: 1161.

Cikes, M., and Friberg, S. (1971). *Proc. Soc. Natl. Acad. Sci. U.S.* **68**: 566.

Cikes, M., and Klein, G. (1972). *J. Natl. Cancer Inst.* **48**: 509.

Claesson, M. H., Ahrons, S., and Jørgensen, O. (1971). *Tissue Antigens* **1**: 94.

Colombani, J., Colombani, M., and Dausset, J. (1964). *Ann. N.Y. Acad. Sci.* **120**: 307.

Colombani, J., Colombani, M., Benajam, A., and Dausset, J. (1967). In Curtoni, E. S., Mattiuz, P. L., and Tosi, R. M. (eds.), *Histocompatibility Testing*, Munksgaard, Copenhagen, p. 413.

Colombani, J., Colombani, M., and Dausset, J. (1970). In Terasaki, P. E. (ed.), *Histocompatibility Testing*, Munksgaard, Copenhagen, p. 79.

Colombani, J., D'Amaro, J., Gabb, B., Smith, G., and Svejgaard, A. (1972). *Transplant. Proc.* **3**: 121.

Colley, D. G., and Waksman, B. H. (1970). *Transplantation* **9**: 395.

Dausset, J. (1958). *Acta Haematol.* **20**: 156.

Dausset, J. (1971). *Transpl. Proc.* **3**: 8.

Dausset, J., and Hors, J. (1971). *Transplant. Proc.* **3**: 1004.

Dausset, J., Rapaport, F. T., Ivanyi, P., and Colombani, J. (1966). In Amos, D. B., and van Rood, J. J. (eds.), *Histocompatibility Testing*, Williams and Wilkins, Baltimore, p. 63.

Dausset, J., Rapaport, F. T., and Legrand, L. (1968a). In Dausset, J., Hamburger, J., and Mathé, G. (eds.), *Advances in Transplantation*, Munksgaard, Copenhagen, p. 275.

Dausset, J., Colombani, J., Colombani, M., Legrand, L., and Feingold, N. (1968b). *Nouvelle Rev. Franc. Hematol.* **8**: 398.

Dausset, J., Colombani, J., Legrand, L., and Feingold, N. (1969). *Presse Med.* **77**: 849.

Dausset, J., Rapaport, F. T., Legrand, L., Colombani, J., and Marcelli-Barge, A. (1970). In Terasaki, P. I. (ed.), *Histocompatibility Testing*, Munksgaard, Copenhagen, p. 381.

Davies, D. A. L. (1968). In Dausset, J., Hamburger, J., and Mathé, G. (eds.), *Advances in Transplantation*, Munksgaard, Copenhagen, p. 275.

Davis, W. C. (1972). *Science* **175**: 1005.

Davis, W. C., Douglas, S. D., Petz, L. D., and Fudenberg, H. H. (1968). *J. Immunol.* **101**: 621.

Davis, W. C., Alspaugh, M. A., Stimpfling, J. H., and Walford, R. L. (1971). *Tissue Antigens* **1**: 89.

Dick, H. M., and Steel, C. M. (1971). *Lancet* **1**: 1135.

Dick, H. M., Steel, C. M., and Crichton, W. B. (1972). *Tissue Antigens* **2**: 85.

Dorf, M. E., and Metzgar, R. S. (1970). In Terasaki, P. I. (ed.), *Histocompatibility Testing*, Munksgaard, Copenhagen, p. 287.

Einstein, A. B., Jr., Mann, D. L., Gordon, H. G., and Fahey, J. L. (1971a). *Tissue Antigens* **1**: 209.

Einstein, A. B., Jr., Mann, D. L., Gordon, H. G., Trapani, R. J., and Fahey, J. L. (1971b). *Transplantation* **12**: 299.

Engelfriet, C. P. (1966). Ph.D. Thesis, University of Amsterdam.

Engelfriet, C. P., and Britten, A. (1965). *Vox Sanguinis* **10**: 660.

Etheredge, E. E., Franecki, B. H., and Najarian, J. S. (1971). *Tissue Antigens* **1**: 109.

Ferrone, S., Tosi, R. M., and Centis, D. (1967). In Curtoni, E. S., Mattiuz, P. L., and Tosi, R. M. (eds.), *Histocompatibility Testing*, Munksgaard, Copenhagen, p. 357.

Ferrone, S., Sirchia, G., Farina, C., and Dambrosio, F. (1968). *Ric. Clin. Lab.* **7**: 56.

Ferrone, S., Pellegrino, M. A., and Reisfeld, R. A. (1971*a*). *J. Immunol.* 107: 613.
Ferrone, S., Cooper, N. R., Pellegrino, M. A., and Reisfeld, R. A. (1971*b*). *J. Immunol.* 107: 939.
Ferrone, S., Pellegrino, M. A., and Reisfeld, R. A. (1972*a*). *Lancet* 1: 1237.
Ferrone, S., Cooper, N. R., Pellegrino, M. A. and Reisfeld, R. A. (1972*b*). *J. Exp. Med.* (in press).
Ferrone, S., Del Villano, B., Pellegrino, M. A., Lerner, R. A., and Reisfeld, R. A. (1972*c*). *Tissue Antigens* 2: 447.
Ferrone, S., Mittal, K.K., Pellegrino, M. A., Terasaki, P. I., and Reisfeld, R. A. (1972*d*). *Immunol. Commun.* 1: 77.
Ferrone, S., Natali, P. G., Hunter, A., Terasaki, P. I., and Reisfeld, R. A. (1972*e*). *J. Immunol.* 108: 1718.
Ferrone, S., Pellegrino, M. A., Götze, D., Mittal, K. K., Terasaki, P. I., and Reisfeld, R. A. (1972*f*). *Proc. Intern. Symp. Standardization HL-A Reagents. Copenhagen* (in press).
Forbes, J. F., and Morris, P. J. (1970). *Lancet* 2: 849.
Fox, E. N., and Peterson, R. D. A. (1970). *J. Immunol.* 105: 1031.
Frye, L. D., and Edidin, M. (1970). *J. Cell Sci.* 7: 319.
Galper, J. B., and Darnell, J. E. (1971). *J. Mol. Biol.* 57: 363.
Gibofsky, A., and Terasaki, P. I. (1972). *Transplantation* 13: 192.
Glick, A. D., Horn, R. G., Collins, R. D., and Bryant, R. E. (1970). *Exp. Mol. Pathol.* 12: 275.
Götze, O., and Müller-Eberhard, H. J. (1971). *J. Exp. Med.* 134: 90s.
Götze, D., and Ferrone, S. (1972). *J. Immunol. Methods* 1: 203.
Götze, D., Ferrone, S., and Reisfeld, R. A. (1972*a*). *J. Immunol.* 109: 439.
Götze, D., Pellegrino, M. A., Ferrone, S., and Reisfeld, R. A. (1972*b*). *Immunol. Commun.* (in press).
Grothaus, E. A., Rauckman, E. J., and Amos, B. D. (1971*a*). *Transplantation* 11: 145.
Grothaus, E. A., Flye, M. W., Yunis, E., and Amos, D. B. (1971*b*). *Science* 173: 542.
Grumet, F. C., Coukell, A., Bodmer, J. G., Bodmer, W. F., and McDevitt, H. O. (1971). *New Eng. J. Med.* 285: 193.
Harris, R., and Zervas, J. D. (1969). *Nature* 221: 1062.
zur Hausen, H., Diehl, V., Wolf, H., Schulte-Holthausen, H., and Schneider, U. (1972). *Nature (New Biology)* 237: 184.
Haywood, G. R., and McKhann, C. F. (1971). *J. Exp. Med.* 33: 1171.
Haughton, G., and McGehee, M. P. (1969). *Immunology* 16: 447.
Hellström, K. E., and Möller, E. (1965). *Progr. Allergy* 9: 158.
Herberman, R. B. (1970). *J. Immunol.* 104: 805.
Hildemann, W. H. (1957). *Transplant. Bull.* 4: 148.
Hirata, A. A., and Terasaki, P. I. (1970). *Science* 168: 1095.
Hirata, A. A., and Terasaki, P. I. (1972). *J. Immunol.* 108: 1542.
Hirata, A. A., Armstrong, A. S., Kay, J. W. D., and Terasaki, P. I. (1970). In Terasaki, P. I. (ed.), *Histocompatibility Testing,* Munksgaard, Copenhagen, p. 475.
Hoecker G., and Hauschka, T. S. (1956). *Transplant. Bull.* 3: 134.
Ivascová, E., Vybiralová, H., Raue, I., Démant, P., and Ivanyi, P. (1969). *Folia Biol. (Prague)* 15: 26.
Jensen, C., and Stetson, C. A. (1961). *J. Exp. Med.* 113: 785.
Jerne, N. K. (1970). In Smith, R. T., and Landy, M. (eds.), *Immune Surveillance,* Academic Press, New York, p. 345.
Kahan, B. D., Reisfeld, R. A., Pellegrino, M., Curtoni, E. S., Mattiuz, P. L., and Ceppellini, R. (1968). *Proc. Natl. Acad. Sci. U.S.* 61: 897.
Kahan, B. D., Pellegrino, M. A., Papermaster, B. W., and Reisfeld, R. A. (1971). *Transplant. Proc.* 3: 227.
Karb, K., and Goldstein, G. (1971). *Transplantation* 11: 569.
Kidd, J. G., and Friedewald, W. F. (1942). *J. Exp. Med.* 76: 543.
Kissmeyer-Nielsen, F., and Thorsby, E. (1970). *Transplant. Rev.* 4: 1.
Kissmeyer-Nielsen, F., Peterson, V. P., Olsen, S., and Fieldborg, O. (1966). *Lancet* 1: 662.
Kissmeyer-Nielsen, F., Staub-Nielsen, L., Lindholm, A. Sandberg, L., Svejgaard, A. and

Thorsby, E. (1970). In Terasaki, P. I. (ed.), *Histocompatibility Testing*, Munksgaard, Copenhagen, p. 105.

Kourilsky, F. M., Silvestre. D., Levy, J. P., Dausset, J., Niccolai, M. G., and Senik, A. (1971). *J. Immunol.* **106**: 454.

Kourilsky, F. M., Silvestre, D., Neauport-Sautes, C., Loosfelt, Y., and Dausset, J. (1972). *European J. Immunol.* **2**: 249.

Kreisler, N., Naito, S., and Terasaki, P. I. (1971). *Transplant. Proc.* **3**: 112.

Kuhns, W. J., and Bramson, S. (1968). *Nature* **219**: 938.

Kuhns, W. J., Faur, Y., Bramson, S., and Friedhoff, F. (1969). *Proc. Soc. Exp. Biol. Med.* **131**: 67.

Lambertenghi-Deliliers, G., Ferrone, S., Ranzi, T., and Sirchia, G. (1971). *Blood* **38**: 759.

Lee, R. E., and Feldman, J. D. (1964). *J. Cell Biol.* **23**: 396.

Legrand, L., and Dausset, J. (1971). *Nature (New Biology)* **234**: 271.

Legrand, L., Dausset, J., and Rapaport, F. T. (1971). *Transfusion* **11**: 233.

Lerner R. A., Oldstone, M. B. A., and Cooper, N. R. (1971). *Proc. Natl. Acad. Sci. U.S.* **68**: 2584.

Linscott, W. D. (1970). *J. Immunol.* **104**: 1307.

Lucas, D. R., and Peakman, E. M. (1969). *J. Pathol.* **99**: 163.

McDonald, J. C., Jacobbi, L., and Williams, R. W. (1970). *Transplantation* **10**: 499.

MacKintosh, P., Hardy, D. A., and Aviet, T. (1971). *Lancet* **1**: 1019.

Mann, D. L., and Fahey, J. L. (1971*a*). *Ann. Rev. Microbiol.* **25**: 679.

Mann, D. L., and Fahey, J. L. (1971*b*). *Transplant. Proc.* **3**: 234.

Mann, D. L., Rogentine, G. N. Jr., Fahey, J. L., and Nathenson, S. F. (1968). *Nature* **217**: 1180.

Medawar, P. B. (1963). *Transplantation* **1**: 21.

Melief, C. J. M., van der Hart, M., Engelfriet, C. P., and van Loghem, J. J. (1967). *Vox Sanguinis* **12**: 374.

Mercuriali, F., Richiardi, P., Mattiuz, P. L., and Sirchia, G. (1971). *Tissue Antigens* **1**: 290.

Metzgar, R. S., and Seigler, H. F. (1967). *Transplantation* **5**: 210.

Metzgar, R. S., and Seigler, H. F. (1972). In Kahan, B. D., and Reisfeld, R. A. (eds.), *Markers of Biological Individuality: The Transplantation Antigens*, Academic Press, New York, p. 209.

Metzgar, R. S., and Zmijewski, C. M. (1966). *Transplantation* **4**: 84.

Metzgar, R. S., Zmijewski, C. M., and Amos, D. B. (1965). In Russell, P. S., and Winn, H. T. (eds.), *Histocompatibility Testing*, Publ. No. 1229, Natl. Acad. Sci. Natl. Res. Council, Washington, D.C., p. 45.

Metzgar, R. S., Flanagan, J. F., and Mendes, N. F. (1967). In Curtoni, E. S., Mattiuz, P. L., and Tosi, R. M. (eds.), *Histocompatibility Testing*, Munksgaard, Copenhagen, p. 307.

Mickey, M. R., Kreisler, M., and Terasaki, P. I. (1970). In Terasaki, P. I. (ed.), *Histocompatibility Testing*, Munksgaard, Copenhagen, p. 237.

Mickey, M. R., Kreisler, M., Albert, E. D., Tanaka, N., and Terasaki, P. I. (1971). *Tissue Antigens* **1**: 57.

Milgrom, F., Kano, K., Barron, A. L., and Witebsky, E. (1964). *J. Immunol.* **92**: 8.

Mittal, K. K., and Terasaki, P. I. (1972). *Tissue Antigens* **2**: 94.

Mittal, K. K., Mickey, M. R., Singal, D. P., and Terasaki, P. I. (1968). *Transplantation* **6**: 913.

Mittal K. K., Mickey, M. R., and Terasaki, P. I. (1969). *Transplantation* **8**: 801.

Mittal, K. K., Rossen, R. D., Sharp, J. T., Lidsky, M. D., and Butler, W. T. (1970). *Nature* **225**: 1255.

Mittal, K. K., Mickey, M. R., and Terasaki, P. I. (1972*a*). *Proc. Intern. Symp. Standardization HL-A Reagents, Copenhagen* (in press).

Mittal, K. K., Ferrone, S., Mickey, M. R., Pellegrino, M. A., Reisfeld, R. A., and Terasaki, P. I. (1972*b*). *Tissue Antigens* (in press).

Miyakawa, Y., Tanigaki, N., Yagi, Y., Cohen, E., and Pressman, D. (1971). *J. Immunol.* **106**: 681.

Miyajima, T., Hirata, A. A., and Terasaki, P. I. (1972). *Tissue Antigens* **2**: 64.

Möller, E., and Möller, G. (1962). *J. Exp. Med.* **115**: 527.

Moore, G. E., and Woods, L. (1972). *Transplantation* 13: 155.
Morton, J. A., and Pickles, M. M. (1947). *Nature* 159: 779.
Mottironi, V. D., and Terasaki, P. I. (1970). In Terasaki, P. I. (ed.), *Histocompatibility Testing,* Munksgaard, Copenhagen, p. 301.
Neauport-Sautes, C., Silvestre, D., Niccolai, M. G., Kourilsky, F. M., and Levy, J. P. (1972). *Immunology* 22: 833.
Nelson, R. A., Jr., and Biro, C. E. (1968). *Immunology* 14: 527.
Old, L. J., Stockert, E., Boyse, E. A., and Kim, J. H. (1968). *J. Exp. Med.* 127: 523.
Opelz, G., Mickey, M. R., and Terasaki, P. I. (1972). *Lancet* 1: 868.
Papermaster, V. M., Papermaster, B. W., and Moore, G. E. (1969). *Federation Proc.* 28: 379.
Patel, R., and Terasaki, P. I. (1969). *New Engl. J. Med.* 280: 735.
Patel, R., Mickey, M. R., and Terasaki, P. I. (1969). *Brit. Med. J.* 2: 424.
Payne, R., Perkins, H. A., and Najarian, J. S. (1968). In Dausset, J., Hamburger, J., and Mathé, G. (eds.), *Advances in Transplantation,* Munksgaard, Copenhagen, p. 221.
Pegrum, G. D., Balfour, T. C., Evans, C. A., and Middleton, V. L. (1971). *Lancet* 1: 852.
Pellegrino, M. A., Ferrone, S., and Pellegrino, A. (1972*a*). *Proc. Soc. Exp. Biol. Med.* 139: 484.
Pellegrino, M. A., Ferrone, S., and Pellegrino, A. (1972*b*) In Kahan, B. D., and Reisfeld, R. A. (eds.), *Markers of Biological Individuality: The Transplantation Antigens,* Academic Press, New York, p. 433.
Pellegrino, M. A., Ferrone, S., Pellegrino, A., and Reisfeld, R. A. (1972*c*). *Clin. Immunol. Immunopathol.* (in press).
Pellegrino, M. A., Ferrone, S., Pellegrino, A., and Reisfeld, R. A. (1972*d*). *Proc. Intern. Symp. Standardization HL-A Reagents, Copenhagen* (in press).
Pellegrino, M. A., Ferrone, S., Natali, P. G., Pellegrino, A., and Reisfeld, R. A. (1972*e*). *J. Immunol.* 108: 573.
Pellegrino, M. A., Ferrone, S., Mittal, K. K., Pellegrino, A., and Reisfeld, R. A. (1972*f*). *Transplantation* (in press).
Pellegrino, M. A., Pellegrino, A., Ferrone, S., Kahan, B. D., and Reisfeld, R. A. (1972*g*) (in preparation).
Pellegrino, M. A., Ferrone, S., Safford, J. W. Jr., Hirata, A. A., Terasaki, P. I., and Reisfeld, R. A. (1972*h*). *J. Immunol.* 109: 97.
Race, R. R., and Sanger, R. (1958). *Blood Groups in Man,* 2nd Edition, Blackwell Scientific Publishers, Oxford.
Reisfeld, R. A., and Kahan, B. D. (1972). In Inman, F. P. (ed.), *Contemporary Topics in Immunochemistry, Vol. 1,* Plenum Press, New York, p. 51.
Reisfeld, R. A., Pellegrino, M. A., Papermaster, B. W., and Kahan, B. D. (1970). *J. Immunol.* 104: 560.
Reisfeld, R. A., Pellegrino, M. A., and Kahan, B. D. (1971). *Science* 172: 1134.
Rogentine, G. N., Jr. (1967). In Curtoni, E. S., Mattiuz, P. L., and Tosi, R. M. (eds.), *Histocompatibility Testing,* Munksgaard, Copenhagen, p. 371.
Rogentine, G. N., Jr., and Gerber, P. (1969). *Transplantation* 8: 28.
Rogentine, G. N., Jr., and Gerber, P. (1970). In Terasaki, P. I. (ed.), *Histocompatibility Testing,* Munksgaard, Copenhagen, p. 333.
van Rood, J. J. (1971). In Amos, D. B. (ed.), *Progress in Immunology,* Academic Press, New York, p. 1027.
van Rood, J. J., and van Leeuwen, A. (1971). *Transplant. Proc.* 3: 1283.
van Rood, J. J., van Leeuwen, A., Eernisse, J. G., Frederiks, E., and Bosch, L. J. (1964). *Ann. N.Y. Acad. Sci.* 120: 285.
van Rood, J. J., van Leeuwen, A., Schippers, A. A., Ceppellini, R., Mattiuz, P. L., and Curtoni, E. S. (1966). *Ann. N.Y. Acad. Sci.* 129: 467.
van Rood, J. J., van Leeuwen, A., and Bruning, J. W. (1967). *J. Clin. Pathol. Suppl.* 20: 504.
van Rood, J. J., van Leeuwen, A., and van Santen, M. C. T. (1970*a*). *Nature* 226: 366.
van Rood, J. J., van Leeuwen, A., Koch, C. T., and Frederiks, E. (1970*b*). In Terasaki, P. I. (ed.), *Histocompatibility Testing.* Munksgaard, Copenhagen, p. 483.
van Rood, J. J., van Leeuwen, A., and Balner, H. (1972). *Transplant. Proc.* 4: 55.
Rotman, B., and Papermaster, B. W. (1966). *Proc. Natl. Acad. Sci. U.S.* 55: 134.

Sachs, D. H., Winn, H. J., and Russell, P. S. (1971). *Transplant. Proc.* **3**: 210.

Sanderson, A. R. (1968). *Nature* **220**: 192.

Sanderson, A. R., and Batchelor, J. R. (1967). In Curtoni, E. S., Mattiuz, P. L., and Tosi, R. M. (eds.), *Histocompatibility Testing*, Munksgaard, Copenhagen, p. 367.

Sanderson, A. R., and Batchelor, J. R. (1968). *Nature* **219**: 184.

Schultz, J. S., and Shreffler, D. C. (1972). *Transplantation* **13**: 186.

Seigler, H. F., Kremer, W. B., Metzgar, R. S., Ward, F. E., Taung, A. T., and Amos, D. B. (1971). *J. Natl. Cancer Inst.* **46**: 577.

Shulman, N. R., Marder, V. J., Hiller, M. C., and Collier, E. M. (1964). *Progr. Hematol.* **4**: 222.

Shulman, N. R., Moor-Jankowski, J., and Hiller, M. C. (1966). In Amos, D. B., and van Rood, J. J. (eds.), *Histocompatibility Testing*, Williams and Wilkins, Baltimore, p. 113.

Silvestre, D., Kourilsky, F. M., Levy, J. P., and Senik, A. (1969). *C. R. Acad. Sci. (Paris)* **268**: 1145.

Silvestre, D., Kourilsky, F. M., Niccolai, M. G., and Levy, J. B. (1970). *Nature* **228**: 67.

Singal, D. P., Mickey, M. R., Mittal, K. K., and Terasaki, P. I. (1968). *Transplantation* **6**: 904.

Singal, D. P., Mickey, M. R., and Terasaki, P. I. (1969). *Transplantation* **7**: 246.

Singer, S. J., and Nicolson, G. L. (1972). *Science* **175**: 720.

Sirchia, G., and Dacie, J. V. (1967). *Nature* **215**: 747.

Sirchia, G., and Ferrone, S. (1970). *Blood* **37**: 563.

Sirchia, G., Ferrone, S., and Mercuriali, F. (1965). *Blood* **25**: 502.

Stastny, P., and Ziff, M. (1971). *Clin. Exp. Immunol.* **8**: 543.

Svejgaard, A. (1969). *Nature* **222**: 94.

Svejgaard, A., and Kissmeyer-Nielsen, F. (1968). *Nature* **219**: 868.

Takasugi, M. (1971). *Transplantation* **12**: 148.

Taylor, R. B., Duffus, W. P. H., Raff, M. C., and de Petris, S. (1971). *Nature (New Biology)* **233**: 225.

Terasaki, P. I., and McClelland, J. D. (1964). *Nature* **204**: 998.

Terasaki, P. I., and Mickey, M. R. (1971). *Transplant. Proc.* **3**: 1057.

Terasaki P. I., Esail, M. L., Cannon, J. A., and Longmire, W. P. (1961). *J. Immunol.* **87**: 383.

Terasaki, P. I., Marchioro, T. L., and Starzl, T. E. (1965). In Russell, P. S., and Winn, H. J. (eds.), *Histocompatibility Testing*, Publ. No. 1229, Natl. Acad. Sci. Natl. Res. Council, Washington, D.C., p. 83.

Terasaki, P. I., Vredevoe, D. L., and Mickey, M. R. (1967). *Transplantation* **5**: 1057.

Thorsby, E., and Kissmeyer-Nielsen, F. (1970). *Vox Sanguinis* **18**: 134.

Thorsby, E., Kjerbye, K. E., and Bratlie, A. (1970). *Vox Sanguinis* **18**: 373.

Ting, C. C., and Herberman, R. B. (1971). *Nature (New Biology)* **232**: 118.

Tosi, R. M., Pellegrino, M., Scudeller, G., and Ceppellini, R. (1967). In Curtoni, E. S., Mattiuz, P. L., and Tosi, R. M. (eds.), *Histocompatibility Testing*, Munksgaard, Copenhagen, p. 350.

Turner, M. J., Strominger, J. L., and Sanderson, A. R. (1972). *Proc. Natl. Acad. Sci. U.S.* **69**: 200.

Unger, L. J. (1951). *J. Lab. Clin. Med.* **37**: 825.

Walford, R. L., Gallagher, R., and Sjaarda, J. R. (1964). *Science* **144**: 868.

Walford, R. L., Gallagher, R., and Troup, G. M. (1965). *Transplantation* **3**: 387.

Walford, R. L., Latta, H., and Troup, G. M. (1966). *Ann. N.Y. Acad. Sci.* **129**: 490.

Walford, R. L., Shanbrom, E., Troup, G. M., Zeller, E., and Ackermann, B. (1967). In Curtoni, E. S., Mattiuz, P. L., and Tosi, R. M. (eds.), *Histocompatibility Testing*, Munksgaard, Copenhagen, p. 221.

Walford, R. L., Colombani, J., and Dausset, J. (1969). *Transplantation* **7**: 188.

Walford, R. L., Finnelstein, S., Neerhout, R., Konrad, P., and Shanbrom, E. (1970). *Nature* **225**: 461.

Walford, R. L., Smith, G. S., and Waters, H. (1971). *Transplant. Rev.* **7**: 78.

Warren, L., and Glick, M. C. (1968). *J. Cell Biol.* **37**: 729.

Waters, H., Smith, G. S., Fishkin, B., Tanaka, K. R., and Walford, R. L. (1971). *Transplant. Proc.* **3**: 145.

van der Weerdt, C. M., Veenhoven-von Riesz, L. E., and Engelfriet, C. P. (1970). In Terasaki, P. I. (ed.), *Histocompatibility Testing*, Munksgaard, Copenhagen, p. 339.
Wigzell, H. (1965). *Transplantation* **3**: 423.
Willingham, M. C., Spicer, S. S., and Graber, C. D. (1971). *Lab. Invest.* **25**: 211.
Winn, H. J. (1965). *Ciba Found. Symp. Complement, 1965*, p. 133.
Wood, W. C., and Morton, D. L. (1970). *Science* **170**: 1318.
Yachnin, S., Laforet, M. T., and Gardwer, F. H. (1961). *Blood* **17**: 83.
Yunis, E. J., Ward, F. E., and Amos, D. B. (1970). In Terasaki, P. I. (ed.), *Histocompatibility Testing*, Munksgaard, Copenhagen, p. 351.
Zervas, J. D., Delamore, I. W., and Israels, M. C. O. (1970). *Lancet* **2**: 634.
Zucker-Franklin, D. (1965). *Am. J. Pathol.* **47**: 419.

Chapter 9

Functional Molecular Anatomy of Fibrinogen: Antibodies as Biological Probes of Structure

Thomas S. Edgington and Edward F. Plow

Division of Clinical Pathology
Scripps Clinic and Research Foundation
La Jolla, California

I. INTRODUCTION

Among the more basic and exciting issues in molecular biology is the elucidation of functional molecular anatomy—the relationship between the molecular structure at all levels and the manifest functions of the molecule. Significant advances in elucidation of general protein structure at all levels of organization have been realized in the past two decades, to a great extent as the result of new and incisive analytical approaches. Major contributions by physicochemical and biochemical methods have provided probes of conformation as well as the primary structure of proteins. Conformational analysis has proven most difficult, and early information was to a great extent inferential and derived from hydrodynamic data. Multidisciplinary approaches including X-ray diffraction, high-resolution ultrastructural visualization, light scattering, optical rotatory dispersion, and functional reconstruction have amassed data from which molecular conformation can frequently be deduced. Among the analytical approaches have been those in which the immune response and the products of that response are analyzed and employed as analytical probes of the basic structure and conformation of a subject molecule. Although the major emphasis in molecular immunology and immunochemistry has been the characterization of the immune response, applied immunochemistry has in no little part contributed to our understanding of molecular structure at all levels of organization (Dorrington and Tanford, 1970; Anfinsen, 1959; Kendrew *et al.*, 1960; Scheraga, 1961; Muirhead and Perutz, 1963).

Fibrinogen is among the earliest proteins recognized and studied in a functional context (Hewson, 1771). There is no doubt that prehistoric man must have recognized the dramatic fluid–gel transition of blood, and direct investigative attention was elicited as early as the 18th century (Hewson, 1771). Because of its dramatic and multiple physiological conversions and its major role in biological survival and health, fibrinogen has attracted the attention of both basic and clinical investigators from the earliest days.

This review will be concerned primarily with immunochemical approaches to the structure and conformation of fibrinogen and its multiple physiological derivatives. The use of antibodies as probes with which to explore the structure of fibrinogen (Salmon, 1959; Nussenzweig and Seligmann, 1960; Nussenzweig *et al.*, 1961a,b; Plow and Edgington, 1972a), a complex and conformationally labile protein, has yielded unique information regarding molecular conformation and antigenic expression (Plow and Edgington, 1972a,b,c; Edgington and Plow, 1972; B. Blombäck and Blombäck, 1972). Recent studies have not only provided new insight into the structure of fibrinogen and the pathobiology of this protein in man, but the fibrinogen model has also yielded information of interest to the basic molecular immunologist in regard to molecular events that modulate the expression of native antigens and control the emergence and expression of neoantigens by complex molecules (Plow and Edgington, 1972b).

II. NONIMMUNOLOGIC STUDIES

A. General Properties and Function of Fibrinogen

Fibrinogen plays a highly significant role in biological survival. It is present in high concentration (1.5–3.5 mg/ml) in the blood plasma of man and is found universally and characteristically among vertebrates. This protein literally professes its existence by the dramatic fluid–gel transition that constitutes blood coagulation. Furthermore, investigation of fibrinogen is facilitated by the relative ease with which it can be isolated and highly purified in large quantity (B. Blombäck and Blombäck, 1956). As the focal point of blood coagulation, fibrinogen contributes physically to normal hemostasis, and is subject to a variety of structural and functional modulations in serving its primary and diverse secondary biological roles in health and disease (Brinkhous *et al.*, 1970; Kowalski, 1968).

Activation of the coagulation system is a common event and serves as an intermediary pathological process associated with a broad variety of disease processes. Coagulation mechanisms may be initiated via two classical pathways, both of which culminate in the enzymatic conversion of fibrinogen to fibrin monomer (Macfarlane, 1964; Davie and Ratnoff, 1964; Barton, 1967). The existence of additional independent shunts between other complex mediation systems, such the complement system, with input into specific points in the coagulation system have been recognized. In this respect, the role of complement components on the facilitation of platelet injury and the initiation or facilitation of coagulation *in vivo* and *in vitro* has suggested a new pathway for the provocation of the coagulation system by immunological mechanisms (Zimmerman *et al.,* 1971; Zimmerman and Müller-Eberhard, 1971). An intricate web of interaction between the coagulation system, complement system, immunologic processes, and the inflammatory response is gradually becoming apparent (Ratnoff, 1969).

Regardless of the primary pathogenetic events or the coagulation pathway utilized, activation of the coagulation system culminates in thrombin-induced conversion of fibrinogen to fibrin monomer, and via spontaneous polymerization, covalently cross-linked fibrin fibers are generated (Porter and Hawn, 1949; Szalontai, 1968) (Fig. 1). These events, through complex physiological feedback systems, lead to the conversion of plasminogen to plasmin (Alkjaersig *et al.,* 1959). An effective and compensatory cleavage of fibrin *in vivo* by this enzyme restores vascular integrity and liberates a variety of characteristic fibrin-derived cleavage fragments into the circulation (Astrup, 1956; Sherry *et al.,* 1959) (Fig. 2). Fibrinogen is an equally suitable substrate for plasmin, and cleavage fragments of the parent molecule also may appear in the circulation through a process independent of coagulation, a direct cleavage of fibrinogen by plasmin referred to as a fibrinogenolytic process (Sherry *et al.,* 1959). Fibrinolysis (cleavage of fibrin) and fibrinogenolysis (cleavage of fibrinogen) represent pathophysiologically distinguishable events and the presence of these fragments and

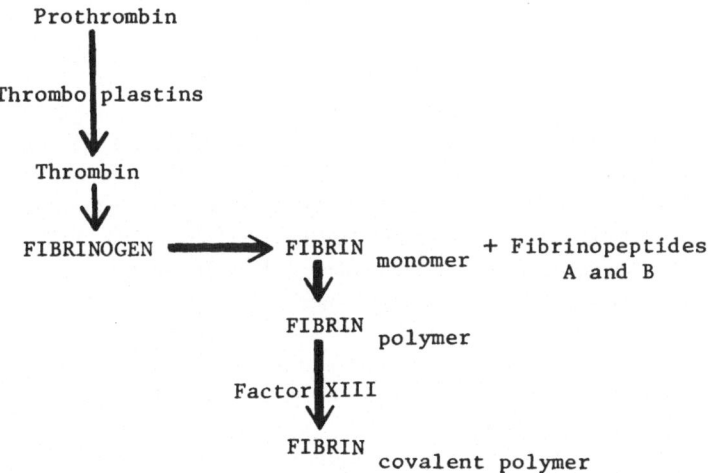

Figure 1. Molecular events associated with the conversion of fibrinogen to fibrin.

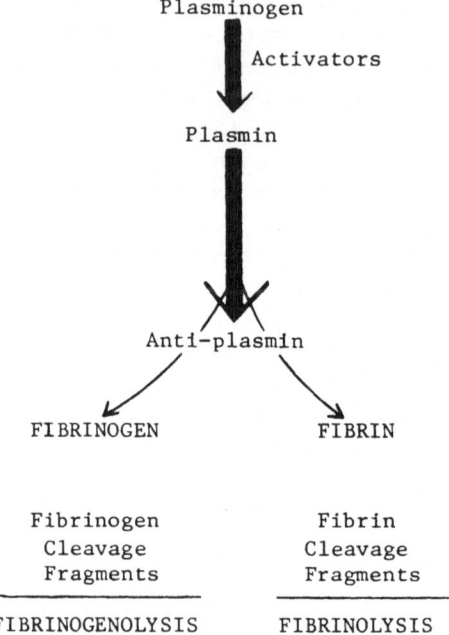

Figure 2. Schematic outline of the plasmin
system. The inactive form of the enzyme, plasminogen, is converted to plasmin by plasminogen activators. The plasmin is in most physiological circumstances inhibited by alpha-2 anti-
plasmin, but if not neutralized can enzymatically hydrolyze either fibrinogen or fibrin.

determination of their origin provides a useful clinical and investigative index of
disease (Merskey *et al.*, 1967; Thomas *et al.*, 1970; Marder *et al.*, 1971).

The various cleavage fragments of fibrinogen and fibrin can each exert
distinctive pathophysiological effects through a variety of basic molecular and
cellular mechanisms (Brinkhous *et al.*, 1970; Kowalski, 1968). Both procoagu-
lant and anticoagulant effects may be observed (D. E. Triantaphyllopoulos *et al.*,
1971). Fibrinogen and fibrin cleavage fragments may not only influence the
deposition and organization of the fibrin network, but they may affect thrombin
formation through antithrombin effects and their capacity to inhibit platelet
aggregation (Niewiarowski *et al.*, 1971). It has also been suggested that cleavage
fragments may directly function in the feedback control of fibrinolysis and
fibrinogenolysis via their capacity to inhibit plasmin activity (Nanninga and
Guest, 1968).

B. Occurrence of Fibrinogen

Proteins capable of undergoing gelation are observed partially distributed among invertebrate phyla. In a teleologic fashion it is attractive to consider that these may serve a role in protection against intrudants. Hemostasis among these organisms appears to be dependent mainly upon cellular mechanisms (Grégoire and Tagnon, 1962). A coagulable protein has been isolated from the lobster *Homarus* which will clot upon exposure to a protein fraction derived from lobster muscle but not on exposure to mammalian thrombin (Duchateau and Florkin, 1954). The horseshoe crab, *Limulus Polyphemus,* also exhibits rapid gelation of plasma upon exposure to endotoxins from several microorganisms (Levine, 1967). In this system, a major protein is activated to undergo gelation by a minor protein (Young *et al.,* 1971). In an analogous fashion, coagulation is also provoked by endotoxins to initiate intravascular coagulation in vertebrates, the Sanarelli-Schwartzmann phenomenon (McKay, 1965). These aggregating molecules are found only in a few members of the phylum *Arthropoda.* In spite of the superficial similarities, upon detailed physicochemical study, the differences are so great as to suggest that the occurrence of coagulable protein among both vertebrates and the phylum *Arthropoda* may be a matter of parallel evolution (Doolittle, 1970).

A protein readily recognizable as fibrinogen and fulfilling all of the criteria for fibrinogen is found universally among vertebrates. A common fundamental scheme is found in which plasma prothrombin is converted to thrombin following the interaction of a variety of procoagulants, and in turn the thrombin enzymatically converts fibrinogen to fibrin (Macfarlane, 1964; Davie and Ratnoff, 1964; Barton, 1967) (Fig. 1). Because of the existence of significant interspecies differences in the primary structure of fibrinogen (Doolittle, 1970; Söderqvist and Blombäck, 1971), interspecies similarities and differences in the structure of fibrinogen have been explored in reference to taxonomic phylogeny and evolution (Mross and Doolittle, 1967; B. Blombäck, 1971).

C. General Structure of Fibrinogen

Following the observation and deductive efforts of Hewson and documentation of his observations in 1771 (Hewson, 1771), little interest in fibrinogen was evident until the naming of the protein by Virchow in 1847 (Virchow, 1847). Through the efforts of Denis (1859) and Hammersten (1880) in the latter 19th century, the initial isolations of this protein were achieved. The detailed efforts of Blombäck and Blombäck (1956) led to effective preparation of fibrinogen in large quantity and high purity suitable for detailed biochemical analysis. Current data supports a molecular weight of approximately 340,000 daltons and the presence of three pairs of polypeptide chains, a, β, and γ (B. Blombäck and

Yamashina, 1958; McKee *et al.*, 1970), linked together by clusters of disulfide bonds (Murano *et al.*, 1972; M. Blombäck *et al.*, 1968) (Fig. 3). It has generally been accepted that organization of the three pairs of chains in the native molecule is symmetrical (Haschemeyer, 1963).

Ultrastructural studies of the structure of fibrin by Porter and Hawn (1947) led to the initial proposal of an oblate ellipsoidal conformation for the molecule. Subsequent studies by Hall and Slayter (1959) led to the proposal of a rodlike molecule measuring 475 ± 25Å in length with a central nodule measuring 50Å and an additional nodule measuring 65Å at each end of the molecule. The three lobular regions when visualized by electron microscopy appear to be attached by thin strands approximately 12 Å thick (Fig. 4). It has been suggested that the characteristic periodicity of fibrin fibers results from end-to-end and side-to-side polymerization of these triglobular rods with a staggered association of proto-fibrils to result in organized fibrin (Porter and Hawn, 1949; Szalontai, 1968).

In 1966, Köppel proposed for fibrinogen a new and unique conformation (Köppel, 1966). Based upon ultrastructural visualization of the fibrinogen mon-

FIBRINOGEN

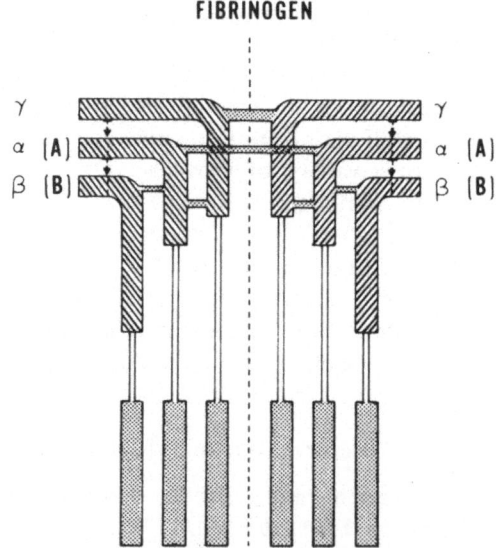

Figure 3. Schematic model of constituent chains and disulfide bridges in the N-terminal disulfide knot (cross-hatched) per B. Blombäck (B. Blombäck and Blombäck, 1972; B. Blombäck *et al.*, 1972) and Wallen (1971). The three pairs of polypeptide chains, α, β, and γ, are indicated as well as the thrombin-susceptible cleavage sites which lead to the release of small N-terminal fibrinopeptides A and B.

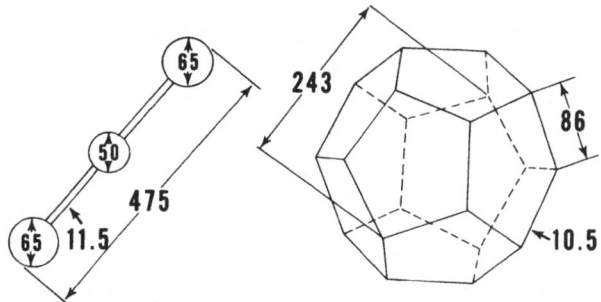

Figure 4. Two widely divergent models of the conformation of fibrinogen: *Left,* the rodlike model, proposed by Hall and Slayter (1959). *Right,* the pentagonal dodecahedral model of Köppel (1966). Intramolecular distances are in angstroms.

omer and the constituent molecules present in fibrin fibers, he proposed a pentagonal dodecahedral organization (Fig. 4). This intriguing conformation will accommodate the indicated 34% alpha-helical structure calculated from optical rotatory dispersion (Budzynski, 1971) and also the observed 226Å·reflex of small angle X-ray diffraction of fibrin fibers (Stryer *et al.,* 1963). Employing the pentagonal dodecahedral model, with an edge length of 76.1–81.2Å, the natural dual periodicity of 200–208Å and 165–170Å of fibrin fibers is readily accommodated. Köppel has also described the hypothetical arrangements of constituent polypeptide chains (Köppel, 1970). More recently Stewart has suggested a large coiled shape for fibrinogen, a rather imprecisely defined model which would embody considerable flexibility (Stewart, 1971). Critical assessment of such a model and its compatibility with various physiochemical and biochemical data is not known; however, the high degree of alpha-helical content of fibrinogen (Budzynski, 1971) would impose some perhaps uncomfortable limits upon the proposed high degree of flexibility.

The constituent polypeptide chains of fibrinogen can be separated after either reduction or oxidation of disulfide bonds (McKee *et al.,* 1970; Murano *et al.,* 1972; Henschen, 1964*a*). Molecular weights of the chains, determined by sedimentation equilibrium, are approximately: a = 64,000–68,000 daltons, β = 56,000–57,000 daltons, and γ = 47,500–48,000 (McKee *et al.,* 1970; Murano *et al.,* 1972). Heterogeneity is found in human fibrinogen and is reflected by the presence of three different a-chain variants with identical N-terminal amino acids but with differing chromatographic behavior and a slight difference in molecular weight of the N-terminal peptides released by thrombin, fibrinopeptide A (Murano *et al.,* 1971; B. Blombäck *et al.,* 1972; McDonagh *et al.,* 1971). The three variants of the fibrinopeptide A occur among fibrinogen from the same individual, and have raised considerable questions regarding the molecular basis of this variation. Heterogeneity of fibrinogen and its composite chains may follow changes introduced *in vivo* or *in vitro* by endogenous proteolytic enzymes (the possibility of more complex molecular biological explanations including transcriptional, translational, and assembly errors must be retained as remote possibilities).

D. The Fibrin Transition

Thrombin, the active physiological enzyme yielded by prothrombin conversion, exhibits considerable specificity for fibrinogen. Thrombin hydrolyzes specific arginyl–glycyl bonds which link the fibrinopeptides A and B to the α and β chains, respectively (Lorand, 1951; Lorand and Middlebrook, 1952) (Fig 3). Fibrinopeptide A (1,519 daltons) consists of the 16 N-terminal amino acids of the α chain (two other random variants known as AY and AP also occur). Fibrinopeptide B (1,555 daltons) represents the 14 N-terminal amino acids of the β chain. Certain other arginyl, and possibly lysyl, bonds are also subject to hydrolysis by thrombin at a much slower rate. Following removal of the fibrinopeptides, the first structural and conformational derivative can be recognized—fibrin monomer. Under physiological conditions, fibrin monomer will spontaneously and rapidly form a very highly ordered and covalently bonded linear polymer (Szalontai, 1968) (Fig. 1).

Local conformational features of the fibrinogen molecule are suggested by the observation that fibrinopeptide A always is initially released and only after a lag phase does free fibrinopeptide B appear (Lorand, 1954). Polymerization is initiated upon removal of the fibrinopeptide A, although it is less efficient than following removal of fibrinopeptide B. The snake venom enzyme reptilase hydrolyzes only the fibrinopeptide A, but complete polymerization can be demonstrated (B. Blombäck, 1958). Differences in the physical behavior of polymers from which only the fibrinopeptide A have been cleaved as contrasted with those from which both fibrinopeptides A and B have been removed (Laurent and Blombäck, 1958) have led to the hypothesis that the thrombin-sensitive peptide bonds on the α chain are more readily exposed and that the thrombin-susceptible site on the β chain is exposed only following cleavage and removal of fibrinopeptide A and the unfolding of the residual α chain (B. Blombäck and Blombäck, 1970). Fibrinogen Detroit, one of the rare hereditary variants of fibrinogen (M. Blombäck *et al.*, 1968), differs in being uncoaguable as a result of a specific molecular defect in the α chain, with substitution of a serine for the arginine normally present in the 19th position (Mammen *et al.*, 1969; Hampton and Garrison, 1972). Although fibrinopeptide A is released, polymerization is ineffective. It has been suggested that local conformational changes associated with hypothesized unfolding of the residual α chain apparently are abnormal and do not lead to formation of a copolymerization site. Apparently local steric effects influence the thrombin-susceptible locus on the β

chain since fibrinopeptide B is only very slowly released from fibrinogen Detroit by thrombin. Thus, this functional manifestation of fibrinogen and an aberration in behavior attributable to a single amino acid substitution provide data from which local intramolecular conformational attributes may be deduced (Fig. 3).

At least 18 hereditary variants of fibrinogen have been described in man (M. Blombäck *et al.*, 1968). Seven of these appear to be functionally incompetent and were associated with abnormal bleeding, two of these aberrant molecules were associated with combined thrombotic and hemorrhagic states suggesting abnormal physical or kinetic responses to thrombin, and one variant was clinically associated with thrombosis, thus suggesting a hypercoagulable molecule.

E. Disulfide Bonds and "Decapitation" of Fibrinogen

One of the more significant and productive strategies in elucidating both the schematic structure of the molecule and also in providing additional conformational information has been the cleavage of fibrinogen with cyanogen bromide to yield the N-terminal disulfide knot (N-DSK) (B. Blombäck *et al.*, 1968; B. Blombäck, 1969). Following cleavage of methionyl bonds of fibrinogen with cyanogen bromide, a great number of fragments are generated. Among these fragments, a dimeric fragment of 52,000–58,000 daltons (B. Blombäck and Blombäck, 1972; Woods *et al.*, 1962) with three pairs of polypeptide chains of 6,200, 12,200, and 11,500 daltons and the fibrinopeptides A and B (Woods *et al.*, 1972) are recovered. Thus, the calculated molecular weight of the N-DSK monomer is 29,000 and of the dimer approximately 58,000. Within each half of the primary fibrinogen molecule the three constituent polypeptide chains are cross-linked by 14 intra- and/or inter-chain disulfide linkages (Henschen, 1962, 1964) whereas in the N-terminal segment of these chains present in the DSK, which represent approximately 16% of the molecule, 5½ disulfide bridges are to be found in each half of the DSK (Murano *et al.*, 1972; B. Blombäck, 1969).

The primary structure of the N-DSK has been deduced and reconstructed in some detail, and a schematic representation of the intermolecular interrelationships of the constituent chains offered by Blombäck (B. Blombäck and Blombäck, 1972; B. Blombäck, 1972) and Wallen (1971) is illustrated in Fig. 3. The molecule is thus visualized as a rather rodlike structure with the fibrinopeptides placed symmetrically around a central axis of symmetry.

F. Plasmin-Cleavage Fragments of Fibrinogen/Fibrin

Plasmin is a trypsinlike enzyme with somewhat more restricted specificity for arginyl–lysyl bonds than trypsin. Theoretically, there are approximately 300 potential cleavage sites present in the fibrinogen molecule; however, only 70% of the trypsin-susceptible bonds are cleaved by plasmin (Wallen, 1971). Following complete digestion of fibrinogen by plasmin, approximately 70% of the molecule is retained in the form of moderate-sized plasmin-resistant fragments, the plasmin-resistant core (Budzynski *et al.*, 1967). The protein fragments present in this core have been separated by ion exchange (Nussenzweig *et al.*, 1961*a*; Nilehn, 1967) or preparative electrophoresis (Marder *et al.*, 1969*a*) into two independent protein fragments termed the D and the E fragments (Nussenzweig *et al.*, 1961*a*; Nilehn, 1967). The D fragments represent 50–55% of the original nitrogen content of the fibrinogen, while the recovered E fragments represent 15–20% (Nussenzweig and Seligmann, 1960; Budzynski *et al.*, 1967; Marder *et al.*, 1967, 1969*b*). In addition to these two stable terminal cleavage fragments of both fibrin and fibrinogen, discrete intermediate fragments can be recognized. High-molecular-weight fibrinogen derivatives, approximately 20% smaller than the parent molecule, have independently been described by Fletcher *et al.*

Table I. Major Characterized Plasmin-Cleavage Fragments of Fibrinogen

Molecule or fragment	Degree of plasmin cleavage	$S_{25,w}$*	Estimated molecular weights	
			(daltons)	(references)
Fibrinogen	None	8.8–8.9	340,000	McDonagh *et al.*, 1971; Caspary and Kekwick, 1957
Fibrinogen, early derivatives	Early	8.5–8.8	269,000–320,000	Fletcher *et al.*, 1966; Mills, 1972; Mosesson *et al.*, 1967*b*
Fragment X	Intermediate	7.9	240,000–270,000	Plow and Edgington, 1972*a* Marder *et al.*, 1967, 1969*b*; Pizzo *et al.*, 1972*a*
Fragment Y	Intermediate	6.8	155,000–205,000	Marder *et al.*, 1967, 1969*b*; Mills and Karpatkin, 1971; Mills, 1972
Fragment D	Late	4.8-5.7	73,000–96,000	Budzynski *et al.*, 1967; Marder *et al.*, 1967; Catanzaro *et al.*, 1972
Fragment E	Late	3.3-3.8	28,000–55,000	Budzynski *et al.*, 1967; Marder *et al.*, 1967; Dudek *et al.*, 1970
D:E complex	Late	3.6	106,000–130,000	Edgington and Plow, 1972; Budzynski *et al.*, 1967; Plow and Edgington, 1973*a*

* Fletcher *et al.*, 1966; Mosesson *et al.*, 1967; Plow and Edgington, 1973*a*; Marder, 1970.

(1966), Mosesson *et al.* (1967), and Marder *et al.* (1967, 1969*b*). It now appears Mosesson's fraction I-8 represents an earlier stage in the cleavage process than fragment X (Mosesson *et al.*, 1972). Fletcher's "fibrinogen first derivative" may again be an intermediate between fibrinogen and fragment X. There is considerable heterogeneity demonstrable within each of the generic fragments derived during progressive plasmin cleavage of fibrinogen or fibrin (Pizzo *et al.*, 1972*a*; Arnesen, 1971; Catanzaro *et al.*, 1972). Continuous cleavage and release of more than 80 peptides occurs (E. Triantaphyllopoulos, 1972) during progressive plasmin cleavage of fibrinogen or fibrin, and each of the described and characterized intermediate and terminal cleavage fragments (Table I) should be considered only as generic entities. This is most evident in the case of the unstable high-molecular-weight intermediate X fragment (Pizzo *et al.*, 1972*a*). Despite the suggestion of a continuum of cleavage culminating in the production of the plasmin-resistant fragments, when plasmin-cleaved samples of fibrinogen are fractionated by molecular size on columns of Sephadex G-200 (Marder, 1971*a*) or beaded 6% agarose (Plow and Edgington, 1972*a*), four discrete elution peaks, clearly differing in size, can be clearly discriminated (Fig. 5). These appear to represent in order of size from the largest to the smallest: fibrinogen, fragment X, fragment Y, and the D:E complex (Plow and Edgington, 1972*a*, 1973*a*; Edgington and Plow, 1972; Marder *et al.*, 1967; Marder *et al.*, 1969*b*). Furthermore, on the basis of electrophoretic mobility in polyacrylamide gels, characteristic discrete banding patterns corresponding to the generically described X, Y, D, and E fragments are observed (Marder *et al.*, 1971).

Physicochemical analyses of the various cleavage fragments have concentrated on the stable terminal D and E fragments but have been sufficient to

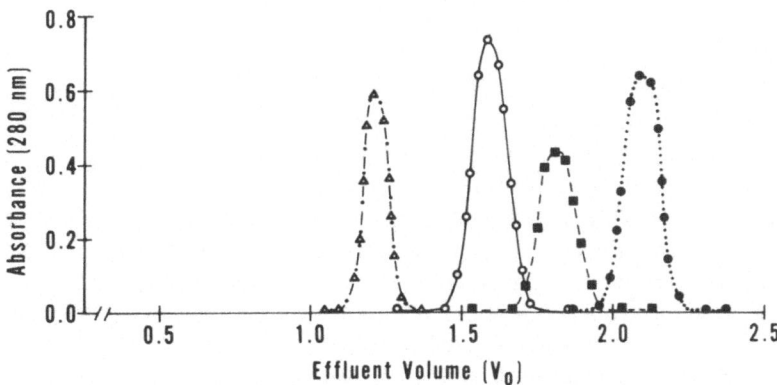

Figure 5. Typical molecular exclusion chromatographic pattern of fibrinogen and plasmin-cleavage fragments. The peaks represent in sequence by size: fg, fg-X, fg-Y, and the D:E complex (Plow and Edgington, 1972*a*). Chromatography on A-1.5 (Biorad) beaded agarose.

characterize each of the fragments. The plasmin-cleavage fragments are generally similar whether derived from fibrinogen or fibrin (Marder et al., 1969b), although a variety of fine differences in structure and some major differences in physicochemical behavior have been demonstrated (Dudek et al., 1970; Lewis and Wilson, 1964). Minimally degraded fibrinogen can be recovered from plasma and appears to reflect minimal cleavage of α and, to lesser extent, β chains (Fletcher et al., 1966; Mosesson et al., 1972). Molecular weight estimates of 269,000–320,000 have been offered for these species.

The X fragment of fibrinogen or fibrin can be isolated after brief plasmin cleavage. This generic product is rather heterogeneous, suggesting multiple species (Pizzo et al., 1972a). Analytical ultracentrifugation of rather homogeneous X fragment has given an $S_{25,w}$ of 8.8–7.9 as compared with 8.34 for fibrinogen (Marder et al., 1969b). Estimates of its molecular weight vary from 270,000 to 240,000 daltons (Marder et al., 1967, 1969b; Fletcher et al., 1966; Mosesson et al., 1967), and it appears to represent nearly 80% of the mass of the parent fibrinogen or fibrin molecule. The X fragment differs from other cleavage fragments in that the fibrinogen-derived variety is slowly clotted upon exposure to thrombin and it is capable of then complexing with itself, fibrin, and certain other cleavage fragments (Niewiarowski et al., 1970). Recent studies of this fragment by Furlan and Beck (1972) and by Marder et al. (1972) have suggested that plasmin cleavage of fibrinogen to yield X may be asymmetrical.

Only very limited studies of the Y fragments have been reported. Estimated molecular weights of 155,000–165,000 daltons have been proposed (Marder et al., 1967, 1969b); however, recent SDS polyacrylamide gel electrophoresis studies yielded a direct molecular-weight estimate of 205,000 daltons (Mills and Karpatkin, 1971). The calculated corrections of the observed value from 205,000 to 155,000 (Mills, 1972) follows the suggestion of McDonagh (1971); however, the degree of correction required may vary with the nature of the subject molecule or fragment.

Estimates of molecular weight of D fragments have ranged from 68,000 to 85,000 daltons (Budzynski et al., 1967; Marder et al., 1967). Recent estimates in our laboratory have given 78,000 ± 3,900 upon analysis of the intact molecule as well as by independent summation of its constituent polypeptide chains (Catanzaro et al., 1972). This is in general agreement with other recent studies (Dudek et al., 1970). This cleavage fragment appears homogeneous by ultracentrifugation and immunoelectrophoresis; however, upon isoelectric focusing or polyacrylamide gel electrophoresis in the absence of SDS, as many as eight hyperfine bands differing only slightly in R_m are recognized (Arnesen, 1971; Jamieson and Gaffney, 1968). Further analysis has suggested that the hyperfine banding represents charge isomers of similar molecular size rather than polymers of molecules of differing size (Catanzaro et al., 1972). Reduction of the D fragment yields three polypeptide chains of molecular weights of 44,000 ± 2,700, 25,350 ± 900, and 10,400 ± 720. Through simple conservation of mass it has been deduced that two D fragment regions must be present in the parent fibrinogen or fibrin molecule (Marder *et al.*, 1969*b*). Conservation of alpha-helical conformation or refolding to generate new alpha-helical regions is observed with an estimated 40% alpha helix in the D fragment as contrasted with 34% for the whole molecule (Budzynski, 1971).

The E fragments of fibrinogen and fibrin do not exhibit microheterogeneity typical of the other fragments. Estimated molecular weights, utilizing a variety of methods, have yielded data indicative of molecular weights ranging from 28,000 to 56,000 daltons (Budzynski *et al.*, 1967; Marder *et al.*, 1967). Recent data, based upon amino acid composition, has suggested a molecular weight of approximately 48,000 (Dudek *et al.*, 1970). Although originally thought to be homogeneous, Niewiarowski and Nandi (1971) have demonstrated three apparent progressively degraded species of E by polyacrylamide gel electrophoresis. Reduction of the E fragment was originally thought to yield a single polypeptide chain (Budzynski *et al.*, 1967), but the presence of three chains of 10,000–15,000 daltons has more recently been suggested (Pizzo *et al.*, 1972*b*). Estimated molecular weights of the constituent polypeptide chains vary from approximately 16,000, 14,000, and 10,500 (Edgington and Plow, 1972), to 5,000, 8,000, and 10,000 (Pizzo *et al.*, 1972*a*; Furlan and Beck, 1972). Because of the limit of the techniques, additional small peptides could be lost from analysis. In order to achieve conservation of mass, the generation of only one mole of E fragment per mole of fibrinogen or fibrin has been proposed (Marder, 1968); however, satisfactory conservation of mass also can be accomplished with a yield of two E fragments (Edgington and Plow, 1972) (Table VII). Wallen (1971) has suggested from peptide mapping that the N-DSK and E fragment overlap, and similar conclusions have been forwarded by N-terminal amino acid analysis (Marder *et al.*, 1972).

It has been suggested that the D and E fragments may exhibit mutual affinity for one another and be recovered as a noncovalently associated bimolecular core from terminal plasmin digests of fibrinogen (Budzynski *et al.*, 1967). Physicochemical studies are limited (Edgington and Plow, 1972; Budzynski *et al.*, 1967), but support immunochemical data (Plow and Edgington, 1972*a*, 1973*a*; Edgington and Plow, 1972) for the existence of this complex.

III. MOLECULAR IMMUNOLOGY

A. Biological Perspective

It is well recognized that the antigenic expressions of protein molecules are determined at multiple levels of molecular organization. Amino acid sequences may serve directly as sequential antigenic determinants analogous to small peptide antigens such as angiotensin (Dietrich, 1967; Benjamini *et al.*, 1972) or

Table II. Biological Basis for Structural Features of Fibrinogen
Responsible for Native, Modulated Native, and Neoantigenic Expressions

Levels of biological organization	Possible parallels with the fibrinogen model
I. *Information* (DNA)	
a) Primary information (genome)	
Heredity	1) Normal fibrinogen
Mutation	2) Heredity abnormal fibrinogens
b) Control	3) Acquired abnormal fibrinogens?
Gene repression	
Gene derepression	
II. *Synthesis*	
a) Transcription	
b) Translation	1) Normal fibrinogen
c) Post-translational modification and assembly	2) Acquired abnormal fibrinogens?
III. *Function*	
Conformational and/or structural changes associated with function	Fibrinogen–Fibrin transition
IV. *Catabolism*	
a) Enzymatic cleavage, degradation	
Physiological	1) Heterogeneity of fibrinogen
Pathological	2) Fibrinogenolysis, fibrinolysis
b) Denaturation, aggregation	

the synthetic polypeptides of defined sequence (Sela *et al.*, 1967; Sela, 1970). Alternatively, the tertiary conformation and quaternary organization may be equally if not more significant in the genesis and control of antigenic expression (Pressman and Grossberg, 1968; Sela, 1969; Goodman, 1969). The latter features may be related not only to the remarkable stereospecificity of antibodies (Pressman and Grossberg, 1968) but also to local spatial features of the surface of proteins that influence exposure of antigenic determinants (Plow and Edgington, 1972*b*). Functional relationships between conformation and antigenic expression have frequently been considered in terms of antigenic deficiency of molecules altered in tertiary conformation (Brown *et al.*, 1959; Javid and Yingling, 1968); however, new antigenic expressions, *neoantigens.* also may be engendered by modification of molecular structure (Bartel and Campbell, 1959; Ishizaka *et al.*, 1960; Williams and Kunkel, 1962; Lehrer and Van Vunakis, 1965).

The molecular basis for distinctive and differential antigenic expression by proteins must be considered in reference to the structure, conformation, and modification of molecules. These molecular parameters are subject to events at four levels of biological organization: (1) *information*, (2) *synthesis*, (3) *function*, and (4) *catabolism* (Table II). Within this conceptual framework, the molecular immunology of fibrinogen may be explored.

B. Species Differences

Informational or genetic prescription of the structural basis of antigenic expression is well exemplified by recognized genetic and antigenic differences between species. In 1912, Bauer and Engel (1912) utilized complement fixation to demonstrate apparent species differences between fibrinogens of beef and swine; however, Kato (1924) subsequently observed broad cross-reactivity of heterologous antisera to fibrinogens. Hektoen and Welker (1927) also substantiated broad antigenic cross-reactivity among mammalian and avian fibrinogens and they again demonstrated only limited interspecies differences. Species differences in native antigenic expression of the intact molecule were systematically established by a number of investigators (Kyes and Porter, 1931; Demanez, 1932; Kenton, 1933). Nussenzweig and DeSouza (1962), explored differences and cross-reactions between the D and E fragments of human fibrinogen and bovine fibrinogen. Antigenic differences were demonstrable in the D and E regions as well as elsewhere in the fibrinogen molecule. These immunochemical studies suggest broad conservation of genetic information with selective differences between the fibrinogens of different species which are reflected by distinctive differences in immunochemical expression.

C. Abnormal Fibrinogens

The reported hereditary abnormal fibrinogens have been recognized because of aberrant functional features distinguishable from normal fibrinogens. They appear to be transmitted as an autosomal dominant trait (Ménaché, 1970). In all reported cases, the abnormal fibrinogens reacted with antiserum to normal human fibrinogen and exhibited apparent identity with normal fibrinogens by Ouchterlony analysis (Mammen et al., 1969; Ménaché, 1970, 1964; Jackson et al., 1965; Forman et al., 1968). Minor immunoelectrophoretic differences have been noted for two abnormal fibrinogens (Ménaché, 1964). Since inheritance of mutant genes or primary mutation would most likely code for minimal structural differences in the fibrinogen molecule, the observed conservation of major antigenic expressions is to be anticipated. Detailed quantitative immunochemical studies of the abnormal fibrinogens are unavilable, although genetically determined structural differences might yield incisive information concerning the molecular basis of antigenic expression.

An acquired abnormal fibrinogen has recently been recognized in association with an hepatic tumor (Von Felten et al., 1969). Since fibrinogen is synthesized by the liver (Miller *et al.,* 1964; John and Miller, 1960), it has been hypothesized that this abnormal population of fibrinogen molecules may have been produced by the neoplastic liver cells. It is not known whether the apparent structural aberration was secondary to mutation or aberration of control mechanisms at the informational level. It is also possible that this abnormal fibrinogen could have been secondary to systematic synthetic errors (Table II). Although qualitatively similar to normal fibrinogen by Ouchterlony techniques, no detailed quantitative immunochemical studies of this acquired abnormal fibrinogen are available.

D. Influence of Synthesis on Immunochemical Expressions

Limited information is available regarding the influence of synthetic events on the immunochemical expressions of fibrinogen. There are no proven examples of abnormal structural fibrinogen resulting from defective transcription, systematic translational error, or aberrant post-translational modification and assembly; however, the possibility that some of the examples of afibrinogenemia, hypofibrinogenemia, and abnormal fibrinogens, particularly the acquired type (Von Felten *et al.,* 1969), may be due to systematic defects of synthesis has not been entirely excluded. Beck (1971) has recently demonstrated immunologically that several families with inherited abnormal fibrinogens have low fibrinogen concentrations in their plasma. Immunologic assays of cases of hypofibrinogenemia, diagnosed by functional assays, have confirmed that there are indeed reduced plasma concentrations of this protein (Beck, 1971). Fibrinogen is either absent or present only in very low concentration in individuals with congenital afibrinogenemia. Some of these individuals produce antifibrinogen antibodies following parenteral administration of normal fibrinogen (Brönnimann, 1954; DeVries *et al.,* 1961). The intramolecular specificity of these antibodies has not been explored. The possibility of synthetic defects leading to reduced synthesis is an intriguing possibility.

The immunochemical expressions of normal fibrinogen are dependent upon assembly of the three pairs of constituent chains and the conformation imparted by such assembly. Employing antisera to isolated S-carboxymethylated α and β chains in Ouchterlony gel precipitin assays, Blombäck and Blombäck (1972) have reported reactions with intact fibrinogen. This suggests that some of the antigenic determinants of the α and β chains are exposed in the intact native molecule. By contrast, anti-γ-chain antisera did not react in these assays with intact fibrinogen, suggesting interiorization of this chain or major post-assembly conformational differences such as to preclude reactions with antisera to the isolated γ-chain. Interiorization of the γ chain is further supported by the marked susceptibility of the α and β chains to plasmin proteolysis, and the marked resistance of susceptible peptide bonds in the γ chain to similar enzymatic hydrolysis (Pizzo *et al.* 1972*a*; Furlan and Beck, 1972). Blombäck and Blombäck (1972) have also noted that their antifibrinogen antiserum did not visibly react with the isolated constituent chains by Ouchterlony analysis, suggesting that native fibrinogen expressions are to a great extent conformational in character.

Employing quantitative radioimmunochemical assays for native antigenic expression of fibrinogen, association of the amino-terminal and carboxy-terminal aspects of the molecule have been suggested (Edgington and Plow, 1972; Plow and Edgington, 1973*a*). This association is apparently mediated by hydrophobic forces (Plow and Edgington, 1973*a*). A high axial ratio of the D:E complex, and by inference this region of the molecule, is suggested by an observed sedimentation velocity $S_{20,w}$ of approximately 3.6 in the face of an estimated molecular weight of 128,000. These data, coupled with the well recognized influence of fibrinopeptide release from the N terminus upon γ–γ cross-linking sites at the C terminus seems to be inconsistent with the long linear arrangement of fibrinogen proposed by Hall and Slayter (1959) while favoring the more globular arrangements suggested by Köppel (1970) or the oblate ellipsoid model of Hawn and Porter (1947).

E. The Fibrinogen–Fibrin Transition

Salmon (1959) has suggested the existence of subtle antigenic differences between fibrinogen and fibrin by precipitin techniques. Similar results have not been reported by others. Recently, immunochemical assay of fibrinopeptide A has been described by Nossel *et al.* (1971). Detailed exploration of fibrinopeptide antigen expression by fibrinogen, fibrin, and the various fragments have not been reported, although this technique should permit an incisive view of the N terminus of the molecule. Definite, though subtle, differences in antigenic expression between fibrinogen and fibrin have been recognized recently by competitive-inhibition primary binding assays. Rabbit antisera to fibrinogen reacts preferentially with the fibrinogen molecule although the reaction can be completely inhibited by fibrin; and antifibrin antisera reacts preferentially with soluble fibrin although this reaction can also be completely inhibited by fibrinogen. No unique absolute antigenic differences were demonstrated. The observed relative differences may represent conformational influences on the expression of antigenic determinants and the affinity of the primary immunochemical reactions (Edgington and Plow, 1972, 1973). M. Blombäck (1972) has recently suggested that N-DSK-associated antigens are more exposed or effectively expressed by fibrin as compared to fibrinogen. This is also compatible with immunochemical data indicating greater exposure of the E region of the molecule in fibrin (Plow and Edgington, 1973*b*).

F. Catabolic Events and the Intramolecular Distribution
of Antigenic Expression

1. Qualitative Features of Catabolic Fragments

Nussenzweig and colleagues generically segregated fibrinogen antigens in respect to their expression by terminal plasmin-cleavage fragments (Nussenzweig and Seligmann, 1960; Nussenzweig et al., 1961a,b). Employing hyperimmune antifibrinogen antisera, they recognized the presence of two large and antigenically independent fragments which they named D (fg-D) and E (fg-E) and the presence of additional smaller peptide fragments referred to as A, B, and C which were thought to be nonantigenic. The total antigenic expression of fibrinogen was then considered in respect to the D-associated antigens, the E-associated antigens, and those expressions not accounted for by either D or E (Nussenzweig et al., 1961b; Nussenzweig and DeSouza, 1962). They described the immunoelectrophoretic characteristics of fg-D and fg-E and estimated that 20–40% of late hyperimmune antibody responses were directed to D- and E-associated antigens (Nussenzweig et al., 1961b). Marder and colleagues subsequently described the intermediate fragments X (fg-X) and Y (fg-Y) and demonstrated their immunologic properties by Ouchterlony and immunoelectrophoretic techniques employing antifibrinogen antisera (Marder et al., 1967; 1969b; Marder, 1968).

Immunoelectrophoretic analysis has provided an effective means for identification of fibrinogen and the diverse intermediate (X and Y) and terminal (D and E) cleavage fragments. Typical immunoelectrophoretic behavior is illustrated in Fig. 6. The type of agar or agarose and buffer characteristics have a profound effect upon the immunoelectrophoresis pattern, and conditions need be carefully standardized prior to use of this technique (Edgington and Plow, unpublished). Fibrinogen, fg-X, and fg-Y exhibit apparent identity by Ouchterlony analysis, and a long arc without spurs or other evidence of antigenic heterogeneity is observed when analyzed by immunoelectrophoresis (Marder, 1968; Marder and Sherry, 1971). Fg-D and fg-E only exhibit partial identity with fibrinogen, fg-X, and fg-Y by Ouchterlony analysis or immunoelectrophoresis (Marder, 1968). Complete nonidentity is observed between fg-D and fg-E by both precipitin in gel techniques (Nussenzweig et al., 1961b; Marder, 1968). Based upon these observations, the generic distribution of molecular regions can be deduced. Both D and E regions of the molecule must be present in fibrinogen, fg-X, and fg-Y; and the D and E regions represent the smallest antigenic and structural denominators yielded by plasmin cleavage.

The N-terminal disulfide knot (N-DSK) represents a key fragment of nonphysiologic derivation. Within this 52,000–58,000 molecular-weight fragment (B. Blombäck and Blombäck, 1972; Woods et al., 1972) of the N terminus are found fg-E-associated antigens. Apparent immunochemical identity between fg-E

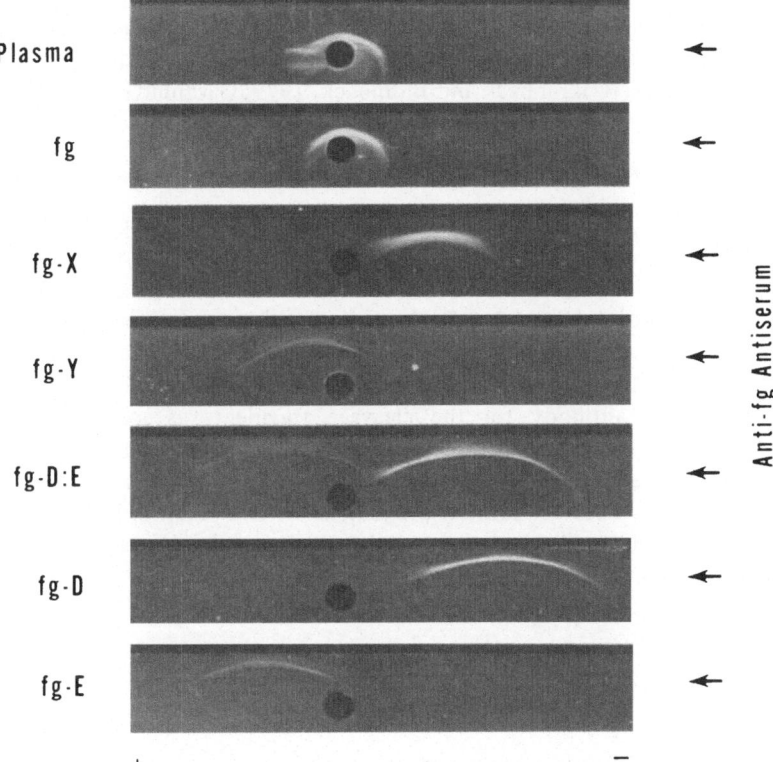

Figure 6. Immunoelectrophoresis of fibrinogen (fg) and each of the plasmin-cleavage fragments including the terminal plasmin-resistant core of D and E fragments (fg-D:E) in 1% Difco agar agar No. 2 in 0.25 M veronal buffer pH 8.6 at 5.5 V/cm for 75 min. Ten-μl samples at 1 mg protein/ml or 5 μl plasma were elctrophoresed and all slides developed with rabbit antifibrinogen antiserum. Note that the relative mobility of the D and E fragments in fg-D:E are reduced by comparison with the individual fg-D or fg-E fragments isolated from fg-D:E.

and N-DSK has been observed in Ouchterlony gel analysis employing antifibrinogen antisera (Marder *et al.*, 1972; Marder and Sherry, 1971). By contrast, only partial identity has been observed when antiserum to N-DSK is employed (B. Blombäck and Blombäck, 1972). Whether the additional antigenic determinants expressed on isolated N-DSK and responsible for eliciting anti-N-DSK antibodies not reactive with fg-E are native or are secondary to denaturation induced by the rather drastic conditions during isolation of N-DSK is not known. To further cloud this problem, anti-fg-E antiserum has been reported to be nonreactive with N-DSK although it precipitates fg-E (B. Blombäck and Blombäck, 1972). It can be tentatively concluded that all or part of the E-fragment region of fibrinogen is present in N-DSK. A recent report suggests that a small part of the D-fragment region of the molecule may also be contained within N-DSK; anti-N-DSK has been observed to react with isolated fg-D as well as with a small disulfide cluster isolated from fg-D (B. Blombäck and Blombäck, 1972; Gardlund *et al.*, 1972).

2. Quantitative Immunochemical Studies of Catabolism

Modulation of antigenic expression during plasmin cleavage of fibrinogen has been investigated by Plow and Edgington (1972*a*). Competitive inhibition profiles illustrated in Fig. 7 show progressive qualitative and quantitative loss of total or native antigenic expression as the molecule is reduced to each of its progressively smaller physiological cleavage fragments. The competitive-inhibition slopes differ significantly, reflecting differences in the binding affinity of antifibrinogen antibody for the cleavage fragments as compared to the radiolabeled native fibrinogen. Progressive absolute antigenic deficiency is indicated by incomplete inhibition with competing antigen in excess. The data have been developed in a tabular fashion utilizing as criteria of antigenic differences: (1) the competitive-inhibition slope and (2) the molar concentration of a fragment required for 50% competitive inhibition (Table III).

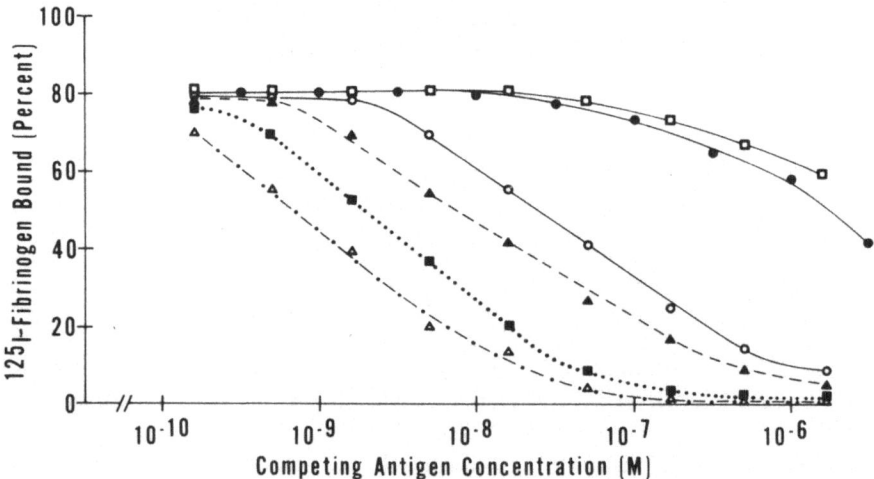

Figure 7. Competitive inhibition radioimmunoassay of native antigenic expression of fibrinogen and derivatives using ^{125}I-fibrinogen (1×10^{-9}M) and anti-native-fibrinogen antiserum in a double antibody type of assay. Competing antigens are introduced at indicated molar concentrations. Note the striking loss of native antigenic expression associated with plasmin cleavage, indicated by the increasing concentration of competing fragment required for 50% inhibition of binding of ^{125}I-fibrinogen. Fibrinogen ($\triangle \cdots \triangle$), fg-X ($\blacksquare \cdots \blacksquare$), fg-Y ($\blacktriangle$----$\blacktriangle$), fg-D:E ($\circ$————$\circ$), fg-D ($\bullet$————$\bullet$), and fg-E ($\square$————$\square$).

Table III. Relative Expression of Native Fibrinogen Antigens by Cleavage Fragments of Fibrinogen[a]

Molecule	Estimated molecular weight	Competitive-inhibition slope	Molar expression of fibrinogen antigen[b]	Fibrinogen antigen per molecule
Fibrinogen	340,000[c]	0.314	1.45×10^{-9} M	1.000
Fg-X	270,000[d]	0.326	3.98×10^{-9} M	0.365
Fg-Y	155,000[d]	0.258	1.88×10^{-8} M	0.077
Fg-D:E	130,000[e]	0.304	5.75×10^{-8} M	0.025
Fg-D	78,000[f]	0.173	$> 10^{-6}$ M	< 0.001
Fg-D	50,000[g]	0.129	$> 10^{-6}$ M	< 0.001

[a] Competitive inhibition radioimmunoassay employing ^{125}I-fibrinogen and anti-fg.
[b] Molar concentration required for 50% inhibition of ^{125}I-fibrinogen binding by anti-fg.
[c] Caspary and Kekwick, 1957.
[d] Marder et al., 1969b.
[e] Estimated from the sum of the molecular weights of fg-D plus fg-E.
[f] Cantanzaro et al., 1972.
[g] Dudek et al., 1970.

The X fragment, possessing approximately 80% of the mass of fibrinogen, exhibited only 36% of the total antigenic expression recognized by the anti-fibrinogen antiserum; the Y fragment, with slightly less than half of the molecular mass, exhibited 7.7% of the total antigenic expression of the parent molecule. This suggests that many of the antigenic determinants may be conformationally dependent or associated with small peptides lost during proteolysis. Relatively few of the recognized native antigenic sites were conserved and expressed by fg-D and fg-E. Antisera resulting from prolonged immunization and differing modes of immunization have given somewhat differing values indicative of differential antigenic selection in the immune response (Plow and Edgington, 1972a, 1973a; Edgington and Plow, unpublished). The profound modulation of native exposed antigenic expression observed with cleavage also suggests that the differences in helical content of fg-D, fg-E, and fibrinogen (Budzynski, 1971) could be explained by changes in conformation engendered by cleavage rather than by conservation of original alpha-helical content of the molecule.

It has generally been considered that the D and E fragments exist in free solution following terminal cleavage, although Budzynski et al. (1967) suggested that these fragments might exist as a noncovalently-associated bimolecular core.

Quantitative immunochemical data (Table III) indicates that the D and E fragments, present in the terminal plasmin digest, must be associated in a complex which conserves or recapitulates greater native conformation than the isolated constituent fragments (Plow and Edgington, 1972a, 1973a; Edgington and Plow, unpublished). Antifibrinogen antisera appear to have a significantly higher binding affinity for the D:E core when compared with either the D or E fragment, and tenfold or greater quantitative expression of native fibrinogen antigens by the D:E core is observed as compared with the sum of free D and free E in equal molar concentrations. Immunochemical exploration has provided definitive evidence for the existence of a native intramolecular constituent region—the D:E-complex region (Edgington and Plow, 1972; Plow and Edgington, 1973a).

Detailed probing of the molecule has been possible by utilizing antibodies to the D fragment of fibrinogen (fg-D). The early antibody response contains a variety of discriminating antibodies. Utilizing quantitative competitive-inhibition techniques, similar to these employed for assay of native determinants, estimation of the D fragment content of the various fragments has been attempted (Plow and Edgington, 1972a). As shown in Table IV, the Y fragment exhibits an almost identical molar expression of D-fragment-associated antigens as the isolated D fragment, indicating the presence of one D-fragment region in fibrinogen Y, whereas approximately two moles of D-fragment-associated antigens are demonstrated in the X fragment. Fibrinogen D antigenic expression is incomplete in the D:E core. This latter behavior suggests that some of the D-fragment determinants are sterically hindered or that conformational differences are

Table IV. Quantitative Distribution of D-Fragment-Associated Antigens in Fibrinogen Cleavage Fragments

Cleavage fragment	Moles D-fragment-associated antigens/mole fragment*	Apparent integer value (D regions/fragment)
Fg-X	1.8	2
Fg-Y	0.9	1
Fg-D:E complex	0.65	1
Fg-D	1.0	1
Fg-E	0	0

* Estimated from molar concentration required for 50% competitive inhibition of a primary binding radioimmunochemical assay employing ^{125}I-fg-D and anti-fg-D. All values referenced to that observed for standard isolated fg-D.

induced which lead to steric hindrance of these sites. These observations further substantiate the existence of the D:E complex. Absolutely no D-fragment-associated antigenic expressions are observed in isolated E fragment, thus confirming the absolute antigenic and structural independence of these two basic constituent regions of the fibrinogen molecule.

3. Cleavage-Associated Neoantigens

The existence of unique cleavage-associated neoantigens in the D fragment was first indicated by Plow *et al.* (1971). Utilizing anti-D antiserum absorbed with fibrinogen in Ouchterlony gel double diffusion, they were able to show a specific reaction with D fragment and not with the parent fibrinogen molecule (Fig. 8). This reaction was observed only following optimal absorption of the anti-D with fibrinogen, and appeared to be dependent upon traces of coprecipitating antifibrinogen antibodies since further absorption with fibrinogen could abrogate the reaction. This cleavage-associated neoantigenic expression was referred to as fg-D_{neo} following more detailed competitive-inhibition studies (Plow *et al.*, 1971). Utilizing a four-compartment competitive-inhibition primary-binding radioimmunoassay, it was shown that anti-D antisera contained antibodies of two generic groups of antigens present on the D fragment. The first group, neutralized by native fibrinogen, consisted of antibodies to the native fibrinogen antigens expressed on the D fragment (X, Fig. 9C). The second group (Y, Fig. 9C), not reactive with native fibrinogen, appeared to represent antibodies to new antigenic moieties (fg-D_{neo}) engendered by or exposed in the

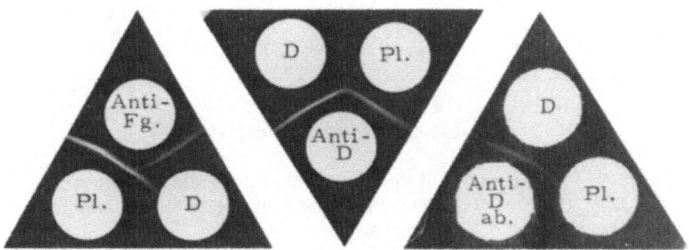

Figure 8. Qualitative demonstration of cleavage-associated neoantigens on the D fragment of fibrinogen (Plow *et al.*, 1971). *Left*, antigenic deficiency of the D fragment compared to the parent fibrinogen molecule is detected with antiserum to fibrinogen. *Center*, apparent identity of the D fragment and fibrinogen is recognized with antiserum to the D fragment. *Right*, anti-D when optimally absorbed with fibrinogen retains its ability to precipitate the D fragment but does not apparently react with fibrinogen even though both fragments are present at equimolar concentration. This suggests the presence of a subpopulation of anti-D antibodies which react with determinants on the cleavage fragment that are not present on the parent molecule.

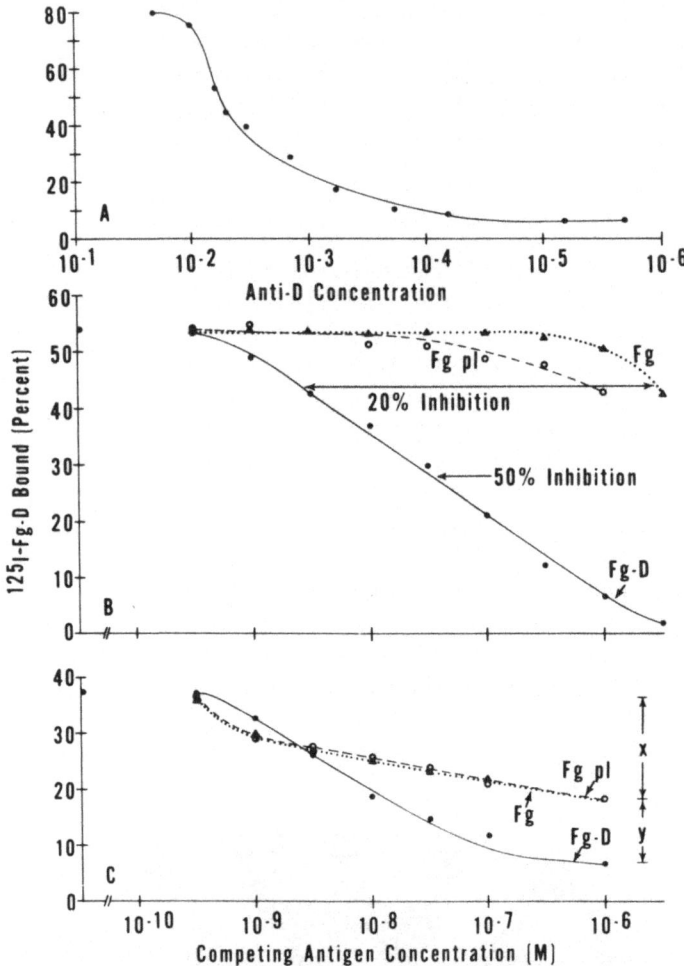

Figure 9. Competitive-inhibition radioimmunochemical demonstration of fg-D$_{neo}$ (Plow *et al.*, 1971). (A) Dependence of ^{125}I-fg-D binding on the concentration of antiserum to the D fragment. (B) Discrimination of fg-D from isolated fibrinogen and plasma fibrinogen by anti-fg-D antibodies. (C) Subpopulation of anti-fg-D antibodies: *x* indicates antibodies reactive with determinants common to fibrinogen and the D fragments, *y* indicates antibodies specific for the fg-D$_{neo}$ determinants expressed only on the D fragment fg-D$_{neo}$

course of plasmin cleavage of fibrinogen. These results indicated that neoantigens may be created or exposed by a *physiological* cleavage mechanism.

Qualitative and quantitative features of fg-D$_{neo}$ site expression by the various plasmin-cleavage fragments have been explored in quantitative competitive-binding experiments (Plow and Edgington, 1972a d; Plow et al., 1972). As summarized in Table V, this neoantigenic determinant(s) is expressed in a qualitatively identical fashion by the X, Y, D:E complex, and D fragments. The relative binding affinity of anti-fg-D_{neo} antibody for fg-D_{neo} sites on each of these cleavage fragments, as reflected by the competitive-inhibition slopes (Table V), appears to be identical, suggesting that the fg-D_{neo} site(s) is presented in a conformationally similar fashion by each cleavage fragment. The lack of expression by fg-E is consistent with the antigenic independence of the D and E fragments. Molar expression of the fg-D_{neo} site by fg-X, fg-Y, fg-D:E complex, and fg-D has been explored and found to be identical within the limits or error imposed by the estimated molecular weights. Employing the fg-D_{neo} expression, it is possible to derive estimated molecular weights of 272,000 for fg-X and 191,000 for fg-Y from the data in Table V.

Quantitative immunochemical studies have demonstrated the presence of two D regions in fg-X, the first major plasmin-cleavage fragment of fibrinogen. Only one of the two potential fg-D_{neo} sites is exposed, however, at this stage of proteolytic degradation (Plow and Edgington, 1972a,d; Plow et al., 1972). This strongly suggests that symmetry inherent in fibrinogen has not been preserved

Table V. Cleavage-Associated Neoantigen, Fg-D_{neo}, Expression by Fibrinogen and Cleavage Fragments of Fibrinogen[a]

Molecule	Estimated molecular weight	Competitive-inhibition slope	Molar expression of fg-D_{neo}[b]	Fg-D_{neo} per molecule
Fibrinogen	340,000[c]	0.013	$> 10^{-5}$ M	0.00
Fg-X	270,000[d]	0.258	8.70×10^{-8} M	0.99
Fg-Y	155,000[d]	0.267	1.07×10^{-7} M	0.81
Fg-D:E	130,000[e]	0.264	9.89×10^{-8} M	0.87
Fg-D	78,000[f]	0.260	8.61×10^{-8} M	1.00
Fg-E	50,000[g]	0.000	$> 10^{-5}$ M	0.00

[a] Competitive-inhibition radioimmunoassay employing ^{125}I-fg-D and anti-fg-D_{neo}.
[b] Molar concentration required for 50% inhibition of ^{125}I-fg-D binding by anti-fg-D_{neo}.
[c] Caspary and Kekwick, 1957.
[d] Marder et al., 1969b.
[e] Estimated from the sum of the molecular weights of fg-D plus fg E.
[f] Catanzaro et al., 1972.
[g] Dudek et al., 1970.

and indicates that the action of plasmin leading to the X fragment is asymmetrical or that it culminates in an asymmetric conformation which permits exposure of only one of the two latent fg D_{neo} sites. Evidence for asymmetric cleavage of fibrinogen by plasmin has been further suggested by analysis of N-terminal amino acids (Marder et al., 1972). Fg-Y and the fg-D:E complex each exhibit unitary fg-D_{neo} expression which is consistent with the number of D regions in each fragment. Thus, further incubation of fg-X with plasmin is associated with further cleavage and exposure of the second fg-D_{neo} site. This interpretation is required by the demonstrated quantitative yield of two moles of fg-D_{neo} per mole of fibrinogen (Edgington and Plow, 1972), and the proposed content of two D fragments per mole of fibrinogen and fg-X (Plow and Edgington, 1972a,d; Marder et al., 1969b). The uniform antigenic expression of fg-D_{neo} by each cleavage fragment except fg-E suggests the feasibility of quantitative molar assay of cleavage in vivo independent of the particular fragment assayed or the differential reactivity of other antisera with different fragments (Plow and Edgington, 1972a; Nussenzweig and DeSouza, 1962; Vermylen and Donati, 1971).

In contrast to the uniform molar expression of fg-D_{neo} by cleavage fragments, a recently recognized neoantigen associated with the E fragment, fg-E_{neo}, is differentially expressed by each fibrinogen cleavage fragment (Plow and Edgington, 1973b). As cleavage proceeds through the intermediate fragments to the terminal cleavage products, the expression of fg-E_{neo} progressively increases. The D fragment exhibits no fg-E_{neo} expression as is to be anticipated, but the X, Y, D:E complex, and the E fragment exhibit differential fg-E_{neo} expression. These results further confirm that conformational modulations are associated with cleavage. The fg-E_{neo} site may provide an additional specific marker for probing these conformational changes.

Although other neoantigenic determinants specifically associated with the intermediate X and Y fragments are readily conceived, no attempt has yet been made to recognize the presence of such determinants. The demonstration of such sites should prove valuable in assessing the extent of cleavage in vivo. Other neoantigenic sites specifically associated with the cleavage of fibrin have been suggested (Plow and Edgington, 1972c; Edgington and Plow, unpublished) and may provide a basis for the discrimination of fibrinogen from fibrin cleavage.

Preliminary evidence from the Blombäcks suggests the presence of some sites on N-DSK that are exposed to a greater degree on fibrin than on fibrinogen (M. Blombäck, 1972). This putative N-DSK$_{neo}$ is expressed to a greater degree on reduced N-DSK than on unreduced N-DSK. The minimal expression on fibrinogen suggests that these sites, exposed during the fibrin transition, are buried in the parent molecule or represent modulation of native determinants that then cross-react with denatured determinants of the N-DSK. The increased expression by fibrin suggests that physiological cleavage of the fibrinopeptides can lead to conformations which allow expression of these antigenic determinants. This expression is in some ways similar to the fg-E_{neo} system. Further studies with both of these neoantigenic markers may further elucidate conformational modulation of the N terminus associated with the fibrin transition and with plasmin cleavage. Early evidence suggests that much of the N terminus (N-DSK and E-fragment regions) may be buried and undergo progressive exposure during the fibrin transition and during plasmin cleavage.

G. Molecular Events Underlying Neoantigenic Expression

Molecular events responsible for the modulation and emergence of the fg-D_{neo} neoantigenic expression have been explored, and similar considerations may apply to neoantigens associated with other molecules and other biological mechanisms including neoplasia. Three hypothetical schematic models have been considered to explain the emergence of fg-D_{neo} (Fig. 10). Each model presents distinct conceptual differences, although conformation modulation may occur in each circumstance. The cleavage-site-specific model postulates that neoantigen is associated with amino acids directly at the site of cleavage. The existence of such a system has been suggested by Lehrer and Van Vunakis (1965) from immunochemical studies of the conversion of procarboxypeptidase to carboxypeptidase. The active enzyme differs in the N-terminal portions created by differential

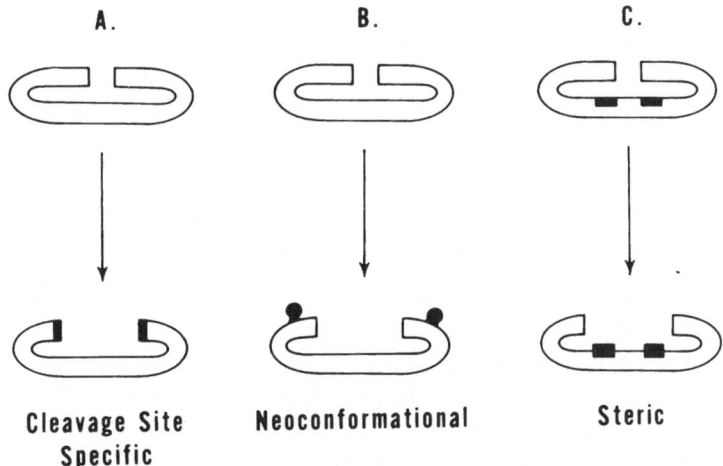

Figure 10. Conceptual models to explain the emergence of a cleavage-associated neoantigen (Plow and Edgington, 1972*b*). (A) The cleavage-site-specific model suggests that determinants are associated directly with amino acid sequences at the site of cleavage. (B) The neoconformational model envisions a localized conformation induced by cleavage. (C) The steric model suggests that sites sterically hindered in the parent molecule are exposed by cleavage.

cleavage and can be distinguished immunochemically. The second or neoconformational model postulates that a neoantigen may be created by new local conformations unrelated to the cleavage site but induced secondary to enzymatic cleavage. Mildly denatured and aggregated bovine serum albumin possesses determinants not expressed in native or denatured albumin (Wolberg et al., 1970), suggestive of a neoconformational genesis. The third approach is embodied in the steric model in which the neoantigenic site is contained by the parent native molecule but is sterically hindered. This site is hypothetically exposed only following appropriate enzymatic cleavage or other events that lead to changes in conformation. The existence of such neoantigenic sites on other molecules, and their exposure by enzymatic cleavage has been suggested by studies of IgG and bovine serum albumin following pepsin cleavage (Ishizaka et al., 1960; Williams and Kunkel, 1962; Osterland et al., 1963). The exact mechanisms involved in these latter expressions have not been defined.

By analysis of the effects of diverse enzymes and denaturants on fibrinogen and the fg-D_{neo} expression, some of the molecular events underlying expression of fg-D_{neo} have been deduced (Plow and Edgington, 1972b). Fg-D_{neo} expression was dependent upon the specificity of the enzyme. Plasmin and trypsin, enzymes of similar specificity, generated identical fg-D_{neo} expressions; whereas fg-D_{neo}-like antigenic expressions of lower competitive-binding affinity were generated by cleavage with enzymes of different specificities. In spite of widely diverse chemical modulation of fibrinogen conformation, in the absence of cleavage, fg-D_{neo} was expressed only following selective oxidation, implying some restrictions upon conditions required for exposure of the neoantigenic determinant(s). The steric model appeared compatible with all data, and both the cleavage-site-specific and neoconformational models could be reasonably excluded (Plow and Edgington, 1972b).

H. Immunochemical Discrimination of Fibrin and Fibrinogen Cleavage Fragments

Subtle physiochemical differences between the plasmin-cleavage products of fibrin and fibrinogen have been reported (Dudek et al., 1970) and it has also been recognized that most fibrinogen-derived cleavage fragments are precipitated at 56°C (Lewis and Wilson, 1964; Beller and Maki, 1967). However, quantitative immunochemical studies appear to provide a firm molecular basis for systematic determination of the molecular origin of cleavage fragments (Plow and Edgington, 1972c,d, 1973c). Utilizing the specific antiserum anti-fgD_{neo} to probe the expression of the fg-D_{neo} site, a consistent differential molecular conformation of the fibrin and fibrinogen fragments has now been recognized. The fg-D_{neo} site is expressed in a qualitatively and quantitatively similar fashion on the X, Y, D:E complex, and D fragments of fibrinogen as previously described (Table V). The corresponding fibrin fragments also express the neoantigen in a generically similar manner, but the competitive-inhibition slope, an indication of the binding affinity of the antibody, is distinctly different for fibrin-derived cleavage fragments as contrasted with the fibrinogen-derived fragments. Thus, the anti-fg-D_{neo} probe clearly demonstrates differences in the local conformation in the vicinity of the fg-D_{neo} site of fibrin and fibrinogen cleavage fragments. This characteristic difference in relative binding affinity is quite precise and provides an approach for the discrimination of (1) *in vivo* coagulative processes which lead to fibrin cleavage fragments from (2) primary fibrinogenolytic processes in which coagulation and the fibrin transition has not been involved. The system permits direct assay of plasma, and the unitary expression of fg-D_{neo} yields quantitative molar results.

An apparent new neoantigenic site present on the D fragment of fibrin, a putative fb-D_{neo}, has recently been recognized (Plow and Edgington, 1972c). The binding of ^{125}I-fb-D by specific anti-fb-D_{neo} antibody is competitively inhibited by fb-D, but fg-D only exhibits minimal inhibitory capacity. While the molecular basis for the fb-D_{neo} expression has not yet been explored, these preliminary results suggest that an entirely unique and specific conformational site may be associated exclusively with the fibrin-derived D fragment.

Concomitant with the differential expression of neoantigens on fibrinogen as contrasted to fibrin cleavage fragments, the native antigenic expressions of the parent fibrinogen and fibrin molecules are also expressed differently by the D-fragments (Edgington and Plow, 1973). Antisera prepared to either parent molecule are capable of discriminating the D fragments of fibrin and fibrinogen. Complex conformational modulation of these native determinants on the D region is indicated by both qualitative and quantitative differences in the expressions of the D fragments. It has also been shown that thrombin treatment of the D fragment of fibrinogen does not alter its immunochemical expression to that of fibrin D. The differential expression of both native and neoantigenic determinants reflect conformational modulations occurring in fibrinogen or fibrin transition which then persist or are characteristically modified by plasmin cleavage. These primary conformational differences appear to directly influence the characteristics of subsequent cleavage and reconformation responsible for: (1) the differential expression of native determinants, (2) the differential exposure of the fg-D_{neo} sites, and (3) the generation of the putative fb-D_{neo} expression.

I. Molecular Reconstruction

Most of the available information relevant to reconstruction of the fibrinogen molecule and its derivatives has been given; however, recent quantitative immunochemical experiments have provided additional perspectives. Experiments were designed to directly assay the number of constituent D and E regions per molecule. The fg-D_{neo} system was utilized for the quantitative molar assay of D regions in the fibrinogen molecule (Edgington and Plow, 1972); 2.15 molecules of fg-D_{neo} expression were yielded per mole of fibrinogen which had been cleaved to completion with plasmin. This is interpreted to indicate the presence of two D regions per fibrinogen molecule. This confirms the D-fragment content proposed by Marder (1968) through summation of estimated molecular weights, and the previous immunochemical data regarding expression of total fg-D-associated antigens and fg-D_{neo} by each of the cleavage fragments (Plow and Edgington, 1972a,d; Plow et al., 1972). Utilizing the characteristic native antigenic expression of the D:E complex, Edgington and Plow (1972) have performed recombinant studies to determine the number of moles of E fragment bound per mole of D fragment in the D:E complex. Exact immunochemical reconstruction of native antigenic expression of the D:E complex was achieved precisely with a 1:1 molar ratio of D fragments to E fragments as shown in Table VI; the molar concentration required for 50% competitive inhibition, and the competitive-inhibition slope of the recombinant species were identical to those of the native complex. Since two moles of D are yielded per mole of fibrinogen, an equal number, or two moles, of E must be present in fibrinogen. Although the precise mechanism of cleavage through the N terminus of the molecule to yield two E fragments has not yet been elucidated, the biochemical and physicochemical data are not contraindicative to this conclusion. Simple nitrogen-balance studies as shown in Table VII are also more compatible with the presence of two E regions rather than one region per fibrinogen molecule. The current data then suggests the presence of two E regions, rather than one, in the N terminus of the molecule. These E regions overlap the N-DSK, and much of the rest of the molecule is represented by the two D regions.

Table VI. Recapitulation of the Native Fibrinogen Antigenic Expression of D:E Complex by Recombinant Species of Fg-D and Fg-E*

Fragment species	Molar ratio fg-E/fg-D	Competitive-inhibition slope	50% competitive inhibition
D:E complex	—	0.225	1.42×10^{-8} M
Fg-D + fg-E	0.5/1.0	0.325	2.98×10^{-8} M
Fg-D + fg-E	1.0/1.0	0.224	1.45×10^{-8} M
Fg-D + fg-E	2.0/1.0	0.287	1.20×10^{-8} M

* Radioimmunoassay employing ^{125}I-fibrinogen at 1×10^{-9} M and antinative fibrinogen (Plow and Edgington, 1973a). Results from Edgington and Plow (1972).

Table VII. Estimation of Constituent D and E Regions from Conservation of Protein Nitrogen

	Residual protein nitrogen of fibrinogen in terminal plasmin digest
Observed	70–80%
*Calculated**	
a) 2 D regions plus 1 E region	60.6%
b) 2 D regions plus 2 E regions	74.7%

* Based on molecular weights of 79,000 daltons for the D fragment, 48,000 daltons for the E fragment, and 340,000 daltons for fibrinogen. From Edgington and Plow (1972).

IV. PERSPECTIVES

The elucidation of molecular structure and conformation can be significantly facilitated by quantitative and qualitative immunologic approaches. The structure of fibrinogen, a large and complex molecule with multiple physiological forms and fragments, is as yet only partially understood. The advances that have been realized have benefited from multidisciplinary approaches that have included not only physicochemical, biochemical, and physiological but also immunologic approaches. Through the use of defined antigenic markers, the segregation of molecular fragments within this molecule has been to a great extent accomplished. Such studies, exploiting not only the quantitative expression of neoantigenic sites but also the qualitative and quantitative expression of native conformationally dependent antigens, have provided new data regarding intramolecular associations and the discrimination of functionally significant forms of the molecule. It is anticipated that recent advances in elucidating the structure and physiological cleavage of fibrinogen will facilitate more incisive investigation of the functional molecular anatomy and pathophysiology of this molecule in health and disease.

ACKNOWLEDGMENT

This work was supported by a Grant-in-Aid from the American Heart Association and with funds contributed in part by the San Diego Heart Association, and by National Institutes of Health Research Grants AM-12920 and HL-15216-01. Dr. Plow is the recipient of U.S. Public Health Service Training Grant 5-T01-GM-00683.

This is Publication No. 633 from the Division of Clinical Pathology, Department of Experimental Pathology, Scripps Clinic and Research Foundation, La

Jolla, California. We readily acknowledge the dedicated assistance of Mrs. Cleo-Mae Mrozek in preparation of the manuscript.

REFERENCES

Alkjaersig, N., Fletcher, A. P., and Sherry, S. (1959). *J. Clin. Invest.* **38:** 1086.
Anfinsen, C. B. (1959). In *The Molecular Basis of Evolution,* Wiley, New York.
Arnesen, H. (1971). *Scand. J. Haematol. Suppl.* **13:** 43.
Astrup, T. (1956). *Blood* **11:** 781.
Bartel, A., and Campbell, D. (1959). *Arch. Biochem.* **82:** 232.
Barton, P. G. (1967). *Nature* **215:** 1508.
Bauer, J., and Engel, S. (1912). *Biochem. Z.* **42:** 399.
Beck E. A. (1971). *Thromb. Diath. Haemorrhag. Suppl* **45:** 315.
Beller, F. K., and Maki, M. (1967). *Thromb. Diath. Haemorrhag.* **18:** 114.
Benjamini, E., Scibienski, R. J., and Thompson, K. (1972). In Inman, F. P. (ed.), *Contemporary Topics in Immunochemistry,* Vol. I, Plenum Press, New York.
Blombäck, B. (1958). *Acta Physiol. Scand. 43, Suppl.* **148:** 1.
Blombäck, B. (1969). *Brit. J. Haematol.* **17:** 145.
Blombäck, B. (1971). In Schoffeniels, E. (ed.), *Biochemical Evolution and the Origin of Life,* North-Holland Publ. Co., Amsterdam.
Blombäck, B., and Blombäck, M. (1956). *Arkiv. Kemi.* **10:** 415.
Blombäck, B., and Blombäck, M. (1970). *Nouvelle Rev. Franc. Haematol.* **10:** 671.
Blombäck, B., and Blombäck, M. (1972). *Ann. N.Y. Acad. Sci.* **202:** 77.
Blombäck, B., and Yamashina, I. (1958). *Arkiv. Kemi.* **12:** 299.
Blombäck. B., Blombäck, M., Henschen, A., Hessel, B., Iwanaga, S., and Woods, K. R. (1968). *Nature* **218:** 130.
Blombäck. B., Hessel, B., Iwanaga, S., Reuterby, J., and Blombäck, M. (1972). *J. Biol. Chem.* **247:** 1496.
Blombäck, M. (1972). *Proc. III Congr. Internat. Soc. Thromb. Haematol.* p. 16.
Blombäck, M., Blombäck, B., Mammen, E. F., and Prosad, A. S. (1968). *Nature* **218:** 134.
Brinkhouse, K. M., Owren, P. A., Wright, I. S., Roberts, H. R., Hinnon, S., and Kiesselbach, T. H. (eds.). (1970). *Fibrinogen: Structural, Metabolic, and Pathophysiologic Aspects,* F. K. Schattauer Verlag, Stuttgart.
Brönnimann, R. (1954). *Acta Haematol.* **11:** 40.
Brown, R., Delaney, R., Levin, L., and Van Vunakis, H. (1959). *J. Biol. Chem.* **234:** 2043.
Budzynski, A. Z. (1971). *Biochim. Biophys. Acta* **229:** 663.
Budzynski, A. Z., Stahl, M., Kopec, M., Latallo, Z. S., Wegrzynowicz, Z., and Kowalski, E. (1967). *Biochim. Biophys. Acta* **147:** 313.
Caspary, E. A., and Kekwick, R. A. (1957). *Biochem. J.* **67:** 41.
Catanzaro, A., Hathaway, G., Strathern, J., and Edgington, T. S. (1972). *Proc. Soc. Exp. Biol. Med.* **139:** 1401.
Davie, E. W., and Ratnoff, O. D. (1964). *Science* **145:** 1310.
Demanez, M. L. (1932). *Compt. Rend. Soc. Biol.* **109:** 553.
Denis, P. S. (1859). *Mémoire Su Le Sang ,* Bailliere, Paris.
DeVries, A., Rosenberg, T., Kochwa, S., and Boss, J. H. (1961). *Am. J. Med.* **30:** 486.
Dietrich, F. M. (1967). *Immunochemistry* **4:** 65.
Doolittle, R. F. (1970). In Brinkhouse *et al.* (eds.), *Fibrinogen: Structural, Metabolic, and Pathophysiologic Aspects,* F. K. Schattauer Verlag, Stuttgart, pp. 25–42.
Dorrington, K. J., and Tanford, C. (1970). *Advan. Immunol.* **12:** 333.
Duchateau, G., and Florkin, M. (1954). *Bull. Soc. Chim. Biol.* **36:** 295.
Dudek, G. A., Kloczewiak, M., Budzynski, A. Z., Latallo, Z. S., and Kopec, M. (1970). *Biochim. Biophys. Acta* **214:** 44.
Edgington, T. S., and Plow, E. F. (1972). *Proc. III Congr. Internat. Soc. Thromb. Haematol.* p. 84.
Edgington, T. S., and Plow, E. F. (1973). *Thromb. Diath. Haemorrhag. Suppl.* (in press).
Edgington, T. S., and Plow, E. F., unpublished.

Fletcher, A. P., Alkjaersig, N., Fisher, S., and Sherry, S. (1966). *J. Lab. Clin. Med.* **68**: 780.
Forman, W. B., Ratnoff, O. D., and Boyer, M. H. (1968). *J. Lab. Clin. Med.* **72**: 455.
Furlan, M., and Beck, E. A. (1972). *Biochim. Biophys. Acta* **263**: 631.
Gardlund, B., Kowalska-Loth, B., Gröndahl, N. J., and Blombäck, B. (1972). *Thromb. Res.* **1**: 371.
Goodman, J. W. (1969). *Immunochemistry* **6**: 139.
Grégoire, C., and Tagnon, H. J. (1962). In Flockin, M., and Moor, H. S. (eds.), *Comparative Biochemistry*, Vol. 4B, p. 435.
Hall, C. E., and Slayter, H. S. (1959). *J. Biophys. Biochem. Cytol.* **5**: 11.
Hammersten, O. (1880). *Pflüger's Arch. Ges. Physiol.* **22**: 431.
Hampton, J. W., and Garrison, D. (1972). *Med. Clin. N. Am.* **56**: 133.
Haschemeyer, A. E. V. (1963). *Biochemistry* **2**: 851.
Hektoen, L., and Welker, W. (1927). *J. Infect. Diseases* **40**: 706.
Henschen, A. (1962). *Acta Chem. Scand.* **16**: 1037.
Henschen, A. (1964a). *Arkiv. Kemi.* **22**: 375.
Henschen, A. (1964b). *Arkiv. Kemi.* **22**: 1.
Hewson, W. (1771). *An Experimental Inquiry into the Properties of the Blood*, Printed for T. Cadell in the Strand, London.
Ishizaka, T., Campbell, D., and Ishizaka, K. (1960). *Proc. Exp. Biol. Med.* **103**: 5.
Jackson, D. P., Beck, E. A., and Charache, P. (1965). *Federation Proc.* **24**: 816.
Javid, J., and Yingling, W. (1968). *J. Clin. Invest.* **47**: 2290.
Jamieson, C. A., and Gaffney, P. A., Jr. (1968). *Biochim. Biophys. Acta* **154**: 96.
John, D. W., and Miller, L. L. (1960). *J. Biol. Chem.* **241**: 1817.
Kato, K. (1924). *Centralbl. Bakteriol. I.* **75**: 353.
Kendrew, J. C., Dickerson, R. E., Strandberg, B. E., Hart, R. G., Davies, D. R., Phillips, D. C., and Shore, V. C. (1960). *Nature* **185**: 422.
Kenton, H. B. (1933). *J. Immunol.* **25**: 461.
Köppel, G. (1966). *Nature* **212**: 1608.
Köppel, G. (1970). In Brinkhouse *et al.* (eds.), *Fibrinogen: Structural Metabolic, and Pathophysiological Aspects*, F. K. Schattauer Verlag, Stuttgart, pp. 71–73.
Kowalski, E. (1968). *Sem. Hematol.* **5**: 45.
Kyes, P., and Porter, R. (1931). *J. Immunol.* **20**: 85.
Laurent, T. C., and Blombäck, B. (1958). *Acta Chem. Scand.* **12**: 1875.
Lehrer, H., and Van Vunakis, H. (1965). *Immunochemistry* **2**: 255.
Levine, J. (1967). *Federation Proc.* **26**: 1707.
Lewis, J. H., and Wilson, J. H. (1964). *Am. J. Physiol.* **209**: 1053.
Lorand, L. (1951). *Nature* **167**: 992.
Lorand, L. (1954). *Physiol. Rev.* **34::** 742.
Lorand, L., and Middlebrook, W. R. (1952). *Biochem. J.* **52**: 196.
McDonagh, J., Messel, H., McDonagh, R. P., Jr., Murano, G., and Blombäck, B. (1971). *Biochim. Biophys. Acta* **257**: 135.
Macfarlane, R. G. (1964). *Nature* **202**: 498.
McKay, G. D. (1965). In *Disseminated Intravascular Coagulation: An Intermediary Mechanism of Disease*, Hoeber-Harper, New York.
McKee, P. A., Mattock, P., and Hill, R. L. (1970). *Proc. Natl. Acad. Sci. U.S.* **66**: 738.
Mammen, E. F., Prosad, A. S., Barnhart, M. I., and Au, C. C. (1969). *J. Clin. Invest.* **48**: 235.
Marder, V. J. (1968). In Laki, K. (ed.), *Fibrinogen*, Marcel Dekker, New York, p. 339.
Marder, V. J. (1970). *Thromb. Diath. Haemorrhag. Suppl.* **39**: 187.
Marder, V. J. (1971a). *Scand. J. Haematol. Suppl.* **13**: 21.
Marder, V. J. (1971b). *Scand. J. Haematol. Suppl.* **13**: 62.
Marder, V. J., and Sherry, S. (1971). *Thromb. Diath. Haemorrhag. Suppl.* **45**: 269.
Marder, V. J., Shulman N. R., and Carroll, W. R. (1967). *Trans. Assoc. Am. Physicians* **80**: 156.
Marder, V. J., James, H. L., and Sherry, S. (1969a). *Thromb. Diath. Haemorrhag.* **22**: 234.
Marder, V. J., Shulman, N. R., and Carroll, W. R. (1969b). *J. Biol. Chem.* **244**: 2111.
Marder, V. J., Matchett, M. O., and Sherry, S. (1971). *Am. J. Med.* **51**: 71.

Marder, V. J., Budzynski, A. Z., and James, H. L. (1972). J. Biol. Chem. 247: 4775.
Ménaché, D. (1964). Thromb. Diath. Haemorrhag. Suppl. 13: 173.
Ménaché, D. (1970). Thromb. Diath. Haemorrhag. Suppl. 39: 307.
Merskey, C., Johnson, A. J., Kleiner, G. J., and Wohl, H. (1967). Brit. J. Haematol. 13: 528.
Miller, L. L., Hanavan, H. R., Titthasiri, N., and Chowdbury, A. (1964). Chemistry 44: 17.
Mills, D. A. (1972). Biochim. Biophys. Acta 263: 619.
Mills, D. A., and Karpatkin, S. (1971). Federation Proc. 30: 1076.
Mosesson, M. W., Alkjaersig, N., Sweet, B., and Sherry, S. (1967). Biochemistry 6: 3279.
Mosesson, M. W., Finlayson, J. S., Umfleet, R. A., and Galanakis, D. (1972). J. Biol. Chem. 247: 5210.
Mross, G. A., and Doolittle, R. F. (1967). Arch. Biochem. 122: 674.
Muirhead, H., and Perutz, M. F. (1963). Nature 199: 633.
Murano, G., Wiman, B., Blombäck, M., and Blombäck, B. (1971). FEBS Letters 14: 37.
Murano, G., Wiman, B., and Blombäck, B. (1972). Thromb. Res. 1: 161.
Nanninga, L. B., and Guest, M. M. (1968). Thromb. Diath. Haemorrhag. 19: 526.
Niewiarowski, S., and Nandi, M. (1971). Brit. J. Haematol. 21: 71.
Niewiarowski, S., Stewart, G. J., and Marder, V. J. (1970). Biochim. Biophys. Acta 221: 320.
Niewiarowski, S., Gurewich, V., Senyi, A. F., and Mustard, J. F. (1971). Thromb. Diath. Haemorrhag. Suppl. 47: 99.
Nilehn, J. E. (1967). Thromb. Diath. Haemorrhag. 18: 89.
Nossel, H. L., Younger, L. R., Wilner, G. D., Procupez, T., Canfield, R. E., and Butler, V. P., Jr. (1971). Proc. Natl. Acad. Sci. U.S. 68: 2350.
Nussenzweig, V., and DeSouza, E. (1962). Intern. Arch. Allergy Appl. Immunol. 21: 294.
Nussenzweig, V., and Seligmann, M. (1960). Rev. Hematol. 15: 451.
Nussenzweig, V., Seligmann, M., Pelmont, J., and Grabar, P. (1961a). Ann. Inst. Pasteur 100: 490.
Osterland, C. K., Harboe, M., and Kunkel, H. G. (1963). Vox Sanguinis 8: 133.
Pizzo, S. V., Schwartz, M. L., Hill, R. L., and McKee, P. A. (1972a). J. Biol. Chem. 247: 636.
Pizzo, S. V., Schwartz, M. L., Hill, R. L., and McKee, P. A. (1972b). Federation Proc. 31: 261.
Plow, E. F., and Edgington, T. S. (1972a). J. Clin. Invest. 52: 273.
Plow, E. F., and Edgington, T. S. (1972b). Proc. Natl. Acad. Sci. U.S. 69: 208.
Plow, E. F., and Edgington, T. S. (1972c). Proc. III. Congr. Internat. Soc. Thromb. Haematol., p. 32.
Plow, E. F., and Edgington, T. S. (1972d). Federation Proc. 31: 653.
Plow, E. F., and Edgington, T. S. (1973a). Thromb. Res. (in press).
Plow, E. F., and Edgington, T. S. (1973b). Federation Proc. 32 (in press).
Plow, E. F., and Edgington, T. S. (1973c). Proc. Natl. Acad. Sci. U.S. 70 (in press).
Plow, E. F., Hougie, C., and Edgington, T. S. (1971). J. Immunol. 107: 1496.
Plow, E. F., Hougie, C., and Edgington, T. S. (1972). Blood 38: 794.
Porter, K. R., and Hawn, C. V. Z. (1947). J. Exp. Med. 86: 285.
Porter, K. R., and Hawn, C. V. Z. (1949). J. Exp. Med. 90: 225.
Pressman, D., and Grossberg, A. L. (1968). In The Structural Basis of Antibody Specificity, Benjamin, New York.
Ratnoff, O. D. (1969). Advan. Immunol. 10: 146.
Salmon, J. (1959). Clin. Chim. Acta 4: 767.
Scheraga, H. A. (1961). In Protein Structure, Academic Press, New York.
Sela, M. (1969). Science 166: 1365.
Sela, M. (1970). N.Y. Acad. Sci. 169: 23.
Sela, M., Schechter, B., Schechter, I., and Borek, F. (1967). Cold Spring Harbor Symp. Quant. Biol. 32: 537.
Sherry, S., Alkjaersig, N., and Fletcher, A. P. (1959). Physiol. Rev. 39: 343.
Söderqvist, T., and Blombäck, B. (1971). Naturwissenschaften 58: 16.

Stewart, G. (1971). *Scand. J. Haematol. Suppl.* **13**: 63.
Stryer, L. C., Cohen, R., and Langridge, R. (1963). *Nature* **197**: 793.
Szalontai, S. (1968). In Laki, K. (ed.), *Fibrinogen.* Marcel Dekker, New York, p. 131.
Thomas, D. P., Niewiarowski, S., Myers, A. R., Bloch, K. J., and Colman, R. W. (1970). *New Engl. J. Med.* **283**: 663.
Triantaphyllopoulos, D. E., Triantaphyllopoulos, E., and Chandra S. (1971). *Thromb. Diath. Haemorrhag. Suppl.* **47**: 121.
Triantaphyllopoulos, E. (1972). *Federation Proc.* **30**: 141.
Vermylen, J., and Donati, M. B. (1971). In Losito, R., and Longpre, B. (eds.), *Current Concepts of Coagulation and Hemostasis,* F. K. Schattauer Verlag, Stuttgart, p. 187.
Virchow, R. (1847). *Arch. Pathol. Anat. Physiol.* **1**: 547.
Von Felten, A., Straub, P. N., and Frick, P. G. (1969). *New Engl. J. Med.* **280**: 405.
Wallen, P. (1971). *Scand. J. Haematol. Suppl.* **13**: 3.
Williams, R., and Kunkel, H. (1962). *Arthritis Rheumat.* **5**: 665.
Wolberg, G., Liu, C. T., and Adler, F. L. (1970). *J. Immunol.* **105**: 797.
Woods, K. R., Horowitz, M. S., and Blombäck, B. (1972). *Thromb. Res.* **1**: 113.
Young, N. S., Levin, J., and Prendergast, R. A. (1971). *Federation Proc.* **30**: 340.
Zimmerman, T. S., and Müller-Eberhard, H. J. (1971). *J. Exp. Med.* **134**: 1601.
Zimmerman, T. S., Arroyave, C. M., and Müller-Eberhard, H. J. (1971). *J. Exp. Med.* **134**: 1591.

Index